An Atlas of Surgical Exposures of the Lower Extremity

An Atlas of
Surgical Exposures of the Lower Extremity

Alain C Masquelet MD

Consultant Orthopaedic Surgeon, Hôpital Avicenne and Hôpital Trousseau, Paris
Professor, Faculty of Medicine, University of Paris

Christopher J McCullough MA, FRCS

Consultant Orthopaedic Surgeon, Northwick Park Hospital, Middlesex

Raoul Tubiana MD

President de l'Institut Français de la Main, Paris
Associate Professor, Faculty of Medicine, University of Paris

Ian Fyfe MB BCh, FRCS, FRCS Orth (Ed)

Consultant Orthopaedic Surgeon, Northwick Park Hospital, Middlesex

Leslie Klenerman MB BCh, ChM, FRCS

Professor and Head of the Department of Orthopaedics and Accident Surgery, University of Liverpool

Emile Letournel MD

Consultant Orthopaedic Surgeon, Centre Medico-Chirurgical de la Porte de Choisy
Professor, Faculty of Medicine, University of Paris

With illustrations by Léon Dorn

MARTIN DUNITZ

© **Alain C Masquelet, Christopher J McCullough, Raoul Tubiana 1993**

Artwork and design © Martin Dunitz Ltd 1993

First published in the United Kingdom in 1993
by Martin Dunitz Ltd, The Livery House, 7–9 Pratt Street, London NW1 0AE

A CIP catalogue record for this book is available from the British Library.

ISBN 1 85317 003 8

Photoset by Scribe Design, Gillingham, Kent
Colour origination by Imago Publishing Ltd
Printed and bound in Singapore by Toppan Printing Company (S) PTE Ltd

Contents

Contents

Contents

Preface

Until recently all the books dealing with surgical approaches were divided up according to the traditional specialized fields of research. However, the modern concept of reconstructive surgery implies for each case a holistic vision of the treatment which transcends the various individual academic disciplines: the reconstructive surgeon is no longer involved in the repair of one specific tissue (such as vessels, skin or bone structures) but should tackle compound lesions that are from a physiological point of view included in a regional entity. For that reason this atlas of surgical approaches to the lower limb comprises not only several chapters devoted to bone and joint structures, but also chapters on vessels, nerves, and skin and muscle flaps.

In some very specialized fields where great experience is required we have appealed to world-renowned authors whose scientific authority is well established. The chapters on the pelvic girdle and hip have been written by Professor Emile Letournel, that on the knee by Mr Ian Fyfe, and that on the foot and ankle by Professor Leslie Klenerman. Multiple discussions have been for us (and, we hope, for the reader also) extremely fruitful.

All the surgical approaches described have been performed at the operating theatre of the Ecole de Chirurgie des Hôpitaux de Paris, and were often repeated to allow M Léon Dorn to achieve original and accurate artwork. We dedicate this book to all the anonymous persons whose cadavers have permitted this work.

ACM
CJM
RT

Artist's preface

I have in the past tried to evoke the role of the medical illustrator by an analogy from the theatre, comparing the surgeon to an author and the illustrator to a producer. I have also noted the artistic techniques necessary for medical illustration to be comprehensible and didactic: the elimination of superfluous detail in order to emphasize the main point, and the correct use of contrasting colours to distinguish the variety of human tissues (if necessary, in an almost caricatural manner).

One further very important function remains: the artist must suggest the continuity and movement inside the surgical procedure. There is, of course, one medium of medical illustration which can capture movement — namely the video recording, which can faithfully transmit all the necessary phases of the surgical approach; but against it can be laid the charge that one would make against photography in general, that it does not give sufficient importance to certain details and parts of the image that one would like to emphasize. Moreover, a video recording of the entire procedure lacks the effect of staging, a natural aid to the presentation of the image. Finally, the transience of the image does not facilitate perception of the key message that should be communicated to the future practitioner.

The desire to evoke the notion of continuity by highlighting crucial points was understood by the sculptors of Greece and the artists of the Renaissance who would use in their works a set gesture to suggest an entire movement. In a similar manner the medical illustration is not only the reflection of a particular moment in the surgical procedure but also the evocation of the sequence of stages in the operation. This impression is created by an 'unrealistic' picture in which, for example, the surgical field is more extensive than in reality, there are more retractors than are necessary, and other instruments demonstrating steps that would follow each other in the surgical procedure itself are displayed at the same time. By these artificial means, then, the careful choice of the exact moment to represent the stage should suggest the whole sequence of the procedure to that point.

I have tried to promote the artistic or aesthetic aspects of the illustrations without jeopardizing the scientific accuracy indispensable for a medical illustration. I wish to thank Professors Masquelet and Letournel for their understanding and their help in this task.

LD

1

Pelvic girdle

Introduction

Detailed anatomy of the hip and pelvis is well covered by standard anatomical texts. In this introduction practical anatomical points will be described to aid the surgeon in the practice of surgery of the hip and pelvis. The anatomy in surgery differs in many regards from that described by traditional anatomists who work on cadavers, where tissues are modified in texture and size. Anatomical approaches are often extensive, with the prime aim of displaying the anatomy, whereas surgical approaches are often much more restricted. The information in this chapter is given on the basis of many years of practical experience of surgery of the hip and pelvis.

Surface anatomy of the hip (**A,B,C,D,E**)

The ease of identification of these landmarks depends to an extent on the obesity of the patient.

The anterior superior iliac spine and the pubic tubercle

These structures are easily palpated in slim patients and lie at either end of the cutaneous inguinal fold which corresponds nearly perfectly to the line of the inguinal ligament. In obese patients the abdominal skin and subcutaneous tissues must be drawn proximally in order to expose the landmarks. With the patient prone, the anterior superior iliac spine lies two fingers' breadth medial to the lateral limit of the thigh. Tensor fasciae latae is palpated relatively easily, lying distal and lateral to the anterior superior iliac spine. Immediately medial and separated by a shallow depression is the belly of sartorius which arises directly from the anterior superior iliac spine. Crossing the subcutaneous tissues within this depression are the branches of the lateral cutaneous nerve of thigh. The

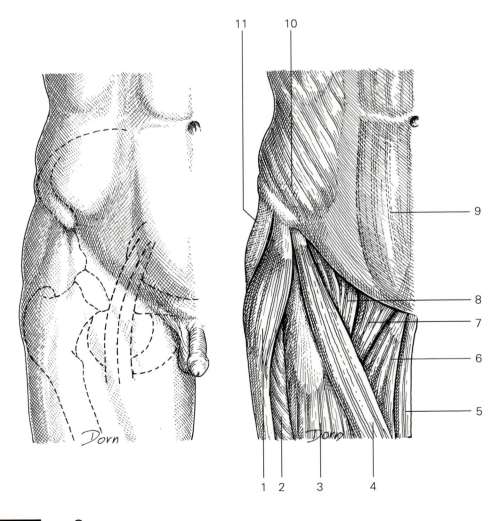

A Landmarks and muscles

1 tensor fasciae latae
2 vastus lateralis
3 rectus femoris
4 sartorius
5 gracilis
6 adductor longus
7 pectineus
8 iliopsoas
9 rectus abdominis
10 external oblique
11 gluteus medius

B Landmarks and muscles

1 gracilis
2 adductor magnus
3 semimembranosus
4 semitendinosus
5 biceps femoris
6 iliotibial tract
7 gluteus maximus
8 tensor fasciae latae
9 gluteus medius
10 external oblique
11 latissimus dorsi

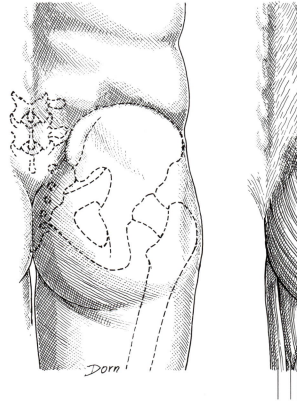
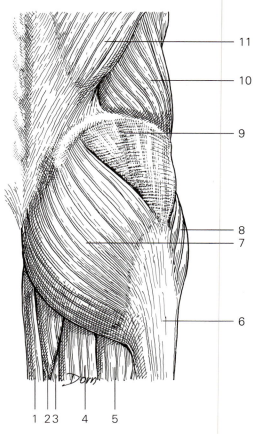

C Landmarks and muscles

1 gluteus maximus
2 biceps femoris
3 vastus lateralis
4 rectus femoris
5 sartorius
6 tensor fasciae latae
7 external oblique
8 latissimus dorsi

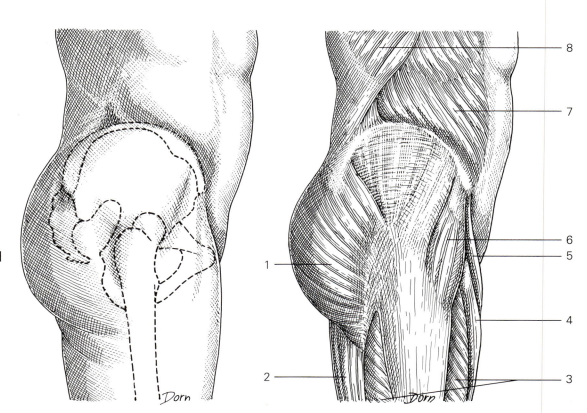

3

Pelvic girdle

identification of this shallow depression between the two muscles is a prerequisite before making the incision for the anterior and anterolateral approaches to the hip, thus avoiding unnecessary damage to the lateral cutaneous nerve.

The superior border of the pubic symphysis is palpated by identifying the abdominal midline and tracing it distally. It is palpated one or two fingers' breadth distal to the superior limit of the pubic hair. If the mons pubis is palpated between thumb and index finger, the pubic spines can be palpated lateral to the superior border of the body of the pubis on either side.

The iliac crest

This is easy to palpate in slim patients, but can be difficult to locate in obese ones. Often the abdominal wall will overlie the iliac crest, so it can be difficult to position an incision accurately. Skin and subcutaneous tissues must be retracted proximally and medially in order to identify the crest. On occasion in more obese individuals the abdominal muscles themselves overlie the iliac crest and are recognized during the subcutaneous dissection. As soon as the superficial aspect of the muscles is reached they must be retracted proximally and medially to identify the iliac crest and an incision into the overlying fascia can then be made. If a transverse line is drawn across the abdomen from the most proximal point of the iliac crest on either side, it will cross the body of the fourth lumbar vertebra.

The greater trochanter

The greater trochanter is not always easy to palpate because of the adiposity of the patient. Following pelvic or hip trauma it may be displaced. However, the greater trochanter can usually be palpated, and its anterior and posterior borders identified, allowing an incision to be placed over its lateral aspect. On occasions a screw may need to be passed percutaneously into the femoral neck along the proximal border of vastus lateralis as it inserts into the trochanteric crest. This point can usually be palpated as a depression just distal to the prominence of the greater trochanter. The superior border of the greater trochanter is a useful landmark over which are centred most of the lateral or posterior approaches to the hip.

Posterior superior iliac spine

The posterior superior iliac spine may be recognized by palpating the iliac crest posteriorly. It forms the posterior limit. There is an overlying dimple in the skin visible even in obese patients some two fingers' breadth lateral to the posterior midline. Sometimes two dimples are visible: the proximal one is also more lateral and corresponds to the insertion of the erector spinae muscles into the iliac crest. The line joining the posterior superior iliac spines will cross in the midline the second posterior sacral foramina. Between the two dimples overlying the posterior superior iliac spine and at the proximal part of the natal cleft is a triangular depressed area overlying the posterior aspect of the inferior sacrum and coccyx. In the midline of the triangle in the sagittal plane the median sacral crest can be palpated.

The gluteal muscles

Gluteus maximus gives the shape to the buttock. The gluteal fold, which is a cutaneous skin fold running horizontally, crosses the oblique inferior border of gluteus maximus. The ischial tuberosity can be palpated 5 cm lateral to the midline and 5 cm proximal to the gluteal fold.

The surgical dissection: anatomical considerations

The anterior midline incision

The linea alba is not always easy to identify, particularly distally between pyramidalis on either side. Often in error the anterior sheath of one rectus abdominis is opened and the posterior sheath must then be divided vertically in order to expose the pubic symphysis. Rectus abdominis inserts into both the superior and the anterior aspects of the body of the pubis. To gain access to the superior aspect of the pubis we may need to divide the tendon of insertion of rectus abdominis 1 cm proximal to the bone or elevate the posterior part from the superior aspect of the pubis from a dorsal direction anteriorly, leaving the anterior tendon in continuity with the bone. If a plate is to be inserted it can be positioned on the superior aspect of the pubis deep to the muscle.

The bladder is adjacent to the posterior aspect of the pubis and should be separated from it by blunt finger dissection and from the obturator internus fascia. The inferior aspect of the pubic symphysis can be reached and the urethra can then be palpated since it lies immediately beneath it, particularly when a catheter has been inserted as an essential preoperative step. Moving laterally from the inferior border of the symphysis the inferior pubic rami can be palpated; the muscles can

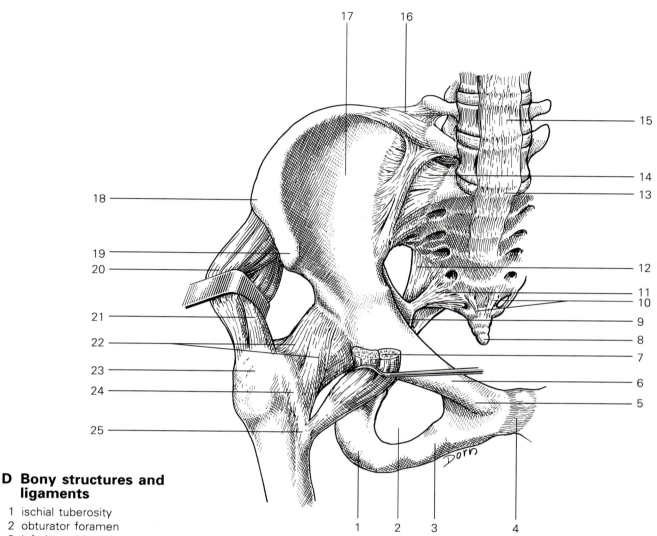

D Bony structures and ligaments

1 ischial tuberosity
2 obturator foramen
3 inferior pubic ramus
4 pubic symphysis
5 pubic tubercle
6 superior pubic ramus
7 iliopsoas
8 coccyx
9 ischial spine
10 anterior sacrococcygeal ligaments
11 sacrospinous ligament
12 sacrotuberous ligament
13 sacral promontory
14 anterior sacroiliac ligament
15 anterior longitudinal ligament
16 iliolumbar ligament
17 iliac fossa
18 tubercle of iliac crest
19 anterior superior iliac spine
20 gluteus medius
21 gluteus minimus
22 iliofemoral ligament (Y ligament of Bigelow)
23 greater trochanter
24 trochanteric line
25 lesser trochanter

be stripped from them and if necessary the bone can be osteotomized. The obturator neurovascular bundle can be identified as it enters the obturator canal just below the superior pubic ramus.

If a transverse incision is used the spermatic cord or the round ligament is identified after division of the external oblique aponeurosis and the rectus femoris sheath. These structures should be protected by a suitable tape.

The pubic rami can be approached in order to fix disruptions of the pubic symphysis internally or to perform an osteotomy. In order to expose the bone the fascia overlying obturator internus should be divided adjacent to the bone along the superior medial and inferior attachments of the muscle. The muscle is then elevated together with the obturator membrane over the medial part of the obturator foramen as far laterally as necessary, with great care being taken not to damage the obturator neurovascular bundle lying within the obturator canal. Access to the superior aspect of the superior pubic rami can be achieved by dividing the fascia overlying pectineus along the pectineal line and sharply elevating pectineus from the superior aspect of the superior

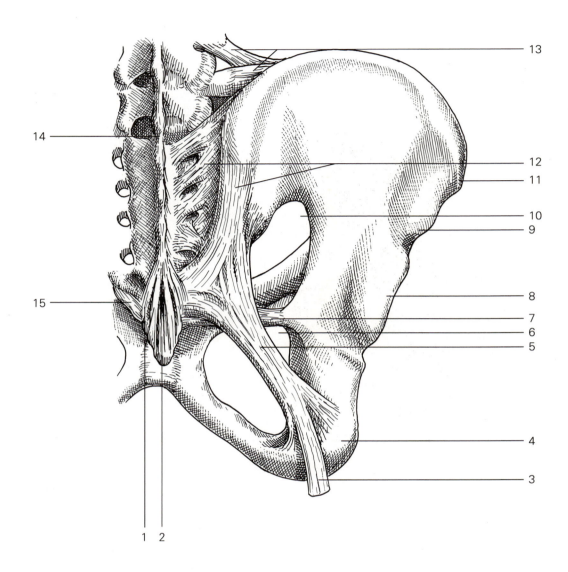

pubic rami. Once all steps have been accomplished one has control of the full circumference of the superior pubic ramus. If the dissection of obturator internus is conducted carefully and carried sufficiently posteriorly the quadrilateral space of the innominate bone and the iliopectineal eminence beneath the external iliac vessels can be reached.

The ilioinguinal approach (**D** and **F**)

The abdominal muscles are sharply incised and stripped from the inner slope of the iliac crest in continuity with iliacus which is elevated from the internal iliac fossa as far as the sacroiliac joint medially and the pelvic brim inferiorly.

The iliopsoas fascia can act as a main obstacle to the approach and requires to be properly divided. The iliopsoas fascia totally covers iliopsoas and is inserted along the medial border of the iliac crest and along the full length of the pelvic brim where it may be reinforced by the tendon of psoas minor if present. Iliopsoas passes beneath the inguinal ligament and is strongly attached to it. Between the inguinal ligament and the iliopectineal eminence the medial

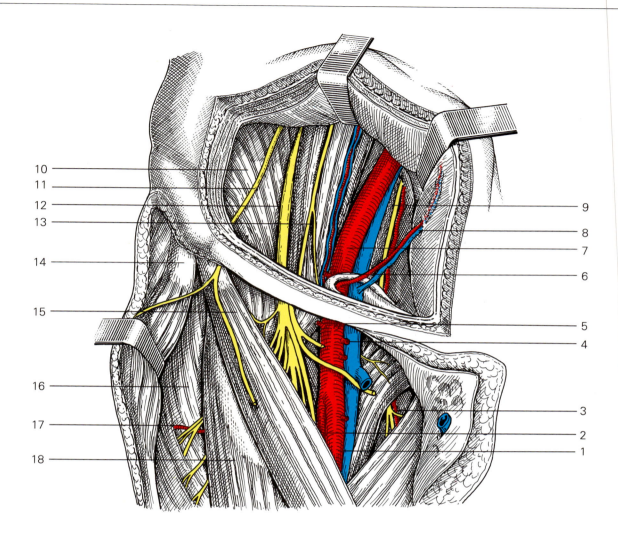

F Soft tissues (anterior aspect)

1 femoral artery
2 profunda femoris
3 obturator nerve and vessels
4 pudendal artery
5 superficial circumflex iliac artery
6 deep circumflex iliac artery
7 external iliac artery
8 epigastric vessels
9 obturator nerve and vessels
10 iliacus
11 lateral cutaneous nerve of thigh
12 femoral nerve
13 genitofemoral nerve
14 tensor fasciae latae
15 sartorius
16 vastus lateralis
17 nerve and vessels to vastus lateralis
18 rectus femoris

free border of the iliopsoas fascia is free and often thickened. It is orientated backwards and medially. The ilipsoas fascia divides the space between the inguinal ligament and anterior edge of the innominate bone into two spaces: the lateral space contains iliopsoas and the femoral nerve, whilst the medial space contains the external iliac vessels and accompanying lymphatic channels. Occasionally the fascia is crossed by a vascular bundle arising from the external iliac vessels which supplies iliopsoas. The thickness of the fascia is variable and it can be palpated by the index finger by laterally

retracting iliopsoas and by bluntly dissecting its medial aspect. Care should be taken not to damage the lymphatics which run adjacent to the external iliac artery.

The external iliac vessels cross the anterior border of the innominate bone, the artery resting on the iliopectineal eminence. When they are dissected it is essential to retain the areolar tissue that surrounds them in continuity in order to protect the lymphatics.

The femoral nerve lies on the superficial aspect of iliopsoas along the gutter separating iliacus from psoas. It is never necessary to dissect the femoral nerve but it is essential to identify it.

Pelvic girdle

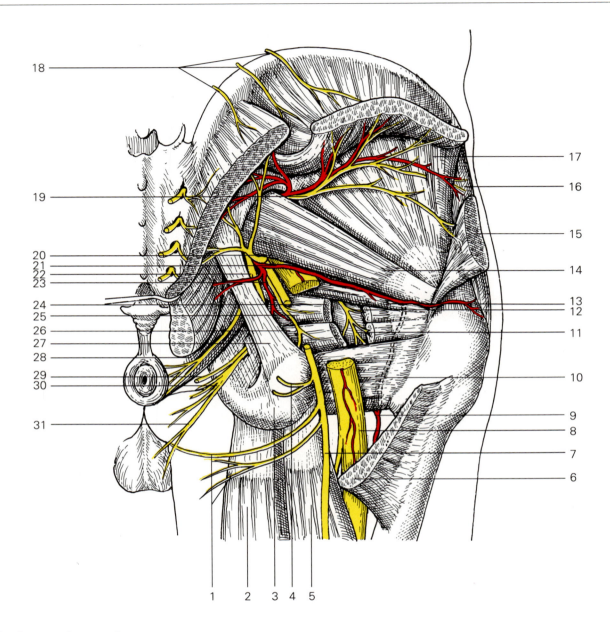

G Soft tissues (posterior aspect)

1 perineal branches of posterior cutaneous nerve of thigh
2 semitendinosus
3 ischial tuberosity
4 inferior clunial nerves
5 biceps femoris (long head)
6 gluteus maximus, cut
7 posterior cutaneous nerve of thigh
8 sciatic nerve
9 medial circumflex femoral artery
10 quadratus femoris
11 nerve to inferior gemellus and quadratus femoris
12 branch to the hip joint
13 superior gemellus
14 piriformis
15 gluteus medius, cut
16 tensor fasciae latae
17 gluteus minimus
18 superior clunial nerves
19 superior gluteal artery and nerve
20 inferior gluteal nerve
21 inferior gluteal artery
22 sacrotuberous ligament
23 pudendal nerve
24 posterior cutaneous nerve of thigh
25 obturator internus
26 gemellus inferior
27 sacrotuberous ligament
28 inferior rectal nerve
29 dorsal nerve of penis/clitoris
30 perineal nerve
31 posterior scrotal (labial) nerves

The lateral cutaneous nerve of thigh is variable in position. Usually it runs adjacent and medial to the anterior superior iliac spine. It can be isolated by carefully dividing the transversus abdominis and internal oblique fibres from the inguinal ligament adjacent to their origins. The ligament itself may need to be divided. The nerve seems to be situated within the aponeurotic origin of these muscles, always accompanied by a small vascular pedicle. Occasionally a little fibrous arcade bordering the nerve medially should be divided. Less commonly, the nerve is situated more medially and may lie 3 cm medial to the anterior superior iliac spine.

The aponeurosis of obturator internus is strongly attached to the pelvic brim in continuity with the insertion of the iliopsoas fascia. The aponeurosis needs to be divided against the pelvic brim in order to elevate the muscle from the quadrilateral space and gain access to the whole surface as far posteriorly as the sciatic notches and as far inferiorly as the superior border of the obturator foramen.

The retropubic anastomosis between the external iliac vessels and the obturator artery is not constant. However, such an anastomosis is frequently encountered and lies against the posterior aspect of the superior pubic ramus running from the obturator vessels to the external iliac vessels. This vascular pedicle can be rolled beneath the fingertip against the posterior aspect of the superior pubic ramus and should be ligated and divided in order to allow dissection and retraction of the external iliac vessels. Occasionally the vessel is much larger and may even be of the same size as the obturator artery. It has been called the corona mortis. It is possible that this is an unusual origin of the obturator

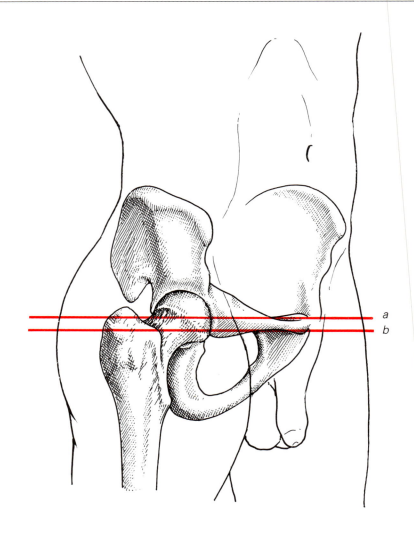

H Cross-section through the hip joint (see **I** and **J**)

artery from the inferior epigastric artery or just a large anastomosis between the two vascular systems.

The anterior approach (F,H,I,J)

The lateral cutaneous nerve of thigh is the only structure which is always at risk during this approach. The nerve has passed beneath the inguinal ligament and appears distal to the anterior inferior iliac spine; it immediately divides into several branches which run in the palpable interval between sartorius medially and tensor fasciae latae laterally. Classical approaches recommended by Hueter (the anterior) and Smith-Petersen (the extended anterior) would result in the division of the majority of these branches; however, we have recommended that the fascia overlying the belly of tensor fasciae latae be divided, sacrificing only one or two branches of the nerve.

Rectus femoris arises by two heads which lie beneath a thin

Pelvic girdle

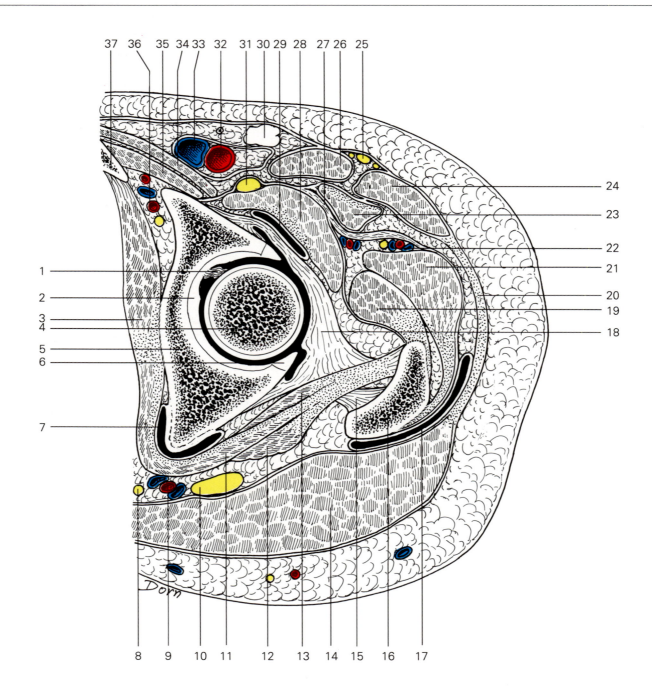

I Cross-section through the hip joint: plane *a*

1 ligamentum teres
2 acetabulum
3 obturator internus
4 femoral head
5 iliac bone
6 acetabular labrum
7 bursa of obturator internus
8 inferior gluteal nerve
9 inferior gluteal vessels
10 sciatic nerve
11 obturator internus

12 gemellus inferior
13 gemellus superior
14 gluteus maximus
15 obturator externus tendon
16 greater trochanter
17 trochanteric bursa
18 joint capsule
19 gluteus minimus
20 fascia lata
21 gluteus medius
22 neurovascular pedicle to quadriceps
23 rectus femoris
24 tensor fasciae latae

25 lateral cutaneous nerve of thigh
26 sartorius
27 deep fascial sheet
28 iliopsoas
29 iliopsoas bursa
30 lymph node
31 femoral nerve
32 femoral artery
33 femoral vein
34 pectineus
35 obturator externus
36 obturator nerve and vessels
37 pubis

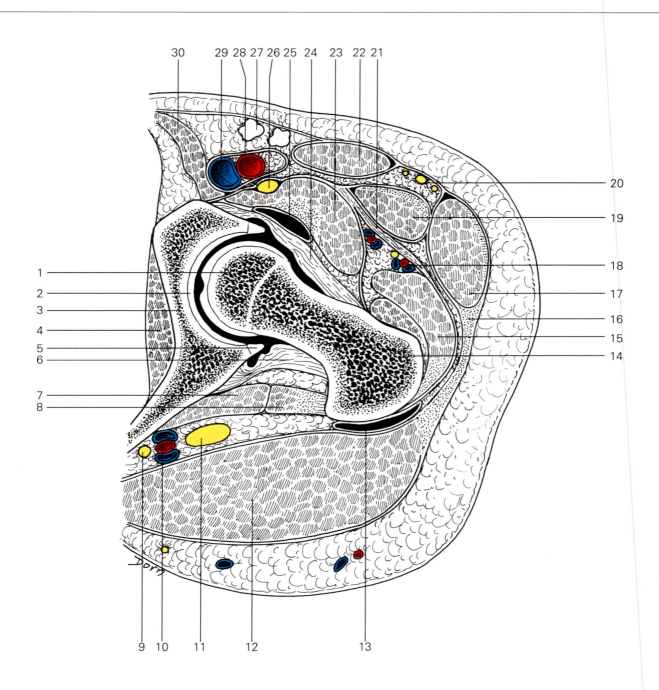

J Cross- section through the hip joint: plane *b*

1 femoral head
2 acetabulum
3 iliac wing
4 obturator internus
5 acetabular labrum
6 joint capsule
7 gemellus inferior
8 obturator externus
9 inferior gluteal nerve
10 inferior gluteal vessels
11 sciatic nerve

12 gluteus maximus
13 trochanteric bursa
14 greater trochanter
15 gluteus medius
16 fascia lata (iliotibial tract)
17 tensor fasciae latae
18 neurovascular pedicle to quadriceps
19 rectus femoris
20 lateral cutaneous nerve of thigh
21 deep fascial sheet
22 sartorius
23 iliopsoas
24 joint capsule

25 iliopsoas bursa
26 femoral nerve
27 lymph nodes
28 femoral artery
29 femoral vein
30 pectineus

and translucent fascial sheet which appears when tensor fasciae latae is retracted laterally. The straight head arises from the anterior inferior iliac spine and is the stronger of the two. The reflected head runs along the superior attachment of the hip capsule to insert 4–5 cm posteriorly adjacent to the acetabular rim. This tendon is flat and may have a free inferior border although usually the border is in continuity with the fascial sheet which lies along the superior aspect of the hip capsule with which it blends. To free the tendon it is necessary to divide this fascial sheet which is thinner than the tendon itself. Deep to the reflected head runs an artery which is closely applied to the bone and follows the depression in the bone in which lies the reflected head. When the tendon of origin needs to be divided it is wise to clamp the tendon and the artery prior to the division since the artery is always divided.

The fascial layers encountered during the anterior approach are remarkably constant. Beginning superficially the fascia covering the belly of tensor fasciae latae is encountered: this is quite thick and arises from the iliac crest running distally. The fascia that surrounds tensor fasciae latae coalesces medially to bridge the gap between that muscle and sartorius and overlies fatty tissue through which runs the branches of the lateral cutaneous nerve of thigh.

The fascia over rectus femoris is a relatively thin and translucent sheet through which can be seen the two heads of the muscle. Once the muscle has been retracted medially the posterior aspect of the rectus femoris sheath is a strong fascial sheet thick in comparison with the others and sometimes opaque. No anatomical name has been given to this structure. Along the anterior border of this fascial sheet is a small vascular pedicle which crosses it arising from the lateral circumflex artery and supplying rectus femoris. By identifying this vessel and tracing it deeply, the lateral circumflex artery can be identified. Deep to this fascial sheet is a layer of fatty tissue crossed by the lateral circumflex vessels which run horizontally and deeper still are the nutrient vessels and nerve to vastus lateralis which run laterally and distally.

Iliopsoas is covered anteriorly by a thin fascial layer which is incised when the circumflex vessels are isolated. Fascia is attached laterally to the hip capsule. The muscle itself has several large strong insertions onto the anterior aspect of the hip capsule (a point not always mentioned by traditional anatomists). The muscle can be sharply dissected from the capsule as far medially as the psoas bursa which lies between the iliopsoas tendon and the hip capsule.

The posterior approaches (G,H,I,J)

Gluteus maximus arises from the posterior part of the external aspect of the iliac wing anterior to the posterior iliac spine: it arises posterior to the posterior gluteal crest and from the posterior 4 cm of the iliac crest. Its superior border runs from the iliac crest to the level of the superior border of the greater trochanter. The proximal limb of posterior approach incisions centred over the greater trochanter can take one of two directions. The incision may run from the greater trochanter to the posterior superior iliac spine or a point distal to it. Deeper dissection will result in splitting the fibres of gluteus maximus which separate the proximal fibres supplied by the superior gluteal artery from the distal fibres supplied by the inferior gluteal artery. However, an incision running from the greater trochanter to the iliac crest more than 4 cm anterior to the posterior superior spine will allow a dissection through the gluteal fascia which avoids gluteus maximus altogether. The distal continuation of the incision will also incise the iliotibial tract, hence subcutaneous dissection is purely transaponeurotic. It must be remembered, however, that whilst the vascularity of the muscle is provided by both superior and inferior gluteal arteries, it is only the inferior gluteal nerve which supplies the muscle. If the muscle is completely split in the line of its fibres there is a risk of damage to the inferior gluteal nerve and hence the proximal part of the muscle will be paralysed. It is vital, therefore, not to continue the splitting of gluteus maximus fibres too far posteriorly.

The superior gluteal neurovascular bundle exits from the true pelvis via the greater sciatic notch above piriformis: it comprises an artery, several veins and the superior gluteal nerve. The pedicle crosses the upper border of the greater sciatic notch which lies against the bone and is separated from it only by a thin translucent fascial sheet which holds it against the gluteal muscles. Anatomists describe ligaments surrounding the pedicle but these are difficult to define at surgery. Once piriformis has been divided through its distal tendon and is retracted proximally, then the superior gluteal pedicle can be seen against the bone. If the greater sciatic notch has been fractured and the fragments are displaced mobilization of the fragments must be conducted very cautiously: one must stick strictly to the bone in order to avoid damage to the pedicle. The pedicle is separated from the bone and the plate passed deep to it. The screws are inserted directly through the muscles above the pedicle.

The sciatic nerve is potentially at risk during the posterior approaches and it is vital to identify and protect it. The nerve exits from the pelvis through the greater sciatic notch beneath piriformis. Following trauma it is not always easy to identify piriformis and the easiest way to identify the nerve is to identify quadratus femoris as it inserts into the trochanteric crest. The horizontal fibres should then be followed proximally into the depths of the wound where the sciatic nerve will be encountered, often lying in adipose tissue. The nerve can then be traced along its lateral border proximally and distally and the lower border of piriformis can be identified, beneath which the nerve disappears into the pelvis. In certain cases the nerve may actually run through the body of the muscle. It is not necessary to place a sling around the nerve but it is essential to identify its position. Accompanying the sciatic nerve are other neurovascular structures, namely the inferior gluteal artery and nerve, the pudendal nerve and the internal pudendal artery, the nerve to obturator internus and the posterior cutaneous nerve of thigh. Regularly encountered at surgery are the inferior gluteal artery and nerve which immediately enter gluteus maximus and are retracted with the gluteal muscles posteriorly. The other structures are rather deeper than the sciatic nerve and are not often encountered. In cases where it is necessary to divide the insertion of the sacrospinous ligament adjacent to the ischial spine the internal pudendal artery may be encountered.

The short external rotators clothe the posterior aspect of the hip capsule and must be divided in order to expose the hip capsule. Piriformis is not easily identified, especially after trauma since its superior border blends with gluteus medius. However, its tendon inserts into the anterior part of the superior border of the greater trochanter and this may be recognized by palpation adjacent to the trochanter above the hip. Piriformis is divided through its tendon to avoid damage to the branches of the ascending branch of the posterior circumflex artery. Between piriformis and quadratus femoris lie obturator internus and the superior and inferior gemelli. The tendons of the two gemelli merge adjacent to their trochanteric insertion and overlie obturator internus. The gemelli arise from the outer aspect of the innominate bone above and below the lesser sciatic notch, whilst obturator internus arises from the inner aspect of the bone from the quadrilateral surface and the obturator membrane and the fibres converge towards the lesser sciatic notch. At the level of the lesser sciatic notch there are five or six continuous musculotendinous units which coalesce at the level of the notch and change direction, forming an angle of approximately 60° as they leave the pelvis. A synovial bursa is present between the tendons and the fibrocartilage of the lesser sciatic notch. The bursa has two parts, one intrapelvic and the other extrapelvic. The bursa is firmly attached to the overlying muscle and is also attached to the limits of the fibrocartilage which covers the lesser sciatic notch. Once the tendon of insertion is divided, approximately 2 cm away from the greater trochanter, the muscle can be elevated from the retroacetabular surface to open the more lateral part of the bursa which allows inspection of the fibrocartilage of the lesser sciatic notch. In addition, the deep aspect of the tendons of obturator internus is seen and it is possible to enter the true pelvis.

The lateral approaches (H,I,J)

These approaches, often extensive, are based on the anatomical fact that the gluteal muscles together with tensor fasciae latae are supplied by the superior and inferior gluteal nerves which exit from the greater sciatic notch. It is possible to elevate these muscles in continuity from anterior to posterior and their nerve supply is left intact.

Gluteus minimus inserts onto the anterior aspect of the greater trochanter. Its inferior fibres are tendinous and form a strong tendon whilst the anterior fibres are fleshy and difficult to suture following their division. If there is difficulty in identifying the insertion of gluteus minimus the dissection can commence distal to the trochanter: one should identify vastus lateralis whose tendinous fibres are attached to the trochanteric line at the inferior aspect of the greater trochanter and also along the inner border of the anterior aspect of the trochanter. By tracing these fibres proximally the tendon of gluteus minimus is easily identified.

Gluteus medius has a comma-shaped insertion, which is rather long and narrow, into the lateral aspect of the trochanter. It runs obliquely distally and anteriorly, the strongest part being posterior.

The trochanteric bursa is constant and separates the fascia lata from the lateral and anterior aspects of the greater trochanter into which insert gluteus medius and gluteus minimus. The bursa is usually thick-walled and complex in shape. In order to gain complete access to the greater trochanter it is necessary to incise the bursa.

The superior gluteal neurovascular bundle is frequently encountered in the lateral approaches. In the lateral 'U' approach or the triradiate approach the pedicle is left undisturbed and protected by the posterior part of gluteus

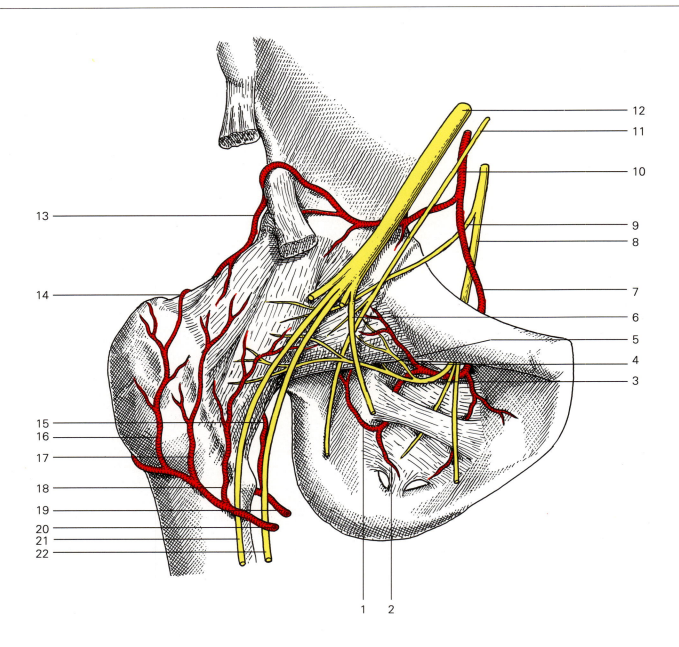

K Vascular and nerve supply

1 ramus acetabularis
2 posterior branch of obturator artery
3 articular nerve of hip joint
4 nerve to acetabular labrum
5 nerve to acetabulum
6 nerve to pectineus
7 obturator artery
8 obturator nerve
9 articular branch from obturator nerve
10 obturator artery
11 accessory obturator nerve (inconstant)

12 femoral nerve
13 artery to roof of acetabulum
14 anastomoses between circumflex arteries
15 inferior artery of femoral neck
16 anterior artery of greater trochanter
17 anterior arteries of femoral neck
18 anterior arteries of femoral neck
19 medial circumflex femoral artery
20 lateral circumflex femoral artery
21 nerve to vastus lateralis
22 nerve to rectus femoris

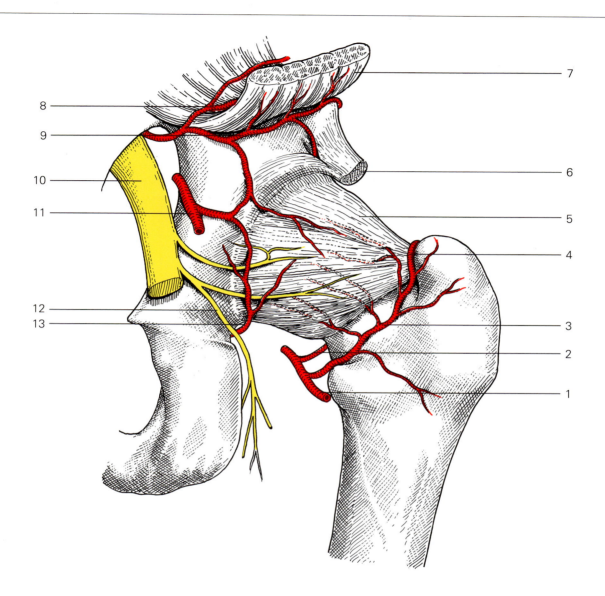

L Vascular and nerve supply

1 medial circumflex femoral artery
2 inferior artery of femoral neck
3 posterior vascular branch to greater trochanter
4 anastomoses between circumflex arteries
5 capsule of hip joint
6 tendon of rectus femoris
7 gluteus minimus
8 deep branch of superior gluteal artery
9 artery to roof of acetabulum
10 sciatic nerve
11 inferior gluteal artery
12 nerve to gemellus inferior and quadratus femoris (articular nerve)
13 arterial ramus from posterior branch of obturator artery

maximus. However, the pedicle is encountered in the extended iliofemoral approach. The gluteal muscles are reflected from the iliac wing and retracted proximally and posteriorly to expose the upper border of the greater sciatic notch. Terminal branches of the superior gluteal pedicle have been mobilized with the muscle mass. The pedicle passes through the greater sciatic notch close to the bone and must not be damaged. Finger dissection is safe and effective and can separate the pedicle from the bone by dividing the fibrous connections, leaving intact the thin fascial sheath

which holds the vessels against the deep aspect of the gluteal muscles. The pedicle is mobilized and freed as far proximally as possible by use of the finger.

The short external rotator muscles are frequently encountered in the lateral approach and are handled in exactly the same way as in the posterior approach, as already described.

The sacroiliac approaches (see D,E,G)

The fibres of gluteus maximus have strong connections with the subcutaneous tissue. Once the muscle fibres are seen sharp dissection is required to dissect the muscle medially, first to the posterior iliac crest and then towards the medial sacral crest. In order to have a viable and thick muscular flap it is recommended that the muscle be elevated from the outer border of the iliac crest from the posterior part of the iliac wing and from its superior and medial attachments to the aponeurosis covering erector spinae. Muscle origins are sharply divided and the muscle is stripped from the aponeurosis of erector spinae and from the posterior aspect of the sacrotuberous ligament. Following this, an 'L'-shaped muscular flap has been created which can be perfectly reattached to its origins. Upon retraction of gluteus maximus the sacrotuberous ligament and, above it, piriformis can be identified as they exit from the pelvis. Further medially and lying against the superior border of the greater sciatic notch lies the superior gluteal neurovascular bundle.

The sacrotuberous and sacrospinous ligaments are arranged in two distinct layers. During the exploration of malunited pelvic fractures it is evident that these ligaments have frequently contracted and would prevent an anatomical reduction of the fracture. It is necessary to divide these tight structures. The superior border of the sacrotuberous ligament is easy to identify when it crosses the posterior aspect of piriformis. It is possible to introduce a narrow malleable blade beneath it to allow its division adjacent to the sacral border. Further distally the sacrospinous ligament is encountered and separated in an identical manner. All tight fibres are divided.

The sacroiliac joint is easy to identify. Gluteus maximus is elevated and retracted as described above and the sacrotuberous and sacrospinal ligaments are divided, beginning from the inner aspect of the posterior part of the iliac crest and continuing between the posterior iliac spines from dorsal to anterior. The joint may then be opened and a lamina spreader can be inserted into the joint to allow identification anteriorly of the anterior sacroiliac ligament. The index finger can be inserted into the joint and it can free the inferior border of the ligament, allowing it to be divided. The L5 nerve root is usually at least 1 cm medial to the sacroiliac joint.

Vascular and nerve supply to the hip joint (**K,L**)

Vascular supply

The arterial supply of the hip joint is provided by several main trunks:

- The circumflex arteries arising from the femoral artery.
- The lateral branch of the obturator artery.
- Branches from the superior and inferior gluteal arteries.

The lateral circumflex femoral artery arises from the deep femoral artery and reaches the joint passing between iliopsoas and rectus femoris. It gives off the anterior artery of the neck of the femur and an anterior branch to the greater trochanter. Finally it anastomoses with the medial femoral circumflex artery on the posterolateral aspect of the greater trochanter.

The medial circumflex femoral artery arises from the deep femoral artery and runs between obturator externus and adductor magnus. It anastomoses with the lateral circumflex femoral artery to form a vascular circle around the neck of the femur. The artery gives off the inferior artery of the femoral neck and several branches to the femoral head.

The lateral branch of the obturator artery supplies the roof of the acetabulum and acetabular labrum. An additional branch is the ramus acetabularis which supplies the artery of the ligamentum teres. The artery supplies the femoral head by running within the ligament.

The superior and inferior gluteal arteries supply branches to the posterior aspect of the joint and particularly to the artery of the roof of the acetabulum. Branches arising from the two gluteal arteries and from the obturator artery constitute a vascular circle around the acetabulum.

Nerve supply

The hip joint is supplied:

- Anteriorly by branches from the femoral and obturator nerves.
- Posteriorly by the sciatic nerve and the nerve to quadratus femoris.

The femoral nerve provides several small branches arising from the nerves to pectineus and the quadriceps.

The obturator nerve supplies a large branch which is the anterior inferior articular nerve of the joint. This branch divides into three rami, one to the acetabular labrum, one to the acetabulum and one to the anterior aspect of the capsule.

The nerve to quadratus femoris and gemellus inferior supplies one or two rami to the posterior aspect of the joint.

The sciatic nerve supplies an articular branch to the inferior part of the posterior aspect of the joint.

Acetabulum: ilioinguinal (Letournel) approach

Indications

The main indication is the surgical treatment of fractures of the acetabulum. These are either simple patterns (anterior wall and anterior column fractures — some transverse, mostly displaced anteriorly) or complex patterns (anterior and posterior column fractures not involving the sacro-iliac joint, with the posterior column fracture being simple and not comminuted). It is not necessary to treat an undisplaced posterior column fracture surgically.

Other indications are tumours of the anterior column of the acetabulum, periacetabular osteotomies for acetabular dysplasia, and some Malgaigne fractures combining an anterior lesion and a posterior fracture through the iliac wing.

Position of the patient

A Before the operation a Foley catheter is placed in the bladder. Most frequently the orthopaedic table is used, with the patient lying supine and the pelvic post applied against the contralateral pubic symphysis. The frequent need to extract the femoral head from the pelvis, and to maintain its dislocation during the acetabular reconstruction, often requires lateral traction; this is facilitated by a Sohana screw or a femoral head extractor which is inserted along the long axis of the femoral neck through a short vertical incision over the vastus lateralis origin. Traction can be applied by an assistant, although it is preferable to use a specially designed lateral traction attachment connected to the table. However, if there are associated fractures of the anterior segment of the contralateral pelvis, it is better to use an ordinary table, because traction risks further displacement of the anterior pelvic fracture.

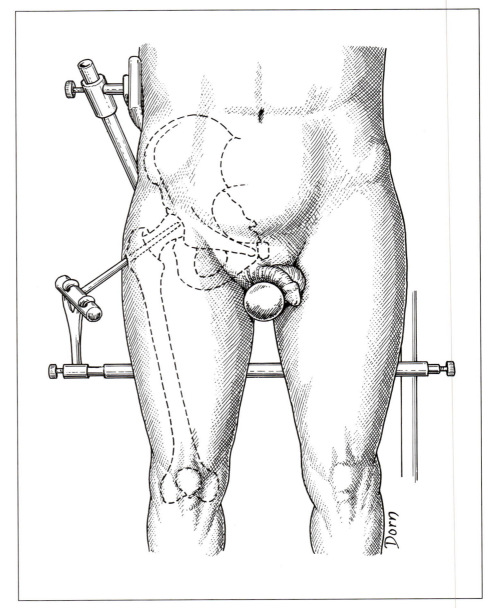

A

Pelvic girdle

Incision

B The incision extends along the anterior two-thirds of the iliac crest and from the anterior superior iliac spine to the midline at a point two fingers' breadth above the pubic symphysis; this incision is slightly concave above and medially. It is essential to extend the incision along the crest beyond its most lateral convexity in order to allow adequate retraction of iliopsoas and the abdominal muscles. By sharp dissection the incision progresses to the iliac crest without injuring the abdominal muscles which sometimes tend to overhang the midportion of the crest.

C The insertions of the abdominal muscles and the origin of iliacus are sharply elevated from the iliac crest; using subperiosteal dissection iliacus is then elevated from the internal iliac fossa — medially as far as the anterior aspect of the sacroiliac joint and distally up to the pelvic brim. The internal iliac fossa is then temporarily packed with wet swabs.

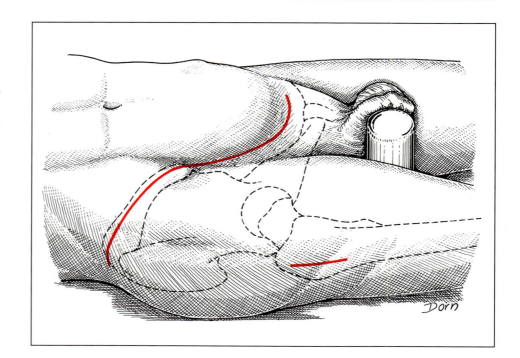

B

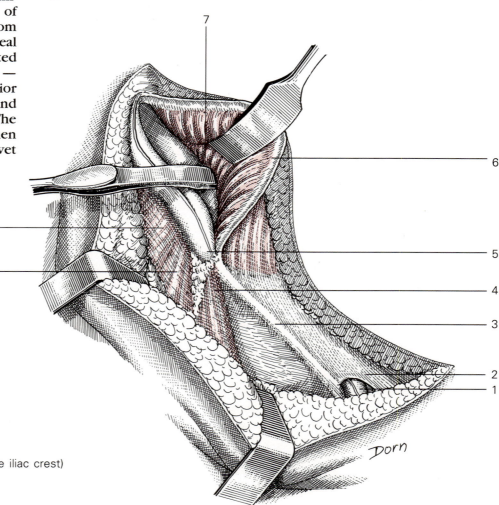

C

1 spermatic cord
2 superficial inguinal ring
3 inguinal ligament
4 sartorius
5 anterior superior iliac spine
6 abdominal muscles (freed from the iliac crest)
7 iliacus
8 gluteus medius
9 tensor fasciae latae

18

D Over the lower abdomen, the incision progresses through the superficial fascia to the aponeurosis of the external oblique and the anterior aspect of the rectus abdominis sheath: these are incised in continuity and in line with the cutaneous incision, passing at least 1 cm above the external inguinal ring.

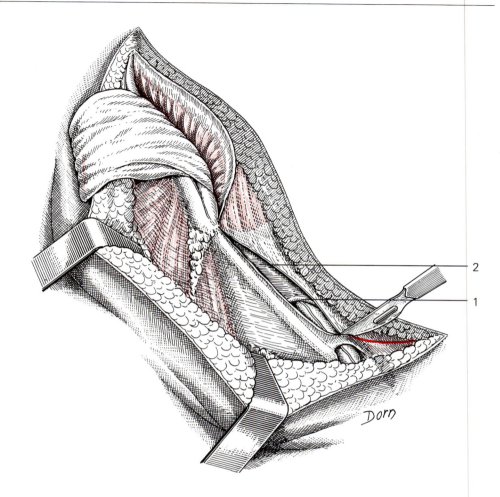

D

1 deep inguinal ring
2 internal oblique

E The edge of the incised aponeurosis is grasped with surgical clamps, the inguinal canal is opened and the inguinal ligament is visualized. A sponge helps to remove areolar tissue from the inguinal ligament.

The spermatic cord or round ligament then becomes visible; a finger is passed posterior to it in order to elevate both it and the adjacent ilioinguinal nerve, and a rubber sling is placed around them so that they can be retracted. At this stage the common origins of the internal oblique and transversus abdominis, and the transversalis fascia, have to be detached from the inguinal ligament; in order to facilitate further reconstruction of the posterior wall of the inguinal canal, it is essential to incise the inguinal ligament itself sharply with a scalpel so that about 1 mm of the ligament remains attached.

Great care should be taken during this step not to injure the structures lying directly beneath the inguinal ligament.

Laterally the psoas sheath is entered directly. Immediately beneath the inguinal ligament the lateral cutaneous nerve is situated in a variable position which may be adjacent to, or up to 3 cm

19

medial to, the anterior superior iliac spine. In the midportion the incision overlies the anterior aspect of the external iliac vessels. Medial to the vessels, and at the level of the pubic tubercle, division of the conjoint tendon of the internal oblique and transversalis allows entry to the retropubic space. If necessary, division of the tendon of rectus abdominis (1 cm above its insertion) is performed. The haematoma of the retropubic space is evacuated and a wet swab used to pack this space. In this way, the anterior aspect of the structures passing under the inguinal ligament is exposed. These structures lie within one of two compartments or lacunae: the laterally situated 'lacuna musculorum' contains iliopsoas, the femoral nerve and the lateral cutaneous nerve of thigh; the medial 'lacuna vasorum' contains the external iliac vessels and lymphatics. The psoas sheath, or iliopectineal fascia, separates the two lacunae and, in order to allow exposure of the quadrilateral surface and the true pelvis, it is essential to divide totally the iliopsoas fascia.

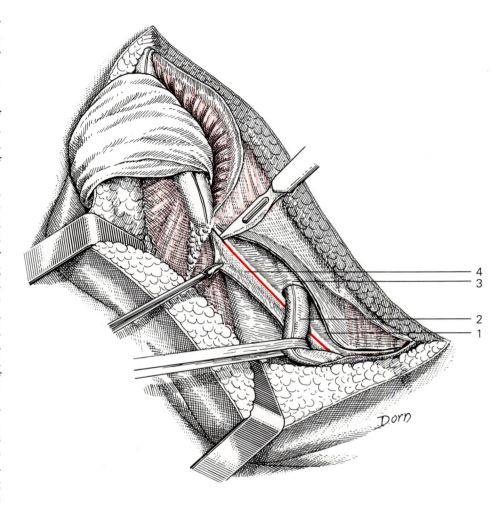

E
1 conjoint tendon (internal oblique and transversus abdominis insertion)
2 spermatic cord
3 deep inguinal ring
4 inguinal ligament

F   To expose the lateral aspect of the psoas sheath, iliopsoas and the femoral nerve are retracted laterally, whereas the external iliac vessels and their satellite lymphatics, medial to the psoas sheath, are carefully dissected from this fascial septum with the use of blunt-tipped scissors or a haemostat. Upon lateral retraction of iliopsoas and medial retraction of the iliac vessels, the iliopsoas fascia is sharply incised by scissors as far as the iliopectineal eminence.

G   Subsequently, the scissors are used to elevate the psoas sheath sharply from the pelvic brim; this manoeuvre is often completed by the use of finger dissection.

A second rubber sling is placed around iliopsoas, the femoral nerve and the lateral cutaneous nerve of thigh for subsequent retraction of these structures.

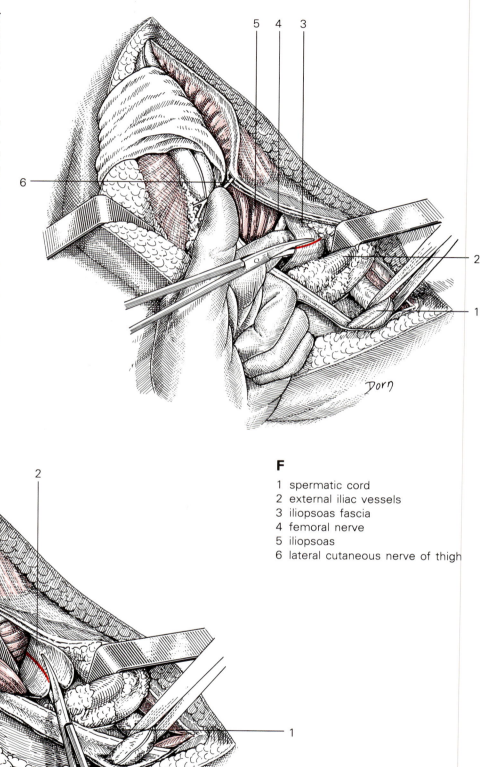

F

1 spermatic cord
2 external iliac vessels
3 iliopsoas fascia
4 femoral nerve
5 iliopsoas
6 lateral cutaneous nerve of thigh

G

1 inguinal ligament (medial border of deep inguinal ring)
2 psoas sheath, being cut along the pelvic brim

21

Pelvic girdle

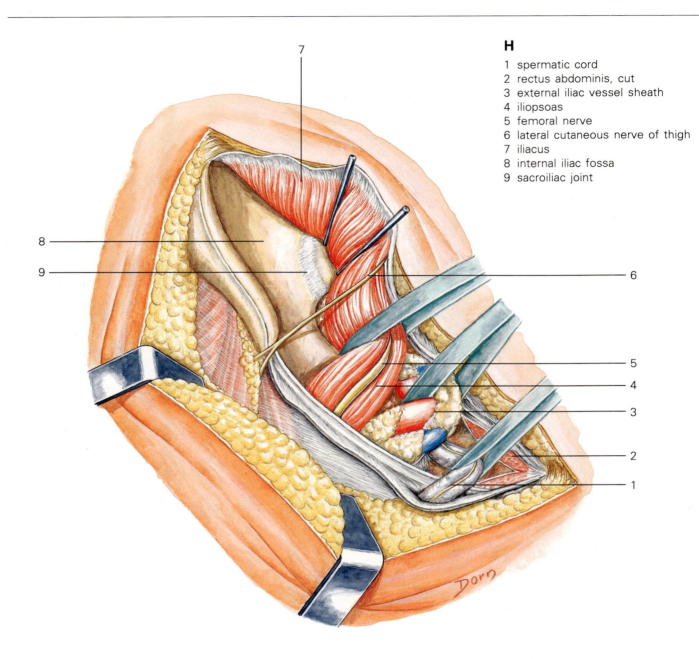

H
1 spermatic cord
2 rectus abdominis, cut
3 external iliac vessel sheath
4 iliopsoas
5 femoral nerve
6 lateral cutaneous nerve of thigh
7 iliacus
8 internal iliac fossa
9 sacroiliac joint

H The insertion of a finger beneath and around the iliac vessels, from lateral to medial, permits the application of a third rubber sling around the external iliac vessels and the adjacent lymphatics. To avoid lymphatic damage it is essential not to dissect too closely to the vessels and to leave as much of the surrounding areolar tissue as possible. Prior to the retraction of the external iliac vessels, a search is made posterior to the vessels for either an anomalous origin of the obturator artery or the presence of an anastomosis between the obturator vessels and the external iliac vessels; the latter is applied closely to the medial aspect of the superior pubis ramus and is recognized easily by finger palpation. If an anastomosis is present, it is clamped, ligated and divided.

The ilioinguinal dissection is now completed. By retraction of the structures held with rubber slings, either medially or laterally, access is gained to the internal aspect of the innominate bone.

Medial retraction of iliopsoas provides access to the entire iliac fossa; distally it provides access along the anterior column as far as the most superior aspect of the iliopectineal eminence. Two Steinmann pins that have been driven into the deepest part of the iliac fossa in front of the sacroiliac joint act as efficient retractors for the abdominal muscles and iliopsoas.

I
1 iliopectineal eminence
2 deep circumflex iliac vessels

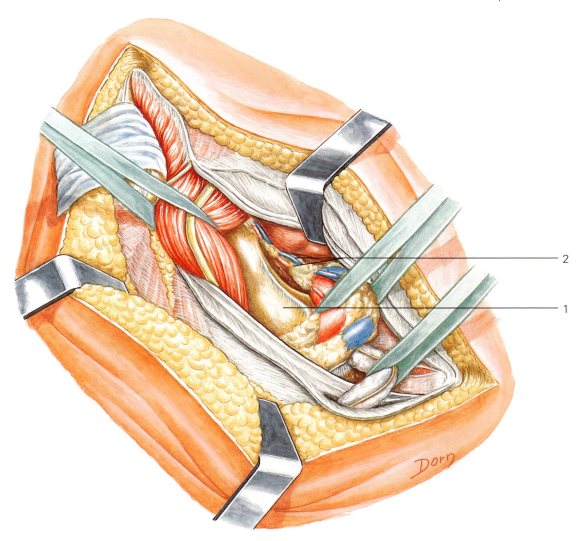

I Lateral retraction of iliopsoas and the femoral nerve, together with medial retraction of the external iliac vessels, opens the medial and probably the most important window of the ilioinguinal incision. This window provides access to a large part of the pelvic brim from the sacroiliac joint to as far distally as the origin of the superior pubic ramus. By subperiosteal elevation of obturator internus, starting at the pelvic brim, access is gained to the whole quadrilateral surface as far as the sciatic notch, the ischial spine and the obturator foramen. Medial retraction is facilitated by the insertion of a malleable ribbon retractor; its tip is placed on the quadrilateral surface and it is moved into the greater sciatic notch. During retraction of the vessels, the pulse of the iliac artery is checked periodically.

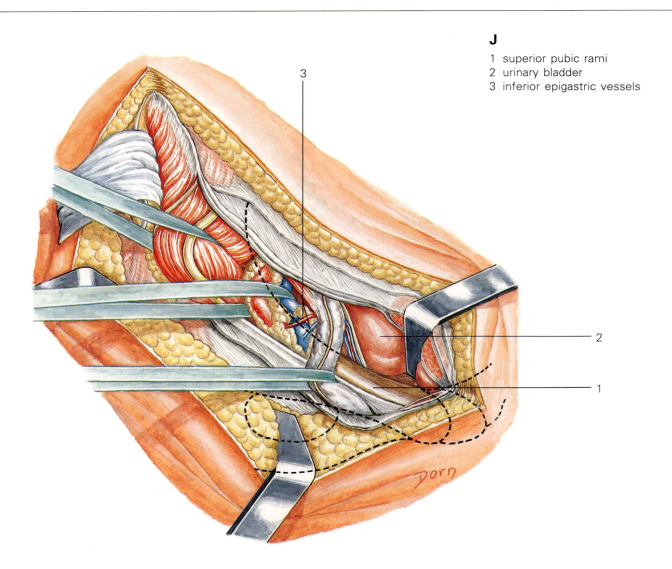

J

1 superior pubic rami
2 urinary bladder
3 inferior epigastric vessels

J Lateral retraction of the vessels with medial retraction of the spermatic cord provides access to the superior pubic ramus, and subperiosteal dissection of pectineus from the superior aspect of the ramus may help to reduce fractures involving this segment.

Lateral retraction of the spermatic cord provides access to the pubic angle and the pubic symphysis.

Extension

Elevation of a greater part of the external aspect of the iliac wing, either to facilitate or to allow the reduction of bone fragments, is possible through the same cutaneous incision, although this increases the risk of significant ectopic bone formation.

It is also possible to facilitate and increase the access to the external aspect of the iliac wing and to the hip capsule by adding an anterior incision to the ilio-inguinal approach: this is started from the anterior superior iliac spine and carried out as described on pages 74-8.

Closure

The closure should be performed very carefully to avoid postoperative abdominal hernias.

Heavy sutures are employed to secure the abdominal fascia to the fascia lata along the iliac crest. If divided, the tendon of rectus abdominis is reattached to its stump. The transversalis fascia and the common origins of the internal oblique and transversus abdominis are reattached to the inguinal ligament, and the narrow strip of inguinal ligament that was retracted with these structures helps in a solid repair. The iliopectineal fascia is not repaired. Closure of the external fascia of rectus abdominis, as well as the aponeurosis of the external oblique, completes the restoration of the integrity of the inguinal canal.

Acetabulum: iliofemoral approach

Introduction

This approach is not dissimilar to the extended anterior approach (see pages 79–82) but differs sufficiently to warrant a specific description.

Indications

The approach is used in isolation for the internal fixation of high anterior column fractures of the acetabulum, and their malunions or non-unions and of fractures of the anterior part of the iliac wing.

It can be used as a combined approach with the posterior approach to the acetabulum to reduce and fix complex acetabular fractures. This approach allows only limited access to the most medial part of the hip capsule which may need to be divided to achieve a perfect reduction of a fractured anterior column.

Position of patient

The patient is positioned supine on either an orthopaedic or an ordinary operating table.

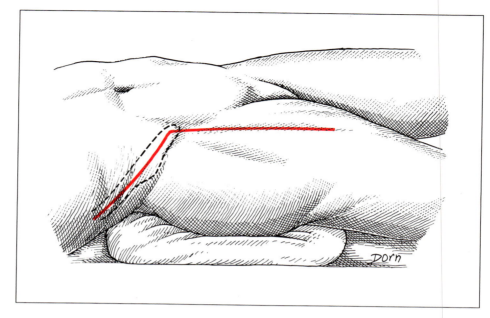

A

Incision

A The incision follows the anterior half or two-thirds of the iliac crest as far anteriorly as the anterior superior iliac spine; it then descends along the lateral border of sartorius for about 15 cm. It runs in a more oblique and medial direction than the extended anterior incision.

Pelvic girdle

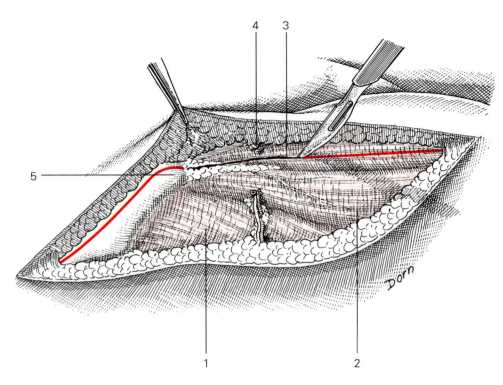

Exposure

B The aponeurosis of the abdominal muscles is sharply incised along the inner lip of the iliac crest and elevated from the inner slope of the crest. In continuity with the abdominal muscles, iliacus is elevated from the internal iliac fossa. From the anterior superior iliac spine the fascial incision follows the line of sartorius.

C At the level of the anterior superior iliac spine, the inguinal ligament is detached together with sartorius which is freed along its lateral border, taking care to preserve its nerve supply. Usually the lateral cutaneous nerve is adjacent to the iliac spine and some of its lateral branches have to be divided.

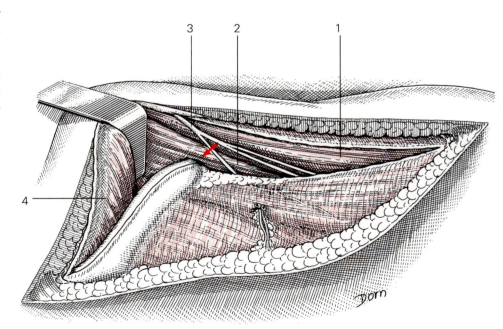

D   Flexion of the thigh facilitates the dissection of the lateral border and the deep surface of iliopsoas. The muscle is raised along the full length of the anterior border of the pelvic bone, running from the anterior inferior iliac spine to the origin of the straight head of rectus femoris. However, the tendon itself is not divided.

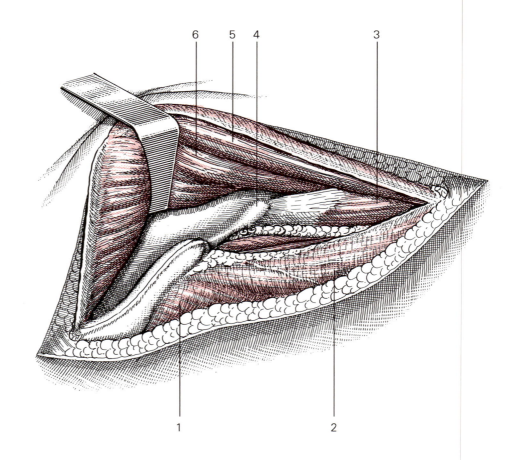

D

1   gluteal aponeurosis
2   tensor fasciae latae
3   rectus femoris
4   anterior inferior iliac spine
5   sartorius
6   iliopsoas

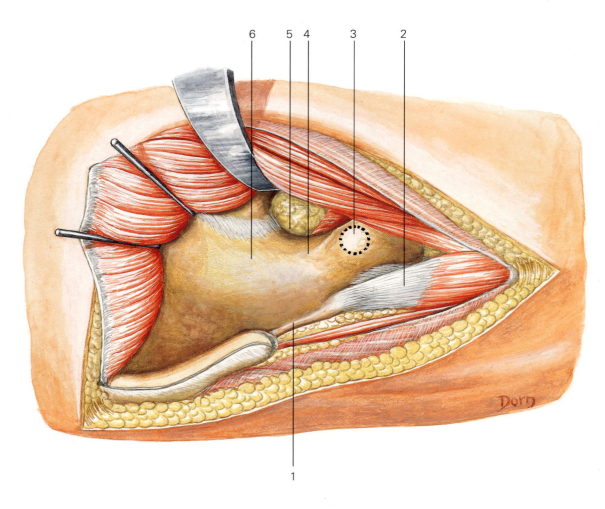

E Iliacus is dissected from the internal iliac fossa as far proximally and medially as the anterior aspect of the sacroiliac joint. Inferiorly, the posterior third or half of the pelvic brim is encountered, together with the iliopectineal eminence; however, the exposure does not go as far distally as the anterior column of the acetabulum.

There have been attempts to enlarge the access by division, under direct vision, of the fibres of the iliopsoas tendon. However, this does not increase the access significantly, and the femoral nerve is thereby exposed to greater risk.

In the region of the interspinous notch at the anterior border of the iliac wing the aponeurotic insertions can be incised at that level and a little of the external iliac fossa can be stripped, thereby enabling a bone-holding forceps to be applied, which affords a solid purchase on the upper part of the anterior column. An artery is always divided at that level and its haemostasis is necessary.

One or two Steinmann pins may be driven into the pelvic brim in front of the sacroiliac joint, or into the sacrum close to its lateral border. They act as very efficient retractors of the abdominal muscles.

Closure

Closure is in anatomical layers. The abdominal muscles are reattached to the aponeurosis of the glutei; sartorius and the inguinal ligaments are reattached to the anterior superior iliac spine, if necessary by transosseous sutures. The aponeurosis of sartorius is closed with interrupted sutures.

E
1 interspinous notch
2 rectus femoris
3 iliopectineal eminence
4 arcuate line
5 greater sciatic notch
6 iliac wing (iliac fossa)

Acetabulum: extended iliofemoral (Judet) approach

Introduction

This extensive surgical approach is based on sound anatomical principles including the wide reflection of muscle groups by preserving their neurovascular pedicles. The muscles supplied by the superior and inferior gluteal nerves are elevated as a unit without jeopardizing their posterior neurovascular pedicles.

This approach embodies 3 main stages:

- The elevation of all the gluteal muscles, together with tensor fasciae latae by dividing both their origins and insertions.
- The division of the short external rotators of the hip exactly as described in the posterior approach.
- An extended capsulotomy along the acetabular margin. When necessary, iliacus can be elevated to expose the internal iliac fossa.

Indications

Complex fractures of the acetabulum, namely:

- Fractures of both columns with posterior column comminution, or involvement of the sacroiliac joint, or when operation is delayed beyond 15–20 days post injury.
- Delayed reconstructions of transverse fractures with or without posterior wall involvement, operated upon beyond 15–20 days, as soon as callus formation is evident on radiographs. All malunions or nonunions of acetabular fractures, except those involving only one column of the acetabulum.

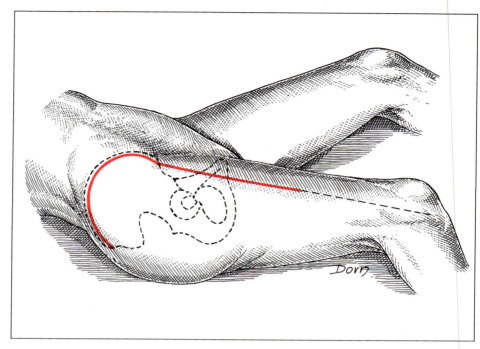

A

- Triple osteotomies of the pelvis to correct acetabular dysplasis.
- Some malunions of pelvic fractures involving the sacroiliac joint.

Position of the patient

Prior to the operation a Foley catheter is placed in the patient's bladder. A standard operating table may be used, the leg being draped separately. The knee is maintained in a flexed position throughout the entire operation to avoid excessive traction on the sciatic nerve. However, it is preferable to place the patient on the Judet fracture table in the lateral position. A Steinmann pin is placed through the distal femur in the supracondylar area to allow longitudinal traction, the knee being flexed at about 45° to relax the sciatic nerve. A pelvic post, which can be moved along a column, is positioned horizontally between the thighs. It can be raised or lowered during the operation from the head of the table. When required, this post can exert pressure on the inner aspect of the thigh and be used effectively to disimpact the femoral head from its centrally dislocated position and to maintain it in the correct position while the reconstruction is performed.

Incision

A The incision is in the form of an inverted 'J' and starts at the posterior superior iliac spine. It is continued along the whole of the iliac crest to the anterior superior iliac spine, and from there descends straight towards the outer border of the patella, halfway down the thigh.

Pelvic girdle

Exposure

B The periosteum is sharply incised along the apex of the iliac crest, and the gluteal fascia is also elevated from the lateral aspect of the crest to facilitate repair at the end of the procedure. The origins of the gluteal muscles are elevated in continuity from the external aspect of the iliac wing subperiosteally. In line with the incision over the iliac crest the fascia overlying the belly of tensor fasciae latae is incised to expose the muscle. During this manoeuvre certain of the branches of the lateral cutaneous nerve of thigh may be divided. Subsequent dissection, however, is deep to the sheath of the muscle and this protects the lateral cutaneous nerve of thigh.

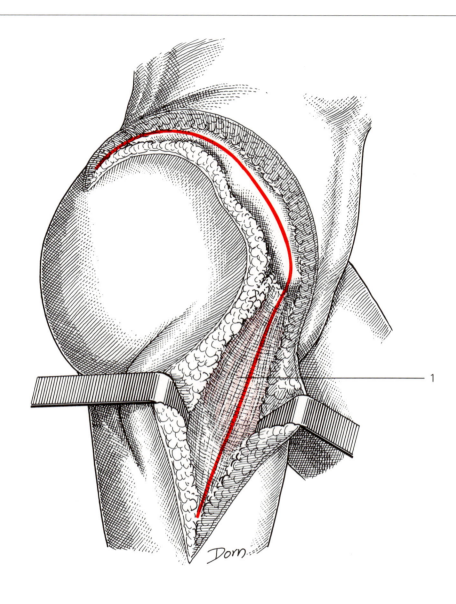

B

1 tensor fasciae latae

C Tensor fasciae latae is freed from its sheath along its anterior border and deep aspect. The gluteal muscles are reflected from the external iliac wing using the periosteal elevator as far posteriorly as the superior border of the greater sciatic notch. As the greater sciatic notch is approached, elevation of the muscles becomes more difficult and it is necessary to incise the strong fibrous origins of gluteus maximus from the posterior gluteal line. The area is then temporarily packed with a large swab. In continuity with the gluteal muscles, tensor fasciae latae is retracted posteriorly and elevated from the iliac wing, allowing division of small vessels arising from the superficial circumflex artery.

The elevation of these muscles continues distally to expose the reflected and straight heads of rectus femoris and the anterior and the superior aspects of the hip capsule.

Further dissection is then required posteriorly to free the superior border of the greater sciatic notch. The dissection here has to be undertaken with great caution as the superior gluteal neurovascular pedicle is adjacent to the bone, and may even be attached to it by a ligament. It is mandatory to protect the neurovascular bundle. On occasions the bundle may be seen within the fracture line, when the fracture of the posterior column extends into the greater sciatic notch. The pedicle can be damaged either directly by the

C

1 rectus femoris
2 lateral femoral circumflex vessels
3 fascial sheet deep to rectus femoris
4 greater trochanter
5 reflected head of rectus femoris
6 straight head of rectus femoris
7 sartorius
8 vessels from the superficial circumflex vessels, ligated
9 anterior superior iliac spine
10 superior gluteal vessels and nerve
11 external iliac fossa
12 iliac crest
13 gluteus medius
14 gluteus minimus
15 tensor fasciae latae

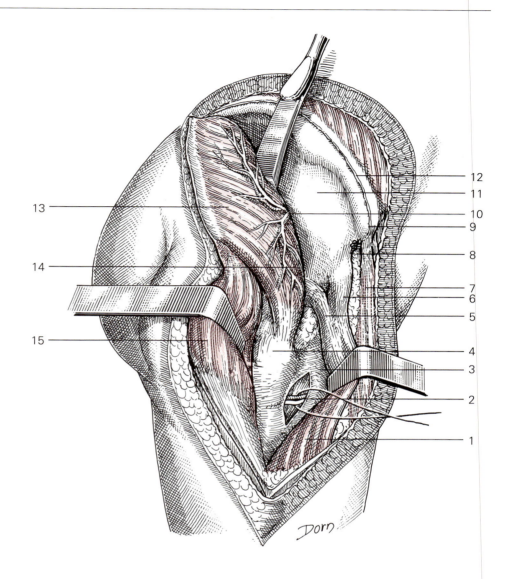

surgical dissection or by the uncontrolled manipulation of the bone fragments which may have a very sharp border. The pedicle should be isolated and protected with a moist swab. Bleeding from the nutrient vessels of the iliac wing can be controlled with bone wax.

Attention is redirected towards the distal part of the incision where posterior retraction of tensor fasciae latae exposes the fascial sheath overlying rectus femoris which is incised longitu-dinally. Rectus femoris is retracted medially and anteriorly to expose a thick aponeurosis which is incised longitudinally to allow identification of the lateral femoral circumflex vascular pedicle which is isolated, ligated and divided. Retraction of rectus femoris will reveal a constant but small vascular pedicle which reaches the lateral border of the muscle: this must be coagulated. This small vessel arises from the lateral femoral circumflex artery and will indicate the position of the parent artery. Following division of the lateral circumflex vessels, fatty tissue can be dissected to expose the sheath covering the iliopsoas muscle and tendon. This fascial sheath is incised, and iliopsoas is reflected from the anterior and inferior aspects of the hip capsule with an elevator and retracted distally. The reflected head of rectus femoris is then incised, and the glutei and tensor fasciae latae are retracted posteriorly together to provide a complete access to the iliac wing.

D The superior and anterior aspects of the hip capsule are completely exposed by incising and excising adipose and fascial tissue. The trochanteric line marks the lateral limit of the anterior capsule of the hip, and by tracing it proximally and laterally the insertion of gluteus medius via its tendon into the anterior aspect of the greater trochanter can be identified. The minimus tendon is dissected free and isolated and divided 3-5 mm from its insertion after placing stay sutures on either side of the proposed line of incision. If there is difficulty in identifying the gluteus minimus tendon, the fibres of vastus lateralis can be traced proximally as they insert into the trochanteric line. Gluteus minimus is retracted to expose the greater trochanter and the deep surface of gluteus medius; the tendon of gluteus medius is divided 3-5 mm from its insertion into the lateral aspect of the greater trochanter (again, stay sutures are placed on either side of the incision).

The origins and insertions of gluteus medius and minimus have now been freed and a massive muscular flap comprising the gluteal muscles and tensor fasciae latae has been retracted posteriorly with their neurovascular pedicles intact, protected by a large moist swab.

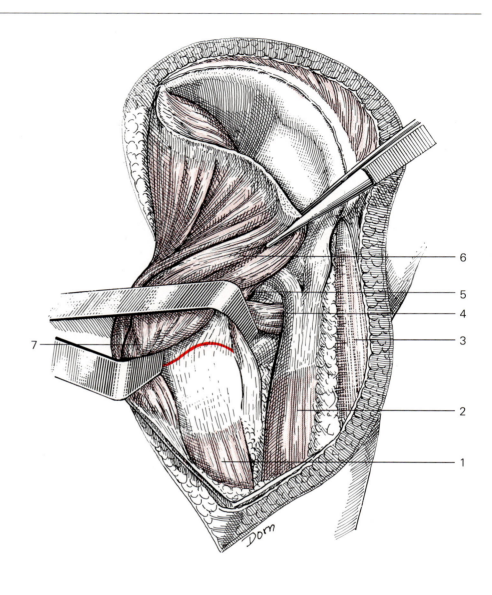

D

1 vastus lateralis
2 rectus femoris
3 sartorius
4 iliopsoas
5 gluteus minimus
6 gluteus medius
7 tensor fasciae latae

E   The muscular flap is retracted posteriorly to expose the posterior aspect of the hip and the short external rotators. The sciatic nerve must be identified by following the line of the fibres posteriorly. The nerve is frequently enclosed in adipose tissue. The tendon of piriformis is divided and the muscle retracted posteriorly and sutured temporarily to the posterior gluteal flap. The superior and inferior gemelli and obturator internus are next divided after placing stay sutures posterior to the line of their incision.

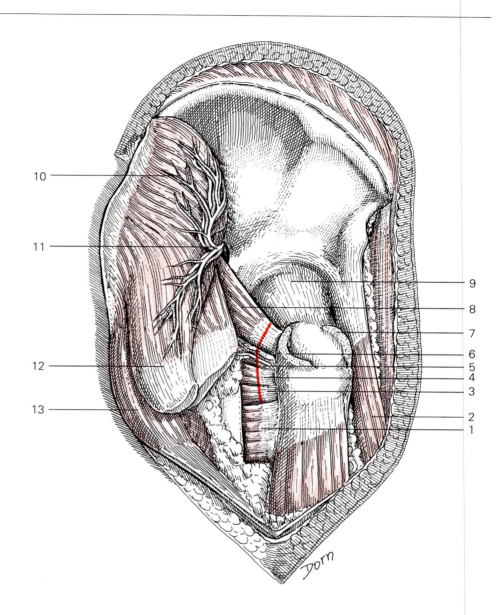

E

1 quadratus femoris
2 rectus femoris
3 gemellus inferior
4 obturator internus
5 gemellus superior
6 tendon of gluteus medius, cut
7 tendon of gluteus minimus, cut
8 piriformis
9 capsule
10 gluteus medius
11 superior gluteal pedicle and nerve
12 gluteus minimus
13 tensor fasciae latae

Pelvic girdle

F Retraction of piriformis posteriorly exposes the sciatic nerve as it leaves the greater sciatic notch and the anterior margin of the notch.

Obturator internus and the gemelli, already divided and held with stay sutures, are dissected from the posterior hip capsule and the posterior acetabulum. The constant synovial bursa between the bone and muscles is opened. The lesser sciatic notch, through which passes obturator internus, is exposed. Access can be gained via the lesser sciatic notch to the interior aspect of the true pelvis. A sciatic nerve retractor is then carefully inserted into the lesser sciatic notch, and gentle traction is applied to the stay suture inserted into obturator internus, thus protecting the sciatic nerve from the retractor. Quadratus femoris is usually left intact since it protects the ascending branch of the medial femoral circumflex artery. If necessary, the muscle is divided in its midportion or alternatively elevated from its origin from the ischial tuberosity in order to best protect the artery.

Extensions

Whenever it is necessary to inspect the interior of the hip joint, either to check the accuracy of reduction, or to look for bone fragments, a capsulotomy along the margin of the acetabulum is performed, and extended as necessary. Then by longitudinal and lateral traction applied with the orthopaedic table the femoral head can be disimpacted or distracted from the acetabulum to allow visualization of the interior of the joint.

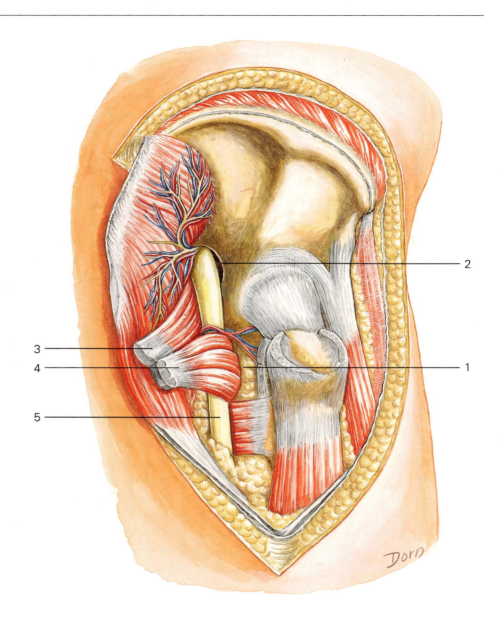

F
1 lesser sciatic notch
2 greater sciatic notch
3 piriformis
4 obturator internus and the gemelli
5 sciatic nerve

G If access to the internal iliac fossa appears necessary, especially for delayed reconstructions, it can be exposed by the elevation of the abdominal muscles from the iliac crest in continuity with iliacus from the internal aspect of the iliac wing. The origins of sartorius and the inguinal ligament are elevated subperiostally from the anterior superior iliac spine. Further anterior exposure is achieved by dividing the straight head of rectus femoris and by elevating iliacus distally to the psoas groove. The elevation of iliacus is carried out inferiorly and medially as far as necessary: at the maximum elevation the sacroiliac joint and the posterior half of the pelvic brim can be reached.

Closure

The hip capsule, if it has been divided (if possible), is repaired, with interrupted sutures. The tendons of obturator internus and piriformis are repaired. The tendons of gluteus medius and minimus are repaired using the stay sutures inserted prior to their division. Abduction of the femur facilitates the repair. If divided, the straight head of rectus femoris, sartorius and the inguinal ligament are reattached by sutures placed through drill holes. The gluteal fascia is reapproximated to the abdominal fascia along the iliac crest and the fascia lata is closed anterolaterally over the thigh. The reattachment of the fascia to the abdominal muscles along the iliac crest can be greatly facilitated by abduction of the hip. If the abdominal muscles have been elevated they are reattached to the iliac crest together with the gluteal fascia by transosseous sutures.

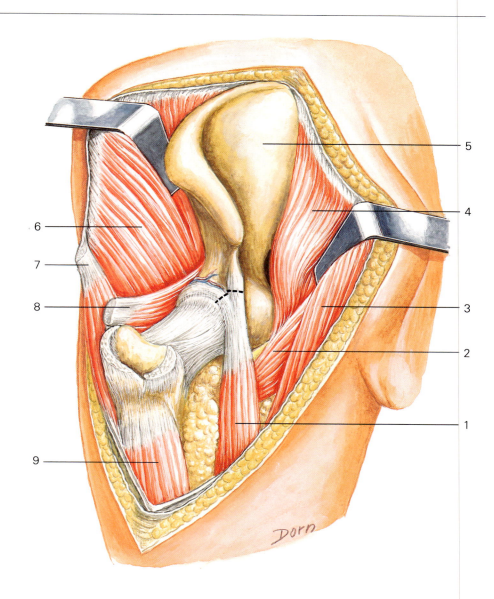

G

1 rectus femoris
2 iliopsoas
3 sartorius
4 iliacus
5 internal iliac fossa
6 glutei
7 tensor fasciae latae
8 piriformis
9 vastus lateralis

Acetabulum: posterior (Kocher–Langenbeck) approach

Introduction

This approach combines two approaches: the transgluteal approach suggested by Langenbeck and the vertical part of the Kocher incision.

The posterior approach provides perfect access to the posterior column of the acetabulum so allowing reconstruction after fracture. Access is also provided to the hip for reconstruction following trauma or for total hip replacement.

However, this approach has two main risks which must be kept in mind during the whole procedure: damage to the sciatic nerve and to the superior gluteal neurovascular bundle.

In the operative field the main trunk of the sciatic nerve can be damaged by a retractor or another instrument. To decrease the risk of damage, the nerve trunk must be identified and protected immediately after splitting gluteus maximus. It is unnecessary to put a sling around the nerve. The sciatic nerve may also be damaged by traction at its origin from the lumbosacral plexus. In this case, postoperative electromyography of the muscles supplied by the femoral and sciatic nerves may show the plexus as the site of damage.

The superior gluteal nerve and the gluteal vessels are particularly at risk during dissection of the superior border of the greater sciatic notch, especially if the fractured posterior column is detached together with the angle of the greater sciatic notch — the fragment may be very sharp. Intraoperative bleeding from the vessels may occur, which could be due to damage of the vessels either by the instruments used or by displacement of a very sharp fragment; also it can result from dissection of the vessels causing a secondary reactionary haemorrhage. If such bleeding occurs it is advisable not to try to control it immediately by suturing, ligation or the use of clips — these manoeuvres put the nerve at great risk. It is better to pack the area with wet swabs and leave them there as long as possible. On removal of the packs the bleeding will either have stopped or be more easily controlled — there will then be a lesser risk of damaging the sciatic nerve.

Indications

The indications include specific fractures of the acetabulum:

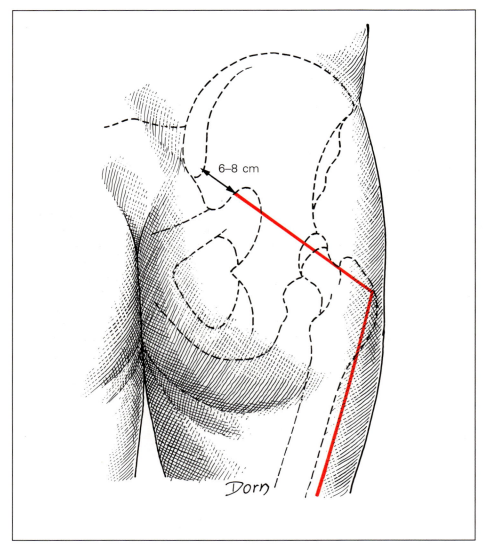

6–8 cm

Dorn

A

- Fractures of the posterior wall of the posterior column.
- Transverse fractures of the roof and proximal acetabulum when operated upon within 15–20 days of the injury.
- Associated transverse and posterior wall fractures operated upon within 15–20 days of the injury. The indications to use the posterior approach instead of the extended iliofemoral approach depend on the amount of callus shown on radiographs and CT scans; if abundant callus is evident, the extended approach is recommended.
- Removal of intra-articular fragments of bone following dislocation of the hip (this approach is recommended when the fragments are still attached to the posterior capsule, and trapped between the head and the roof).
- Total hip replacement or revision arthroplasty (this approach provides an easier access to the medullary canal of the femur than an anterior approach).

Position

There are two possibilities:

1 The patient is placed prone on an orthopaedic table, which allows traction to be applied to the limb via a transcondylar Steinmann pin and a stirrup; the knee is flexed to about 40° to relax the sciatic nerve — if the knee is flexed to a greater degree, the sciatic nerve is increasingly relaxed, but traction is applied to rectus femoris which may be damaged.
2 The patient is placed in the midlateral position with the injured side uppermost. The leg is draped to allow its manipulation during the surgical procedure.

The prone position provides much better access than the lateral position, particularly to the quadrilateral surface.

Incision

A The incision is angled, the angle of the incision being sited lateral to the proximal border of the greater trochanter. The superior limb (the Langenbeck component) is directed towards the posterior superior iliac spine. The skin incision is stopped 6–8 cm from the posterior superior spine — see page 38 for an explanation.

The inferior limb of the incision runs vertically distally, over the lateral surface of the thigh, passing equidistant between the anterior and posterior borders of the greater trochanter.

Pelvic girdle

Exposure

B The superficial fascia is divided in line with the skin incision and the gluteal fascia incised over the greater trochanter. The fascia lata is divided vertically and the fascial incision continued upwards using scissors or blunt section, splitting the fibres of gluteus maximus; this process separates the upper third of gluteus maximus, receiving its blood supply from the superior gluteal artery, from the lower two-thirds, supplied by the inferior gluteal vessels.

The innervation of gluteus maximus is exclusively from the inferior gluteal nerve. The nerve branches which innervate the proximal third of gluteus maximus are encountered when the medial muscle fibres are split and separated. The dissection must stop as soon as the first nerve branch is encountered, thus avoiding postoperative paralysis of the proximal third of gluteus maximus.

The problems resulting from paralysis of gluteus maximus are such that it is imperative that the innervation of the muscle be protected. This is particularly important because after pelvic injury there may have been damage to the other gluteal muscles. If an operation on the posterior iliac crest cannot be avoided, it is wise to use a separate incision.

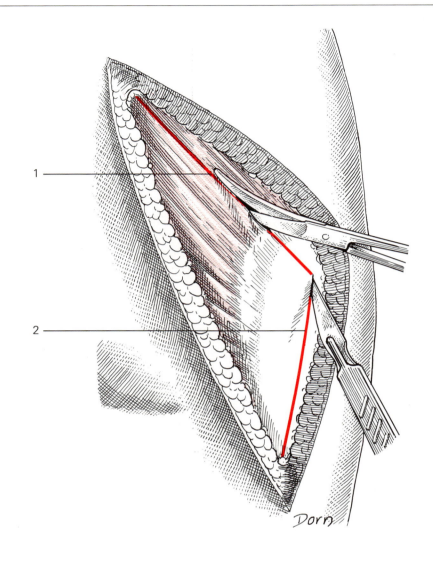

B

1 splitting the fibres of gluteus maximus
2 incision of iliotibial tract

c

1 quadratus femoris
2 greater trochanter
3 piriformis
4 gluteus medius
5 gluteus maximus, split
6 superior gluteal nerve and vessels
   (must be protected)
7 superior gemellus
8 obturator internus
9 inferior gemellus
10 sciatic nerve
11 distal tendon of gluteus maximus
   (to be cut)

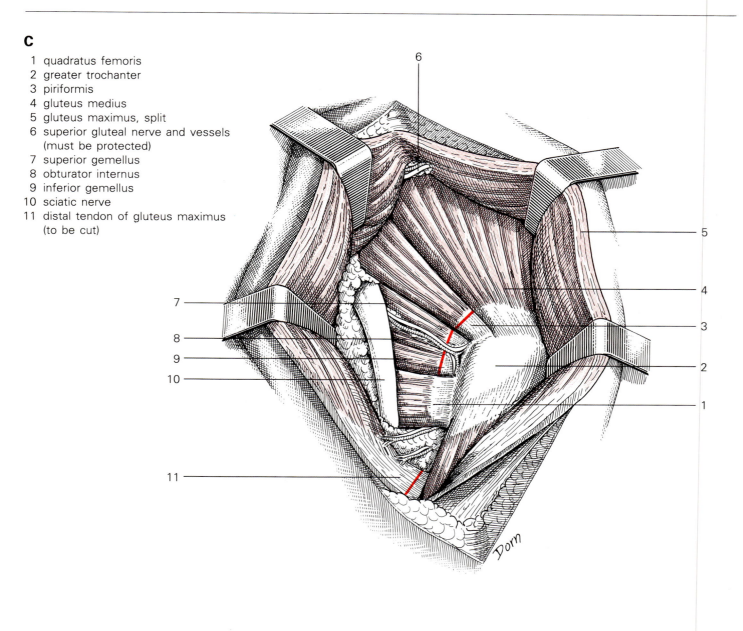

C The trochanteric bursa is opened and divided over the greater trochanter, the margins of gluteus maximus having been retracted. This exposes the deep layer of muscles, and distally the femoral insertion of gluteus maximus. Initially, the plane must be developed from the lower part of the trochanteric crest which is the site of insertion of quadratus femoris. Following the posterior aspect of this muscle medially, the sciatic nerve can be safely identified. The nerve is followed towards the greater sciatic notch and should be exposed throughout its course, especially if a preoperative sciatic palsy has been evident. If necessary it should be freed from haematoma and bone fragments. Frequently the femoral insertion of gluteus maximus is divided adjacent to the femur, at the same time ligating a branch of the posterior circumflex femoral artery — this is divided where it lies just deep to the tendon. The advantage of this is that gluteus maximus is freed and can be retracted more easily, so reducing the chance of damage to the sciatic nerve from retractors and increasing the exposure of the ischial tuberosity. If divided, the tendon must be repaired with interrupted sutures at the time of closure. The essential step comes next: the division of the short external rotators of the hip. These muscles may have been damaged to a greater or lesser extent at the time of injury and their identification may be difficult.

Pelvic girdle

D

1 greater trochanter
2 gluteus medius
3 hip joint capsule
4 superior gluteal vessels and nerve
5 greater sciatic notch
6 piriformis
7 ischial spine
8 obturator internus and gemelli
9 lesser sciatic notch and bursa

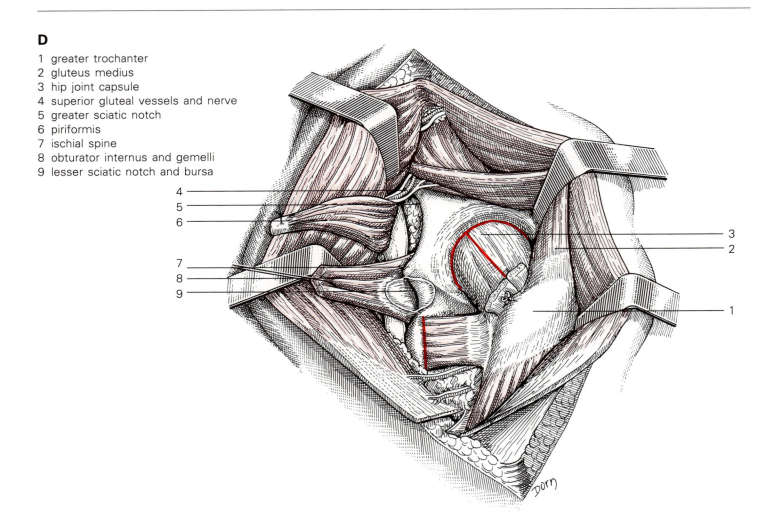

D First, piriformis is divided through its tendon 1 or 2 cm from its femoral insertion. The proximal end is attached to a stay suture which is passed through the lateral cut edge of gluteus maximus for the duration of the operation: retraction of piriformis allows visualization of the sciatic nerve as it emerges from the greater sciatic notch.

The tendons of obturator internus and the gemelli are also divided 2–3 cm from their femoral insertion to protect the posterior circumflex artery; a stay suture is attached to the proximal end and the muscle is elevated by blunt dissection from the capsule and the surface of the posterior acetabulum; the underlying synovial bursa is opened by medial dissection to gain direct and easy access to the lesser sciatic notch which contains distinctive white fibrous tissue. The true pelvis is then entered. Inspection of the deep aspect of obturator internus reveals its separate tendons of origin which converge to form the main tendon. The beak of a Hohmann retractor or a sciatic nerve retractor can easily be inserted into the notch, where it will safely retract the nerve for as long as necessary. The tendon of obturator internus will always be between the retractor and the nerve, so protecting it, provided that the assistant in charge of the retractor pulls constantly on the stay suture attached to the tendon.

If piriformis and obturator internus have been lacerated at the time of injury, their medial ends should be sought and marked with sutures in the same way.

Retraction of obturator internus protects the internal pudendal neurovascular bundle, which is not seen.

When it is necessary to gain access to the ischial tuberosity, it is preferable to strip the origin of quadratus femoris from the pelvis rather than to divide the muscle; this avoids unnecessary damage to the posterior circumflex artery.

By division and elevation of the short external rotators, the capsule and, medially, the retro-acetabular surface of the posterior column are progressively exposed and cleared of soft tissue. Eventually the anterior border of the greater sciatic notch and the ischial spine come into view.

Distally the muscles cushion the sciatic nerve, whereas proximally the nerve rests against the bony edge of the greater sciatic notch.

Next the infra-acetabular gutter is identified. It is necessary to expose the body of the ischium which is covered with dense fibrous tissue that can be difficult to strip. It is essential to keep hard against the bone because the sciatic nerve is tethered somewhat at this point, making retraction difficult; it is a site of potential damage of the nerve. This completes the approach. A Steinmann pin is driven into the upper part of the ischial tuberosity away from the sciatic nerve and acts as an effective retractor of the gluteal muscles.

Access is provided to the whole of the posterior column, to the greater and lesser sciatic notches, to the ischial spine, to all the retroacetabular surface, to the infra-acetabular groove, and to the posterior part of the ischiopubic ramus; the latter structure can be osteotomized, using this route, in the treatment of a malunion of an acetabular fracture.

Through the greater sciatic notch access can be gained to the true pelvis. To achieve this the soft tissues are incised along the medial aspect of the anterior border of the greater sciatic notch, i.e. the aponeurosis of obturator internus; this is then dissected with an elevator, proximally and distally, as far as is needed to allow access to the obturator canal and the midpart of the pelvic brim.

Access within the pelvis can be improved by dividing either the sacrospinous ligament or the ischial spine itself at its base. Either of these procedures further liberates the sciatic nerve which can advantageously be retracted into the pelvis.

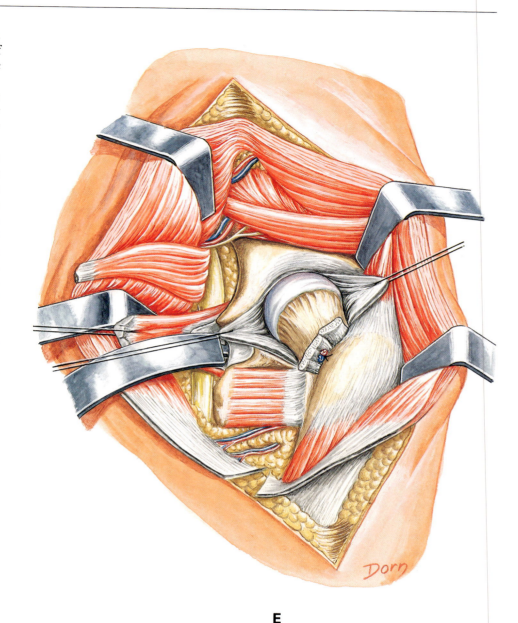

E

E If the hip joint is to be exposed, the capsule may be incised along the acetabular margin both posteriorly and superiorly and, if necessary along the long axis of the femoral neck. This is performed routinely for a total hip replacement using this approach, the femoral head being dislocated posteriorly.

F A cross-section shows the steps of the exposure.

Possible extensions

These extensions are all considered in order to increase access to the iliac wing and to the anterior column.

To improve access to the roof of the acetabulum the distal part of gluteus medius and gluteus minimus may be elevated from the iliac wing above the hip capsule and their tendons partially or totally divided 1 cm from the femur. Despite this, it is still difficult to reach the anterior border of the bone without damaging the muscles.

To improve access proximal to the greater sciatic notch — in order to apply a fixation device — the posterior part of the iliac wing can be exposed but this can only be done by passing beneath the superior gluteal pedicle which puts the pedicle in danger and provides only limited access.

In the case of acetabular fractures, when the initial posterior approach appears to be insufficient, it is probably best to transform it into the triradiate approach (see pages 43-7).

Closure

The closure of the posterior incision is straightforward. It is important to reconstitute a muscular bed deep to the sciatic nerve. The stay sutures placed in obturator internus and piriformis facilitate both identification and suturing of these to the stumps of the tendons remaining attached to the posterosuperior border of the trochanter. Once these tendons are repaired, the neighbouring muscles should also be approximated in order to provide a complete curtain that can protect the nerve. At least two suction drains are inserted, one draining the gluteal region and the other the pelvis via one of the sciatic notches.

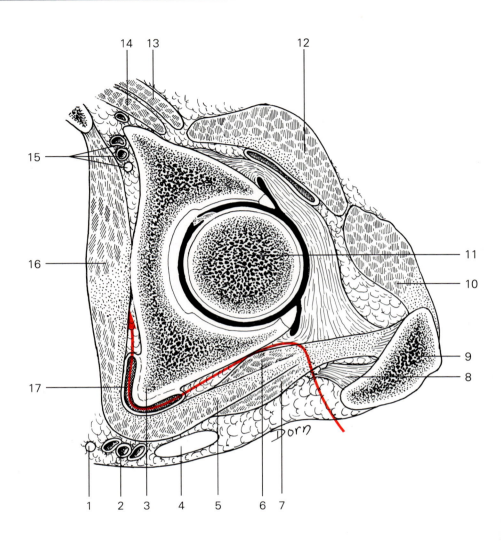

F

1 posterior cutaneous nerve of thigh
2 inferior gluteal vessels
3 ischial spine
4 sciatic nerve
5 obturator internus
6 gemellus superior
7 gemellus inferior
8 obturator externus tendon
9 greater trochanter
10 gluteus minimus
11 femoral head
12 iliopsoas
13 pectineus
14 obturator externus
15 obturator nerve and vessels
16 obturator internus
17 bursa

Acetabulum: triradiate (Dana Mears) approach

Introduction

According to Dana Mears, the triradiate approach is a modification of the approach that John Charnley initially employed for total hip replacement. It can also be considered as the combined development of the lateral 'U'-shaped approach and the additional vertical approach suggested by Mathieu.

The triradiate approach is an extensive approach to the lateral aspect of the innominate bone and to the acetabulum. The access is comparable to that provided by the extended ilio-femoral approach. However, with the triradiate approach the posterior limb splits the fibres of gluteus maximus, and the posterior part of the muscle remains attached to the posterior iliac wing. Here it receives the superior gluteal neurovascular bundle which lies adjacent to the upper border of the greater sciatic notch and is hence difficult to retract. Through the extended iliofemoral approach the whole mass of the gluteal muscles is retracted, including its superior neurovascular pedicle, thus freeing totally the greater sciatic notch. Furthermore, the posterior part of gluteus maximus which remains attached posteriorly impedes access to a disrupted sacroiliac joint, although this is actually possible through an extended iliofemoral approach. If access to the sacroiliac joint is needed, the only way to achieve it, using the triradiate approach, is to elevate the whole of iliacus from the internal iliac fossa, as described in **F**. Even so the exposure is not particularly good.

When an extensive approach is needed for the acetabulum, the choice between the extended iliofemoral and the triradiate approaches is a personal one and depends to an extent on whether or not a good orthopaedic table is available. Nevertheless, if an operation is commenced through a posterior incision which then appears to be insufficient for the reconstruction required, the approach can quite conveniently be extended into a triradiate approach which allows better control and reduction of an anterior column fracture of the acetabulum. It is only necessary to make an incision from the angle of the posterior approach towards the anterior superior iliac spine. The deep dissection is described in **D**.

If feasible for a particular fracture, this extension avoids a subsequent anterior ilioinguinal approach; if the reduction can be perfectly achieved, it carries less risk.

Indications

- Complex fractures of the acetabulum.
- Exposure of the lateral aspect of the ilium, the greater sciatic notch, the external iliac fossa and the internal iliac fossa (access within the pelvis is limited).

Position of the patient

The patient is placed in a full lateral position on a conventional operating table.

Routine preparation and draping are undertaken from the anterior to the posterior midline, including the ipsilateral leg, which is fully exposed and draped to allow intraoperative manipulation.

Pelvic girdle

Incision

A The superficial landmarks for the triradiate incision are the anterior superior iliac spine, the posterior superior iliac spine and the superior border of the greater trochanter, over which the incision is centred.

The longitudinal incision extends distally from the greater trochanter for a distance of about 6–8 cm along the long axis of the thigh.

The anterosuperior limb of the incision runs towards the anterior superior iliac spine which it crosses. The posterosuperior limb is angled towards the posterior superior iliac spine. The angle formed by the two proximal limbs is about 90°.

B The fascia is divided in the line of all three limbs of the incision.

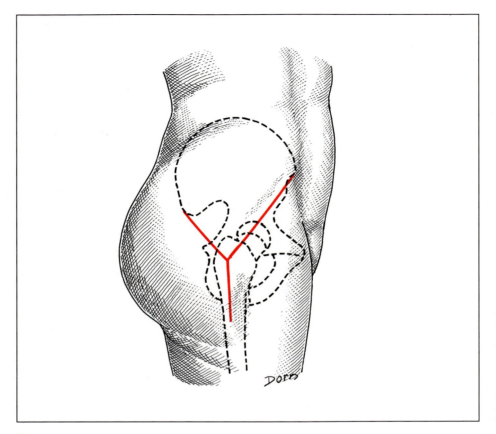

A

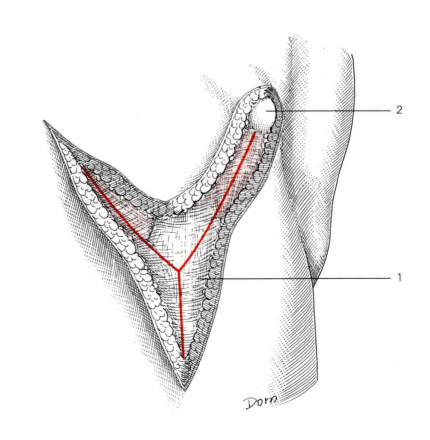

B

1 iliotibial tract
2 anterior superior iliac spine

44

C The fascia lata and the fascia of tensor fasciae latae are incised from the anterior superior spine to the level of the greater trochanter. The anterior border of tensor fasciae latae is sharply incised from its fascia, so that the entire muscle can be retracted proximally and posteriorly along with the cutaneous flap. The origins of tensor fasciae latae, and gluteus maximus and minimus, are incised from the iliac crest; the anterior border of the lateral ilium then becomes evident. Subperiostal elevation of gluteus maximus and gluteus minimus is undertaken from anterior to posterior as far distally as the capsule of the hip joint.

Through the posterior limb of the incision, proximal to the greater trochanter, in the line of the incision of the fascia of gluteus maximus, the muscle fibres are separated by blunt dissection as far medially as the first neurovascular bundle of importance.

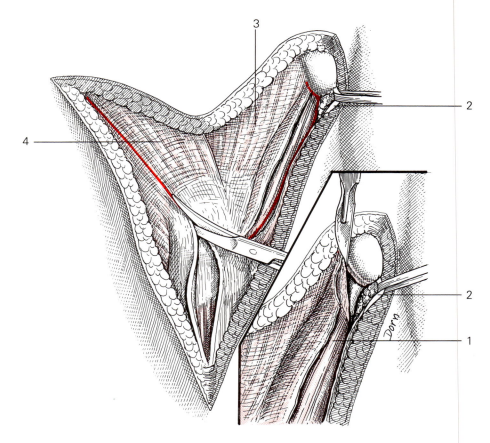

C
1 tensor fasciae latae
2 lateral cutaneous nerve of thigh
3 gluteus medius
4 gluteus maximus

D
1 vastus lateralis
2 line of trochanteric osteotomy

D On the lateral aspect of the proximal femur, the interval between gluteus medius and vastus lateralis is identified and a transverse incision is made in the periosteum. The greater trochanter is osteotomized (using an osteotome or an oscillating saw) and reflected proximally together with the attached gluteus medius and gluteus minimus.

Gluteus minimus is sharply dissected from the capsule of the hip joint using curved heavy scissors and working from proximal to distal and from anterior to posterior; the capsule is carefully preserved. The muscular flap is made up of the three gluteal muscles and tensor fasciae latae.

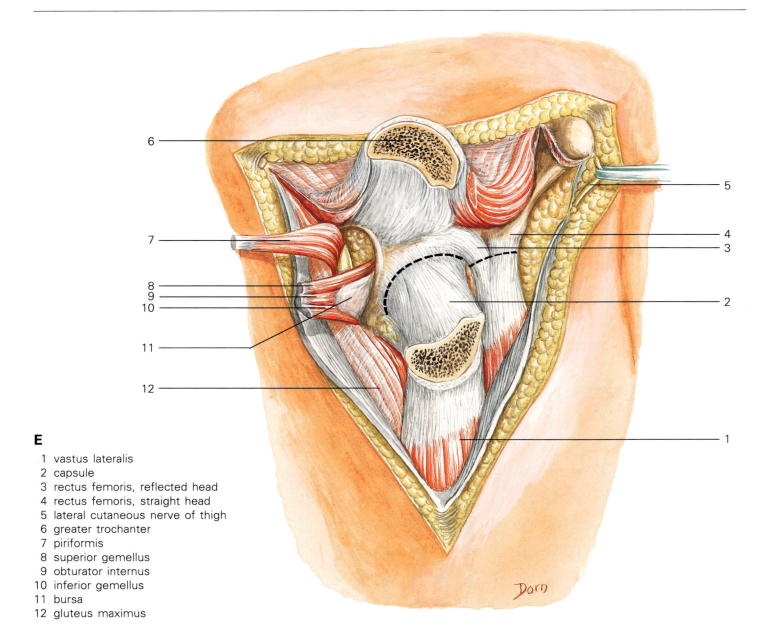

E

1 vastus lateralis
2 capsule
3 rectus femoris, reflected head
4 rectus femoris, straight head
5 lateral cutaneous nerve of thigh
6 greater trochanter
7 piriformis
8 superior gemellus
9 obturator internus
10 inferior gemellus
11 bursa
12 gluteus maximus

E The dissection continues to the greater sciatic notch where the superior gluteal vessels and nerve are identified. Once the sciatic nerve has been identified and protected, the short external rotators of the hip (piriformis, obturator internus and the gemelli) are incised 1 or 2 cm from their insertions into the greater trochanter. Distally, either quadratus femoris can be left or its proximal half can be incised. These muscles are reflected posteriorly with stay sutures to visualize the underlying hip capsule and the adjacent posterior column. They protect the sciatic nerve. Using a combination of sharp and blunt dissection, the posterior column is exposed — from the greater sciatic notch to the upper pole of the ischial tuberosity.

Blunt Hohmann retractors or a sciatic nerve retractor are carefully inserted into either the greater or the lesser sciatic notch in order to maintain the exposure of the posterior aspect of the posterior column.

Gluteus medius and gluteus minimus are reflected and elevated proximally by subperiosteal dissection; the total mass of the abductor muscles is anchored proximally and posteriorly by the use of two Steinmann pins driven into the ilium 2.5–5 cm above the roof of the greater sciatic notch.

To enlarge the access to the ilium, it may be necessary to continue the dissection of the gluteal muscles proximally. In fact the gluteal fascia can even be cut subcutaneously along the iliac crest.

F To obtain better exposure of the anterior column, it is often necessary to extend the dissection medially. The anterior limb of the cutaneous incision is continued 6–8 cm medial to the anterosuperior iliac spine. The origins of sartorius and the abdominal muscles from the anterior iliac crest are sharply incised. Iliacus is then elevated subperiostally from the inner table of the ilium and retracted medially. The dissection may be continued posteriorly to expose the anterior aspect of the sacroiliac joint; almost the entire aspect of the ilium is then exposed.

To increase the anterior exposure, the straight and reflected heads of rectus femoris are released from the anterior inferior iliac spine and the hip capsule.

When the capsule is intact it is incised sharply from its attachments around the acetabular rim to give access to the hip joint.

A possible extension of the triradiate approach is to extend the anterior limb of the incision medially towards the pubic symphysis, as described in the ilioinguinal approach (page 18).

Closure

The lower limb is positioned on a stand with about 30° abduction of the hip joint. The capsule of the hip joint is repaired. Rectus femoris and sartorius often need transosseous sutures (2-mm drill holes) for their reattachment. The greater trochanter is accurately reduced and temporarily held with bone-holding forceps and two 6.5-mm long threaded cancellous screws with washers are used to secure it. Fascial edges, subcutaneous tissues and skin are repaired with interrupted sutures.

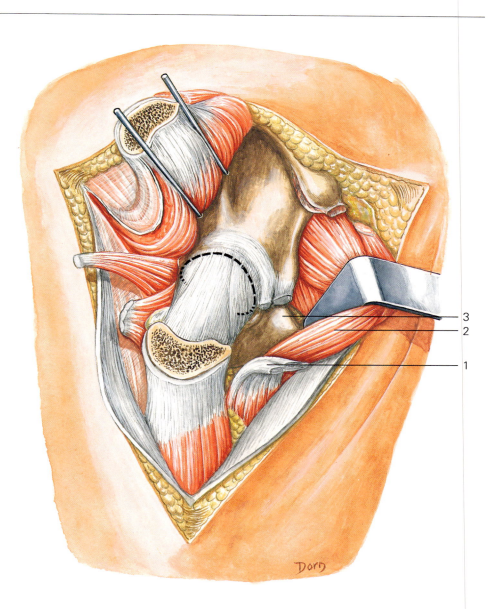

Dorn

F

1 rectus femoris, cut and retracted
2 iliopsoas
3 superior pubic ramus

47

Acetabulum: lateral 'U' (Ollier, modified Sénégas) approach

Introduction

The classic lateral 'U' approach has been modified by Sénégas to improve the access to the acetabulum. The anterior limb of the 'U' has been replaced by a horizontal incision which crosses tensor fasciae latae.

This exposure provides only limited access to the anterior column and exposure of the entire iliac wing is impossible. An exposure of the pelvic cavity is not provided by this surgical approach.

Indication

- Surgical treatment of some acetabular fractures (transverse, associated transverse and posterior wall, 'T'-shaped, both columns).

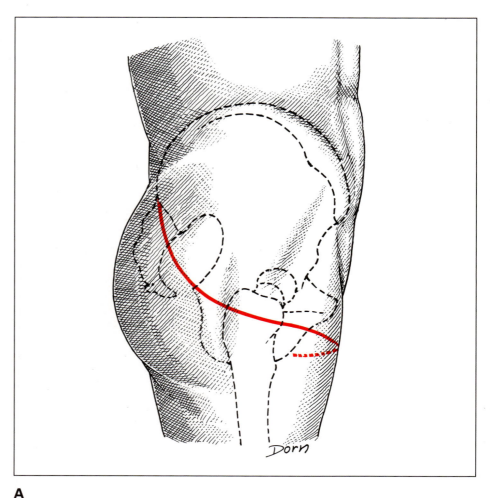

A

Position of the patient

The patient is placed in a modified midlateral position, on an ordinary table, being tilted 60° posteriorly in order to expose the anterolateral aspect of the hip. The leg is fully draped in order to allow its peroperative manipulation.

Incision

A The skin incision begins at the posterior superior iliac spine and reaches the midportion of the lateral aspect of the greater trochanter. From there, its anterior part, instead of turning towards the anterior superior iliac spine, runs horizontally around the anteromedial aspect of the thigh as far as the lateral border of Scarpa's triangle which overlies the belly of sartorius.

B

1 sartorius

B The incision, viewed anteriorly.

Exposure

C In line with the skin incision, the fascia lata is horizontally incised at the level of the midportion of the greater trochanter; then, posteriorly, after division of its superficial fascia, the fibres of gluteus maximus are split. When the first neurovascular bundle is encountered medially, splitting of the gluteal fibres is discontinued in order to avoid the postoperative paralysis of its proximal part. If essential, the muscle can be split as far as the posterior superior spine, but this carries risks. Tensor fasciae latae is then divided in the horizontal plane.

The greater trochanter is then osteotomized; the osteotomy can be performed with a Gigli saw introduced beneath the tendon of piriformis and adjacent to the superior aspect of the hip capsule. The osteotomized trochanter can then be retracted proximally with piriformis and gluteus medius and gluteus minimus. The trochanteric osteotomy can be executed with an osteotome, taking care not to penetrate the joint.

In the most medial part of the posterior incision, the sciatic nerve can be located; it can be found easily by following the fibres of quadratus femoris from anterior to posterior.

C

1 obturator internus and the gemelli
2 greater trochanter (osteotomized with a Gigli saw)
3 tensor fasciae latae, cut
4 piriformis
5 greater sciatic notch
6 gluteus maximus, split
7 sciatic nerve

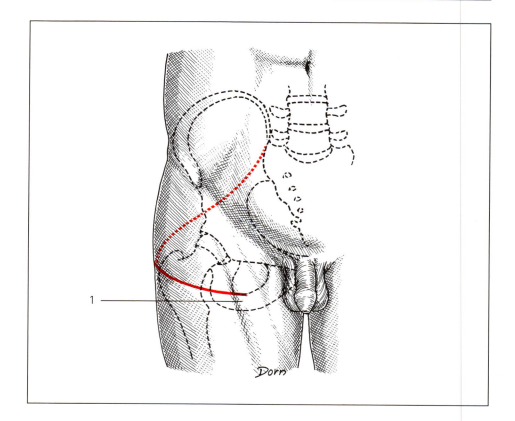

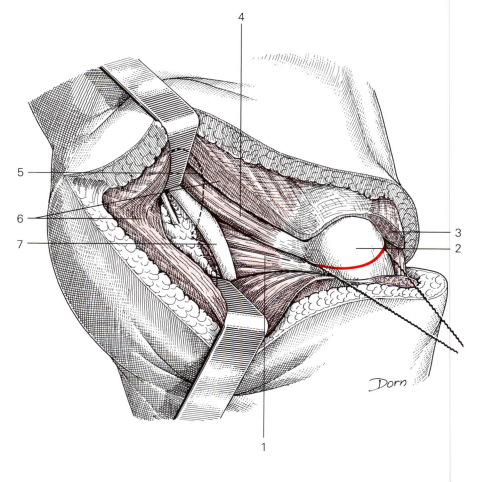

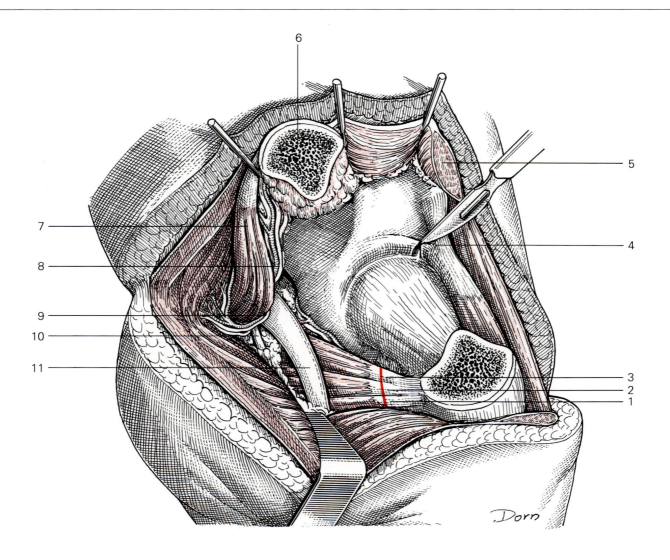

D The osteotomized part of the greater trochanter is retracted upwards together with the gluteal muscles and piriformis; gluteus minimus is dissected from the hip capsule and from the superior acetabular rim; it is then elevated from the iliac wing as necessary. The proximal muscular flap is retracted by several Steinmann pins driven into the iliac wing.

Obturator internus and the gemelli are then divided in the usual manner (see posterior or triradiate approaches), and this allows access to the posterior column as far posteriorly as the upper pole of the ischial tuberosity. To gain or improve access to the anterior column of the acetabulum, the straight head of rectus femoris is detached from the anterior inferior iliac spine and will be reattached at the time of closure by a transosseous suture.

The distal and anterior retraction of rectus femoris reveals iliopsoas which is dissected from its aponeurosis, and held and retracted medially by a Steinmann pin inserted carefully medial to the iliopectineal eminence.

D

1 gemellus inferior
2 obturator internus
3 gemellus superior
4 reflected head of rectus femoris
5 tensor fasciae latae, cut
6 greater trochanter, retracted
7 piriformis
8 superior gluteal nerve and vessels
9 inferior gluteal nerve and vessels
10 posterior cutaneous nerve of thigh
11 sciatic nerve

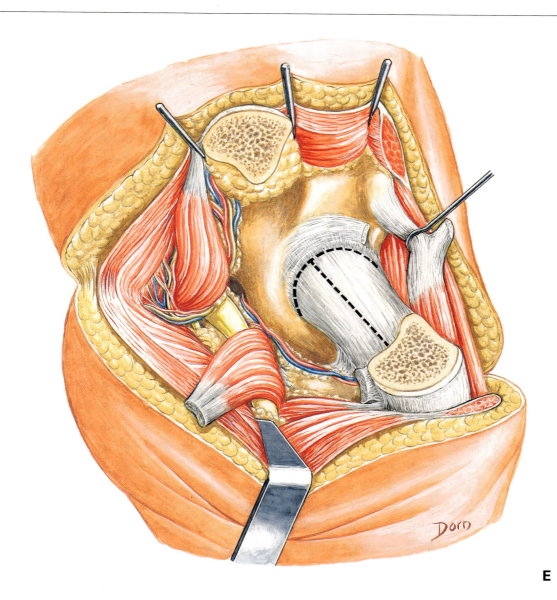

E

E To gain access to the joint, the articular capsule is incised along the acetabular margin as necessary and the capsular flap may be temporarily attached to the tissues adjacent to the base of the trochanter. A longitudinal capsulotomy may be added to improve access to the joint.

Sacroiliac joint: posterior approach

Introduction

Most commonly the sacroiliac joint is approached posteriorly, with the patient lying prone. However, it is also possible to reach the anterior aspect of the sacroiliac joint, with the patient lying supine, via the lateral part of the ilioinguinal approach (see pages 17–24).

The traditional posterior approach to the sacroiliac joint was through an incision which followed the posterior third of the iliac crest and then descended vertically for about 10–15 cm from the posterior superior iliac spine. The main inconvenience of this incision is that, when the patient is lying supine postoperatively, the incision is subject to pressure and skin necrosis may well occur. Furthermore, it is necessary to divide the fibres of gluteus maximus distal to the posterior spine vertically, and the muscle is difficult to repair. A vertical incision, sited 2 cm lateral to the posterior iliac spine, has been found to decrease dramatically the incidence of skin necrosis and is recommended.

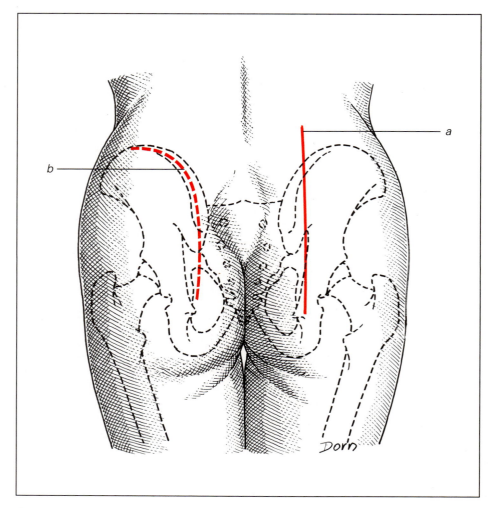

A

a preferred incision
b traditional incision

Indications

- Sacroiliac dislocations.
- Sacroiliac fracture or dislocation, either transiliac or trans-sacral.
- Arthrodesis of an arthritic or infected sacroiliac joint.
- Internal fixation of trans-sacral fractures.

Position of the patient

The patient is placed prone on an ordinary table or on an orthopaedic table, both tables preferably being radiolucent.

It is advisable to operate with the ipsilateral knee flexed at 40–45° to relax the sciatic nerve.

In delayed reconstructions traction is applied to the thigh with a transcondylar Steinmann pin, the knee being flexed at 40°.

Incision

A The incision is strictly vertical, passing 2 cm lateral to the posterior iliac spines, beginning 4–5 cm above the iliac crest and extending downwards for about 15–20 cm. An incision of maximum length is necessary to treat trans-sacral fractures.

Approaches to the pubic symphysis

There are two possible incisions: the midline or the transverse. In the midline incision, the exposure gives access to the pubic symphysis and the adjacent bone, but it does not allow total access to the superior pubic rami.

Pubic symphysis: midline incision

Position of the patient

The patient lies supine on an ordinary table and a Foley catheter is inserted into the bladder.

Indications

- Isolated disruption of the pubic symphysis.
- Exploration of the pubic symphysis.
- Arthrodesis of the pubic symphysis.

Incisions

A The incision follows the midline strictly, for about 10–15 cm, finishing at the level of the upper border of the pubic symphysis or a little lower.

B The linea alba is exposed along the length of the incision.
An attempt is made to divide just the linea alba, but this manoeuvre is not routinely successful, and often the anterior sheath of rectus abdominis is opened. The solution is then to identify the medial border of the muscle and to follow it distally as far as pyramidalis, which presents laterally; finally the superior aspect of the pubic symphysis has to be identified.
To explore or repair the symphysis it is necessary to control its posterior, superior and anterior surfaces.

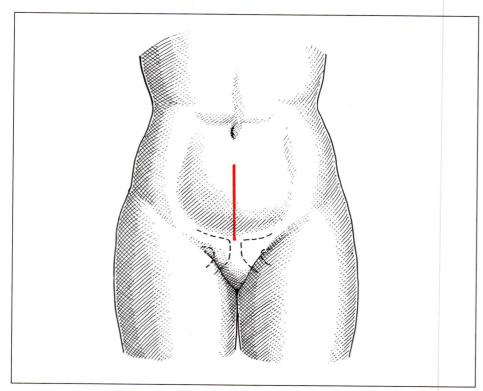

A

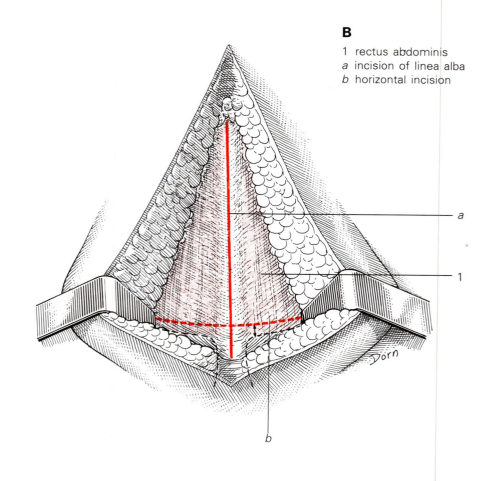

B

1 rectus abdominis
a incision of linea alba
b horizontal incision

a
1
b

C Anteriorly, the subcutaneous fat can be dissected from the anterior aspect of both pubic bones, using sharp or blunt dissection; this separation can go as far distally as necessary.

Posteriorly the retropubic space is opened and entered, and the bladder is retracted posteriorly with a moist wet swab. In the depth of the wound the transurethal Foley catheter can be felt, which allows the surgeon to recognize and safeguard the urethra.

The posterior dissection is then continued by directing an elevator obliquely both distally and laterally to expose the anterior part of the obturator foramen. The dissection is inferior to the obturator pedicle which is not at risk.

Proximal to the pubic symphysis there are several possibilities: one or both tendons of rectus abdominis can be sharply divided 1 cm or more above the bone. This gives a rather wide access to the superior pubic rami, just lateral to both pubic tubercles. Alternatively the posterior insertions of the recti into the pubis can be divided, leaving the anterior insertions of the muscles intact. The exposure thus afforded is limited but is sufficient for positioning of a plate on the superior aspect of the superior pubic rami. Alternatively, one rectus tendon can be completely divided whilst only the posterior fibres of the contralateral muscle are released.

If the pubic symphysis is disrupted, the dislocated joint is exposed immediately, and the soft tissue damage is always found to be asymmetrical: one side is completely denuded of its soft tissue attachments (ligaments and even muscle) whilst on the other side the soft tissues are left undisturbed.

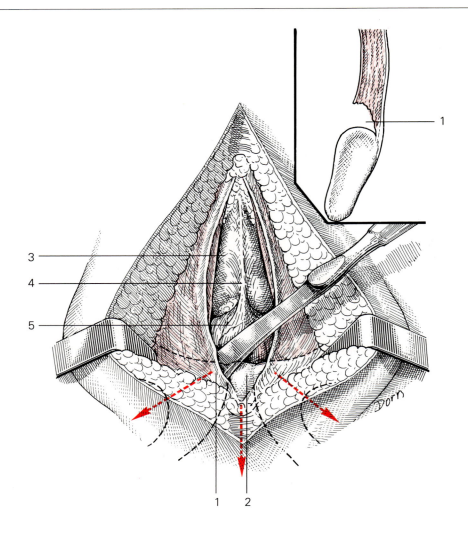

Closure

The rectus sheaths and tendons are reattached to their stumps, if they were cut. The linea aspera is closed.

C
1 partial release of pyramidalis and rectus abdominis
2 pubic symphysis
3 parietal peritoneum
4 median umbilical ligament
5 urinary bladder

Pubic symphysis: transverse (Pfannenstiel) incision

Indications

The transverse skin incision may be chosen for cosmetic reasons. The deep dissection is the same as that following a midline incision.

A true transverse incision is essential when it is necessary to deal with the symphysis and one or both superior pubic rami, or when injury to the urinary tract is associated with the bony lesions.

Position of the patient

The patient lies supine on an ordinary table. A Foley catheter is inserted into the bladder prior to surgery to ensure intraoperative identification of the urethra and the base of the bladder. If urethral damage is suspected, an expert urological opinion should be sought prior to inserting the catheter.

Incision

D About 2 cm superior to the superior pubic rami a curvilinear transverse incision is made, concave from above.

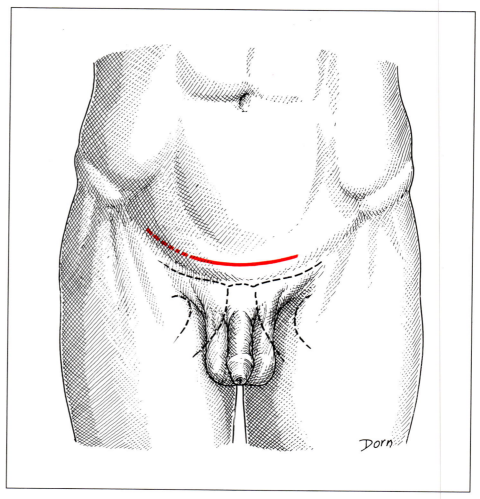

D

Pelvic girdle

E The subcutaneous fat is dissected from the aponeurosis which allows the identification of the external inguinal ring on both sides.

The anterior aspect of the sheath of rectus abdominis, together with the linea alba, is incised at least 1 cm above their insertion to facilitate repair. The muscle fibres of the recti are divided transversely, and the posterior aspect of the sheath divided and marked with stay sutures.

The division of the recti is extended laterally on both sides by section of the aponeurosis of the external oblique parallel to the inguinal ligament, which passes above the external inguinal ring.

The spermatic cord or the round ligament is identified and controlled with a rubber sling.

If it is only necessary to expose the symphysis and one pubic ramus then division of just one rectus is sufficient and the other one can be left intact, at least anteriorly.

F To complete the approach both recti are retracted proximally and the distal stumps are retracted distally. The bladder is retracted posteriorly with a moist swab. If necessary, the medial insertion of the conjoint tendon is incised as far laterally as needed. Access to the superior pubic ramus requires elevation of the pectineal ligament from the pectineal line, and of pectineus from the superior aspect of the ramus. These dissections are extended sufficiently to control the rami fractures. Access to the symphysis requires exposure of its anterior surface and of the pubis on either side. If necessary, the obturator foramen may be identified on both sides with gentle dissection, using scissors or an elevator, in order to allow the subsequent insertion of the jaws of a bone-holding forceps.

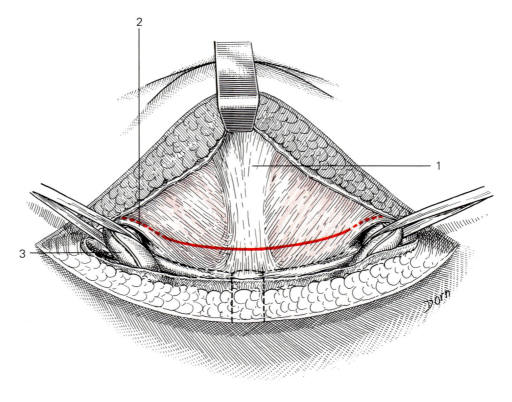

E

1 linea alba
2 superficial inguinal ring
3 spermatic cord

Closure

Closure comprises the repair of the conjoint tendon, if divided. The sheath and tendon of rectus abdominis are reattached (in two layers, posterior and anterior, if possible) with interrupted sutures. The external oblique aponeurosis is repaired.

Extension

G For the treatment of unilateral or bilateral pubic rami fractures adjacent to the acetabulum, this exposure can be extended laterally in the form of a unilateral or bilateral ilioinguinal approach; this allows full visualization of the anterior portion of the pelvic ring.

This extension involves the medial part of the ilioinguinal exposure on one or both sides, necessitating the placement of rubber slings around the spermatic cord and the external iliac vessels. Close dissection of the vessels should be avoided to prevent disruption of the accompanying lymphatics.

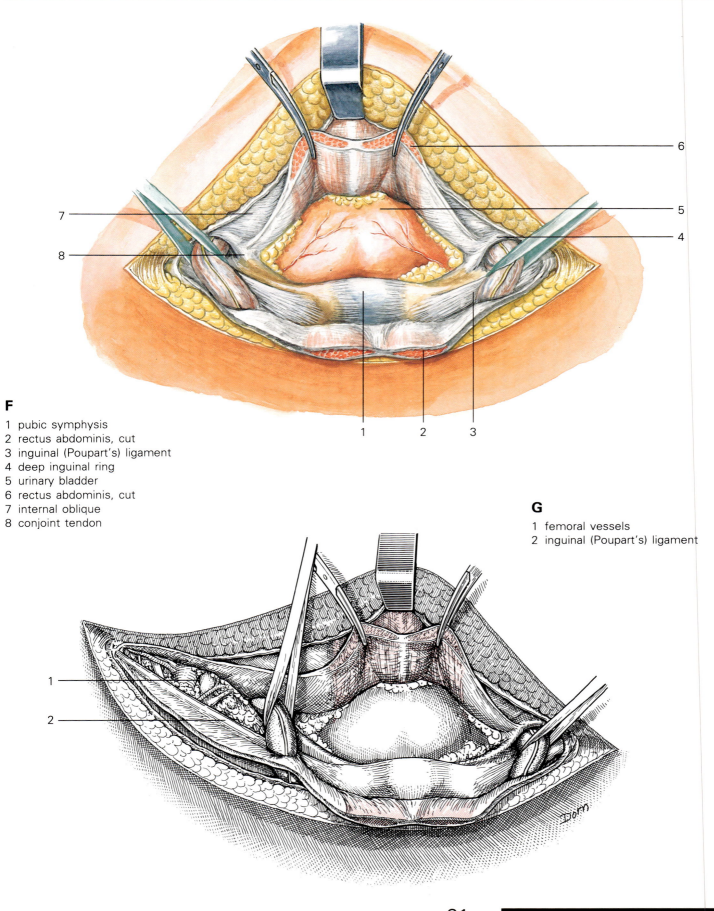

F

1 pubic symphysis
2 rectus abdominis, cut
3 inguinal (Poupart's) ligament
4 deep inguinal ring
5 urinary bladder
6 rectus abdominis, cut
7 internal oblique
8 conjoint tendon

G

1 femoral vessels
2 inguinal (Poupart's) ligament

Obturator foramen and ischium

Indications

- Partial or complete excision of pubis or ischium for neoplasia.
- Surgical treatment of tuberculous or pyogenic osteomyelitis.

Position

The patient is positioned supine with the legs abducted and flexed on appropriate supports, and the buttocks elevated by a sandbag at the end of the table.

Incision

A With a skin marker, indicate the position of the ischial tuberosity, the inferior border of the pubic symphysis and the inferior pubic ramus. The skin incision begins 1 cm distal to the midpoint of the inguinal ligament and proceeds medially parallel to it. At the lateral aspect of the base of the penis or the labium major, curve the incision distal to the scrotum and continue it along the inferior border of the ischiopubic ramus to the ischial tuberosity.

Exposure

B Detach subperiosteally pectineus, adductor longus, obturator externus and gracilis from the pubis and ischiopubic ramus and ischium and from the obturator 'membrane'. This exposes a part of the body of the pubis, the lateral part of the ischiopubic ramus and the ischial tuberosity.

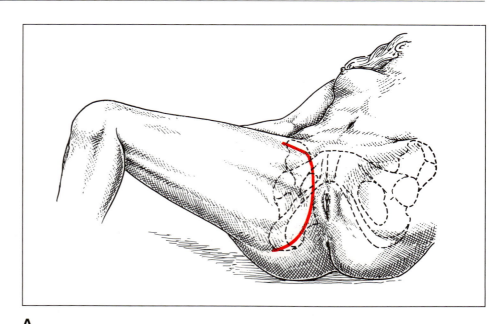

A

B

1 gluteus maximus	6 pectineus
2 ischial tuberosity	7 adductor longus
3 ischiocavernosus	8 gracilis
4 rectus abdominis	9 adductor magnus
5 inguinal ligament	10 semitendinosus

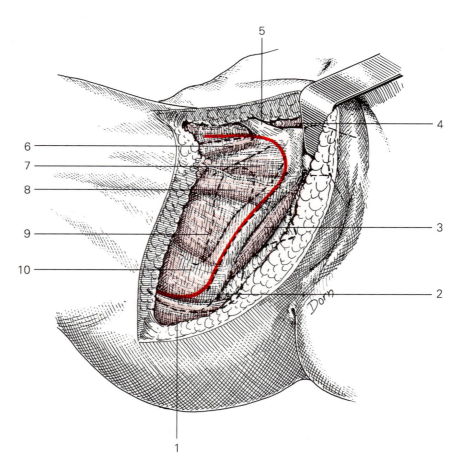

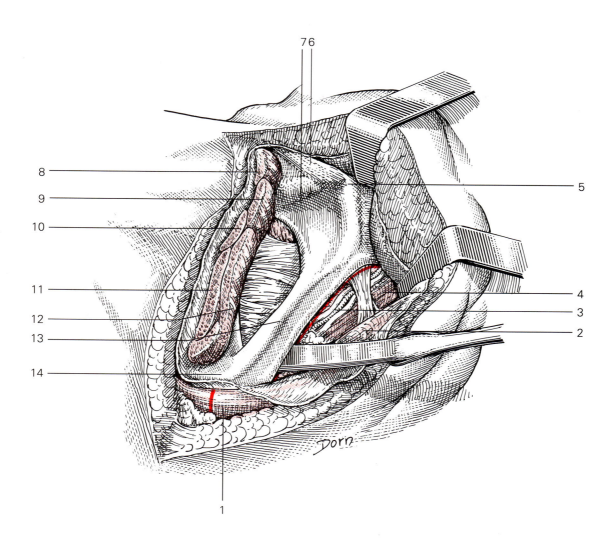

Dorn

C According to the surgical procedure required the exposure can be extended as follows:

1 To expose the ischium, retract or incise the distal edge of gluteus maximus in line with the skin incision, and dissect the hamstrings and quadratus femoris from the lateral aspect of the ischial tuberosity. Free the sacrotuberous ligament from its attachment to the medial aspect of the tuberosity. Protect the pudendal vessels and nerves entering the pelvis via the lesser sciatic notch. Proceed anteriorly and elevate subperiosteally ischiocavernosus and obturator internus from

the inner aspect of the ischiopubic ramus to avoid damage to the pudendal vessels within the pudendal canal.

2 To expose the anterior part of the obturator foramen, elevate subperiosteally the deep and superficial transverse perineal muscles. The crus penis and the constrictor urethrae from the medial borders of the inferior ischial and pubic rami are elevated. Dissect the urogenital diaphragm from the inferior border of the pubic symphysis, avoiding injury to the urethra and the deep dorsal vein, dorsal artery and nerve of the penis/clitoris.

C

1 gluteus maximus
2 superficial transverse perineal muscle
3 internal pudendal vessels and pudendal nerve in Alcock's canal
4 ischiocavernosus
5 pubic tubercle
6 inguinal ligament
7 superior pubic ramus
8 pectineus
9 adductor longus
10 gracilis
11 adductor magnus
12 obturator externus
13 inferior pubic ramus
14 ischium

D Separate rectus abdominis and pyramidalis from the pubis. Divide the insertion of the inguinal ligament and elevate pectineus from its origin along the superior pubic ramus and particularly the pectineal line, avoiding injury to the femoral sheath and its contents which lie on the lateral part of this muscle.

Dissect the obturator internus and externus muscles subperiosteally and if possible preserve the obturator nerve and vessels.

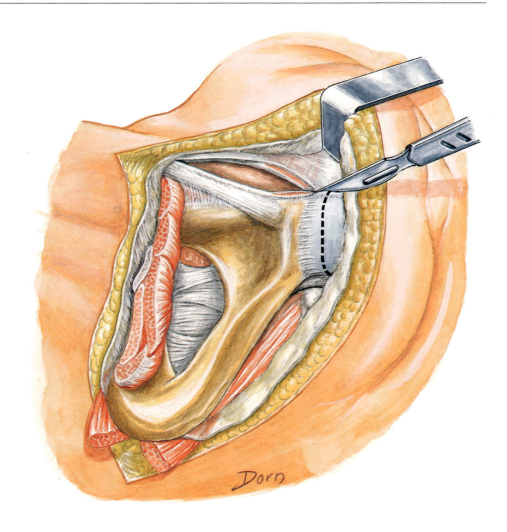

Iliac crest

Introduction

The approach to the iliac crest allows exclusive exposure of the iliac wing along either its outer or its inner aspect.

Indications

- Removal of corticocancellous graft from either aspect of the iliac wing.
- Reduction and fixation of a vertical fracture through the iliac wing.
- Possible access to the anterior aspect of the sacroiliac joint.

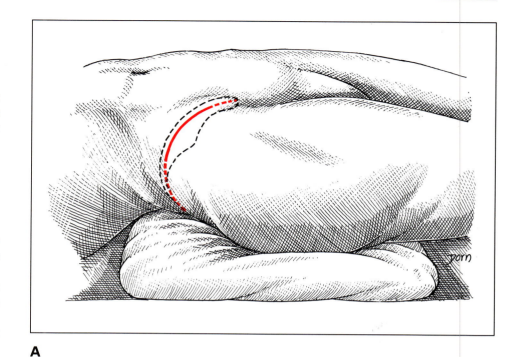

A

Position of the patient

The position of the patient depends on which aspect of the wing needs exposure:
- To approach the outer aspect the patient may be placed in one of the following positions: a full lateral position, a dorsolateral position with a cushion under the buttock (as in **A**) or supine, if only the anterior part of the iliac wing needs to be exposed.

- To approach the inner aspect of the wing it is best to place the patient fully supine on either an ordinary table or an orthopaedic table.

Incision

A The incision runs along the iliac crest and is centred on the area to be exposed. The length of incision depends on the antici-

pated surgical procedure. The incision may start at the anterior superior iliac spine and finish over the posterior iliac spine.

Pelvic girdle

B

1 iliac crest (tubercle)
2 gluteus medius
3 external oblique
4 lateral cutaneous branch of
 hypogastric nerve (L1)

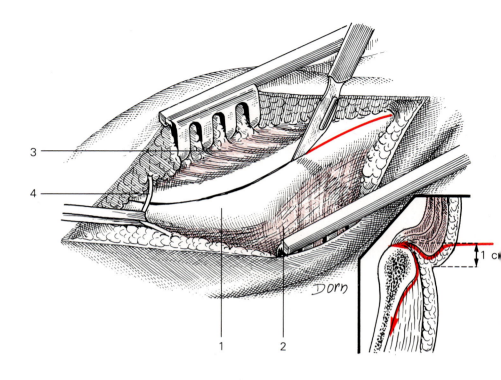

Exposure

B Overhanging abdominal muscles may obscure the iliac crest in obese individuals. Once the skin is incised the abdominal muscles can be identified and the subcutaneous tissues dissected from them in order to identify their origins from the iliac crest.

The aponeurosis covering the iliac crest is incised along its apex and dissected from the underlying bone, using a knife, in order to allow a secure closure.

C Usually the graft is taken from the outer aspect of the wing which is exposed by elevating the gluteal muscles over the desired site.

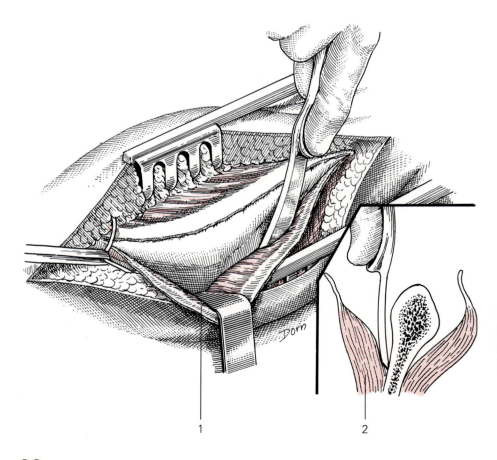

C

1 gluteus medius, released
2 iliacus

D

1 gluteus medius and gluteus minimus, released from ilium
2 hip joint
3 superior gluteal nerve and artery
4 piriformis

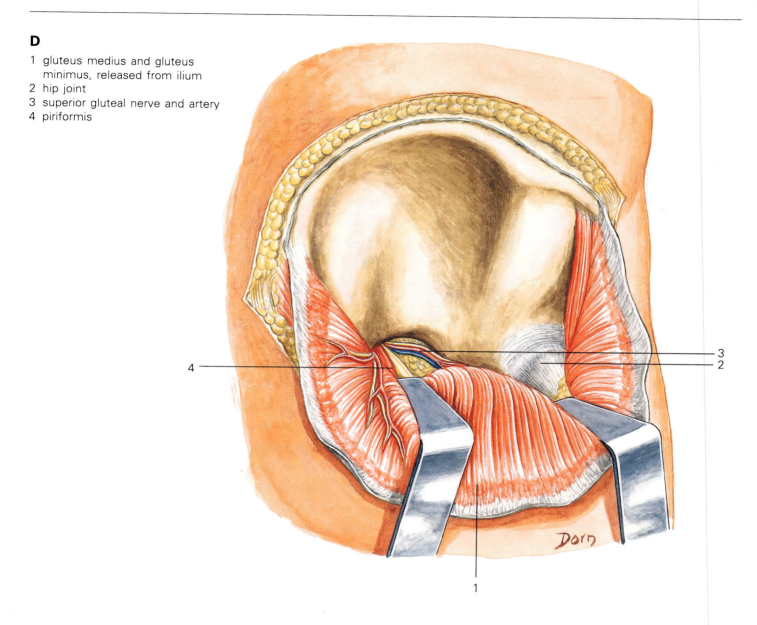

Variations

D For a maximum exposure tensor fasciae latae is elevated with the glutei. Posteriorly the greater sciatic notch can be identified where the superior gluteal neurovascular bundle is encountered; this has to be freed from the notch if a fracture extends into it. Inferiorly the superior hip capsule can be exposed.

These extended incisions will damage some of the vessels and nerves that cross the iliac crest to supply the skin over the lateral aspect of the hip.

In some cases the shape of the iliac graft required is concave and the graft may then be taken from the inner aspect of the iliac wing from its anterior and middle section. The aponeurosis of the abdominal muscles is incised along the iliac crest and sharply elevated away from its inner slope. Iliacus is elevated, in continuity with the abdominal muscles, from the internal iliac fossa over the required area (see **C**).

In order to take a tricortical graft involving the full thickness of the iliac wing, the aponeurosis must be incised along the apex of the iliac crest; both internal and external iliac fossae are then exposed by reflecting iliacus medially and the glutei laterally.

Pelvic girdle

E If the incision is made along the posterior half or two-thirds of the iliac crest, the elevation of iliacus may be continued up to the sacroiliac joint and to the lateral centimetre of the sacrum. Two Steinmann pins inserted into the sacrum close to the sacroiliac joint maintain a good exposure of the joint space. The soft tissues can be elevated as far as the posterior third of the iliopectineal line.

The elevation of the soft tissues close to the sacroiliac joint from the posterior part of the iliopectineal line must be carried out with great care in order not to injure the L5 root which crosses the anterior border of the alar of the sacrum 1 or 2 cm medial to the sacroiliac joint.

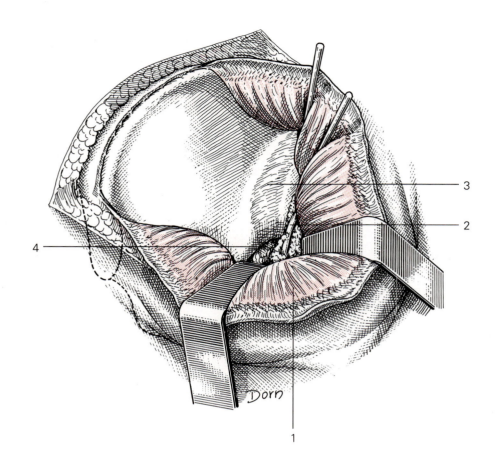

E

1 iliopsoas, retracted
2 L5 root
3 sacroiliac joint
4 greater sciatic notch

Posterior iliac crest bone graft

Introduction

Abundant bone can be harvested from the posterior iliac crest. A corticocancellous graft in one or several pieces can be taken and has the advantage of a thin cortex. Cancellous bone can be readily extracted.

Position of the patient

The patient lies prone or in the midlateral position, with the operated side uppermost.

Incision

A The classic incision (*a*) runs along the posterior iliac crest, starting at the posterior superior iliac spine and its length varies according to the amount of bone required. Damage to the clunial nerves, which cross the posterior iliac crest is avoided by limiting the anterior extent of the incision to within 5 cm of the posterior superior iliac spine. Not infrequently this incision is complicated by skin necrosis resulting from pressure when the patient lies upon it in the early post-operative phase.

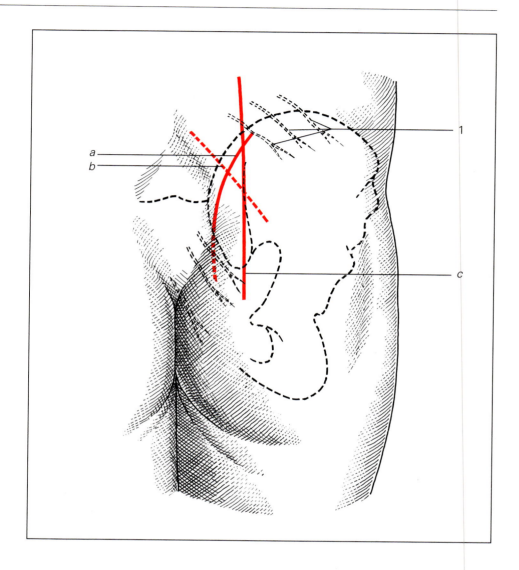

A
1 superior clunial nerves
a classic incision
b oblique incision
c vertical incision

Pelvic girdle

B
1 posterior iliac crest
2 gluteus maximus

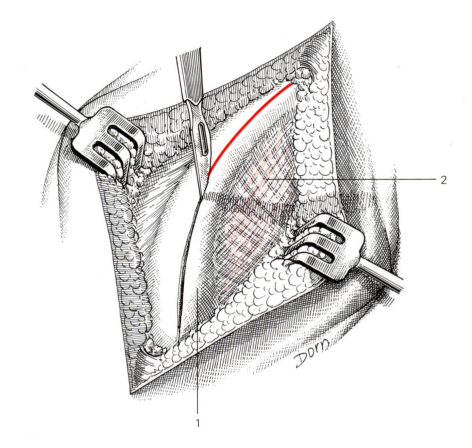

B The gluteal fascia is incised along the apex of the iliac crest and then elevated sharply from the outer slope of the crest.

C Gluteus maximus is dissected with an elevator from the posterior part of the iliac crest over an area that allows the graft to be harvested as required. Reflection of the muscle is easy except at the posterior gluteal line where the tendinous origins of the muscle need sharp dissection.

If a thick graft is needed, it is also possible to dissect the lumbodorsal fascia from the inner slope of the crest. Once the corticocancellous block has been raised, the cancellous bone within the iliac crest can be removed as far as the subchondral bone of the articular surface of the sacroiliac joint, which must not be damaged.

Variations

To try to minimize the risk of skin problems, an oblique incision can be made (as demonstrated in *b* in **A**); this crosses the iliac crest obliquely running in a proximal medial direction. The access provided may be similar, but the incision still crosses the point of pressure over the posterior iliac crest which occurs when the patient is supine.

It is currently preferable to use a vertical incision 2 cm lateral to the posterior spine (*c* in **A**), as described for the approach to the sacroiliac joint (see page 52).

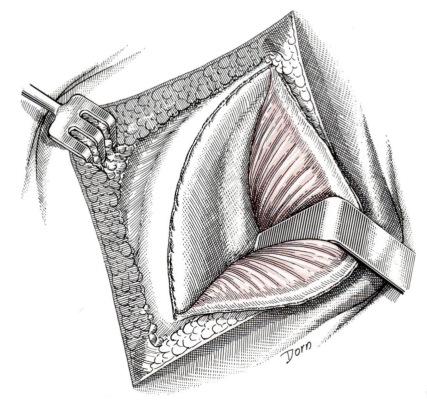

C

D
1 greater sciatic notch
2 superior gluteal artery and nerve

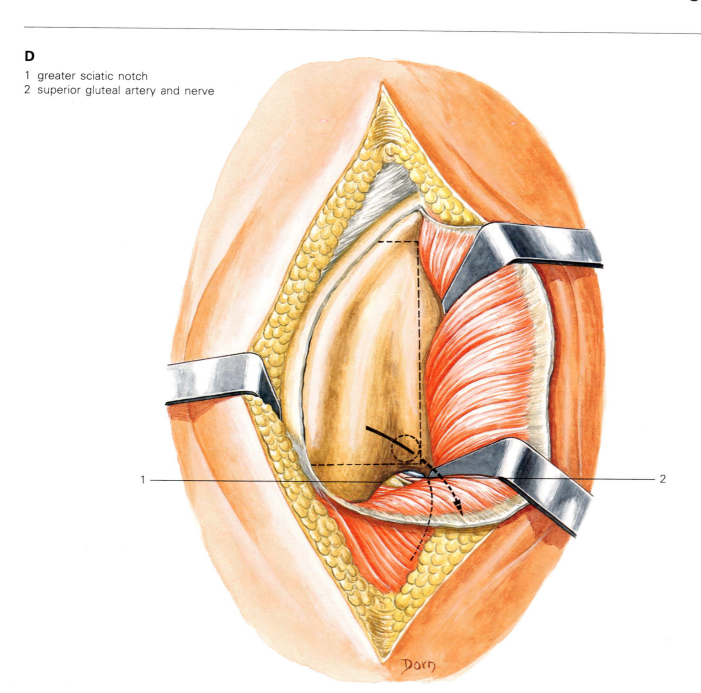

D   The subcutaneous tissues are incised in line with the incision to expose gluteus maximus; they are then dissected from the medial part of the muscle as far medially as the posterior iliac crest, and the posterior and inferior iliac spines. Then, the fascia is incised along the crest, as in **B**, and gluteus maximus elevated from the external iliac fossa. This muscle is reflected according to the amount of bone desired. If a large amount of bone is needed the external iliac fossa can be exposed as far as the superior border of the greater sciatic notch; this is approached with caution, and the superior gluteal neurovascular bundle identified and protected with a moist swab.

A long block of corticocancellous bone can be taken to within 0.5 cm of the superior border of the sciatic notch. When this piece is removed, abundant cancellous bone can be extracted as follows: medially and inferiorly as far as the subchondral bone of the sacroiliac joint, superiorly and laterally from within the iliac crest, inside the sciatic buttress with an angled gauge or a curette. The direction of curettage of the cancellous bone is indicated with dotted lines.

2

Hip

Anterior (Hueter) approach

Indications

- Biopsy of the synovium or synovectomy.
- Surgery of the torn labrum.
- Hip arthroplasty. Note that an orthopaedic table is mandatory.
- Removal of bone fragments from within the acetabulum.

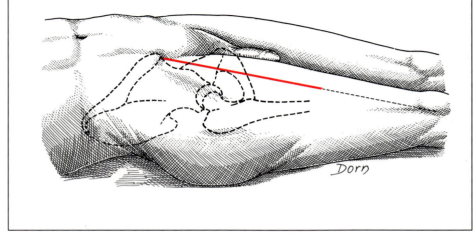

A

Position of the patient

The patient is placed supine. An orthopaedic table is essential if either distraction or dislocation of the hip is planned.

After draping, a rectangular field is exposed extending from two or three fingers' breadth above the anterior superior iliac spine down to the mid-thigh. The width of the field is 15 cm, the midpoint being the anterior superior spine.

Incision

A The straight incision starts at the level of the anterior superior iliac spine and runs distally for about 15–20 cm towards the outer border of the patella anterior to the belly of tensor fasciae latae.

Except in the obese, it is possible to palpate the bellies of tensor fasciae latae and sartorius which are separated by a depression that outlines the classic anterior approach.

It is preferable to incise the skin a little more obliquely than the classic incision along the belly of tensor fasciae latae in order to open its sheath, and by so doing avoid damage to the branches of the lateral cutaneous nerve of the thigh; these are always divided if the interval between tensor fasciae latae and sartorius is dissected.

Exposure

B The fascia covering tensor fasciae latae is incised in line with the skin incision. The belly of the muscle is bluntly separated from its fascial sheath along its medial border, and is retracted laterally. Care has to be taken not to damage the muscle fibres which are sometimes firmly attached to the sheath. The connections between the muscle and the sheath are particularly dense close to the muscle's origin from the iliac crest. In order to achieve maximal exposure it is recommended that the muscle be freed up to this origin.

If in error the knife penetrates the interval between tensor fasciae latae and sartorius, the branches of the lateral cutaneous nerve may be damaged. It is better to stop and look laterally for the belly of the tensor fasciae latae and incise along it.

Tensor fasciae latae is retracted laterally to expose, on its medial border, the fascia beneath which lie the typical fibres of the origin of rectus femoris; this has two heads: one, straight, arising from the anterior inferior iliac spine and the other, reflected, arising from a shallow concavity above the acetabulum.

C The fascia is incised longitudinally with the knife horizontally positioned, and rectus femoris is freed along its lateral border prior to being retracted medially.

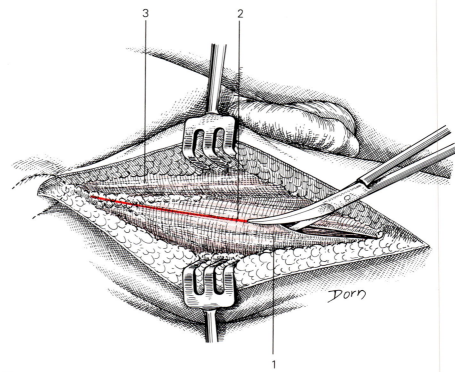

B

1 aponeurosis covering tensor fasciae latae
2 fascia, incised
3 sartorius

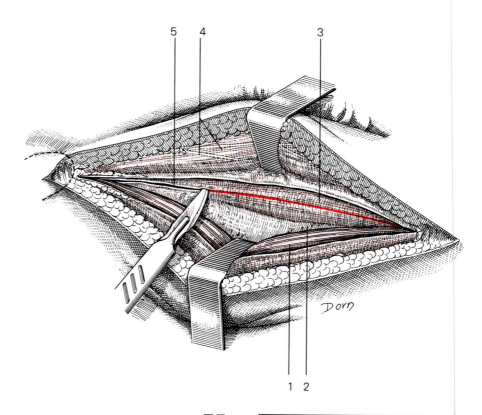

C

1 tensor fasciae latae, retracted laterally
2 deep fascia
3 rectus femoris
4 branches of the lateral cutaneous nerve of thigh
5 incision of the fascia covering rectus femoris

D In the course of this procedure a small vascular pedicle is encountered which enters the lateral border of the muscle about 5 cm from its origin and arises from the anterior circumflex artery. This small vessel indicates the position of the main artery which is soon encountered.

Following the lateral border of rectus femoris proximally, the reflected head is exposed. The lateral border of the reflected head is sometimes free but is quite often attached to the anterior hip capsule by a fibrous membrane – this is divided if present.

A pair of forceps is passed deep to the reflected head adjacent to the straight head. The reflected head can then be divided vertically without cutting the artery of the acetabular roof lying beneath it; this artery would be damaged if not protected. The division of the reflected head will facilitate medial retraction of the belly of rectus femoris.

The medial retraction of rectus femoris demonstrates a very strong fascial sheet, which has no name. However, it may be 0.5 mm thick and is absolutely constant. This fascial sheet is incised longitudinally, always in line with the incision. This is performed carefully in order to avoid injuring the underlying vessels.

The deep fascia is divided approximately at the midpoint of the incision (at the level of cauterization of the small pedicle entering the lateral border of rectus) to expose the anterior circumflex vessels running transversely. In cases of anterior subluxation of the hip these vessels may run proximally and laterally. The circumflex vessels are ligated and divided.

If the incision is prolonged distally the neurovascular bundle to vastus lateralis is encountered, and runs obliquely distally and laterally. It is easily identified because a nerve accompanies the vessels.

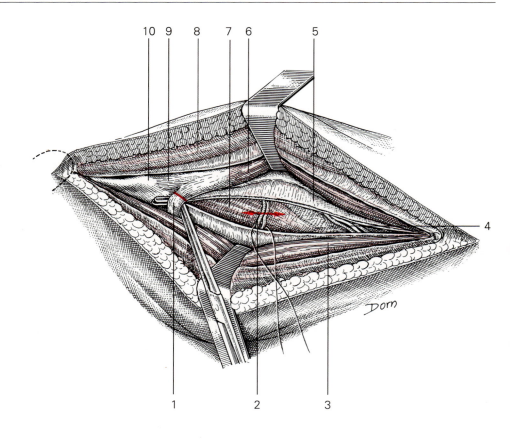

D

1 reflected head of rectus femoris, to be divided
2 anterior circumflex vessels, to be ligated
3 tensor fasciae latae, retracted laterally
4 neurovascular bundle to vastus lateralis
5 deep fascial sheet, incised
6 rectus femoris, retracted medially
7 iliopsoas
8 sartorius
9 straight head of rectus femoris
10 anterior inferior iliac spine

E When the stumps of the anterior circumflex artery are retracted, the fine fascia is seen covering psoas and also the main part of the anterior hip capsule. This thin fascial layer is incised longitudinally and psoas is freed from the hip capsule with an elevator. The arrows indicate the successive directions to be followed by the elevator to reach the anterior lip of the acetabulum, the inferior aspect of the hip capsule and the lesser trochanter.

Finally the elevator divides the fibrous attachments along the superior border of the hip capsule which now appears to be completely freed, except for its posterior aspect.

F Hohmann retractors may be inserted along the superior and inferior borders, while another set retracts rectus femoris and iliopsoas medially.

The anterior hip capsule is then fully exposed and it is now possible to:

- perform an extended anterior capsulectomy if a total hip is to be inserted;
- perform a capsulotomy along the anterior acetabular margin, leaving 2–3 mm of capsule attached to the iliac bone in case closure of the capsule is possible. Most of the time this capsulotomy does not give sufficient access and has to be completed by an incision along the long axis of the femoral neck.

If the exposure of the hip is tight, it is easy to divide tensor fasciae latae adjacent to the iliac crest and retract it laterally to expose the anterior part of the external iliac fossa. The muscle is repaired at the end of the procedure.

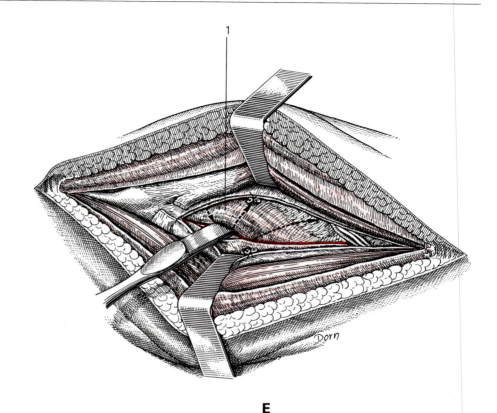

E

1 psoas
arrows: successive directions followed
  by the elevator

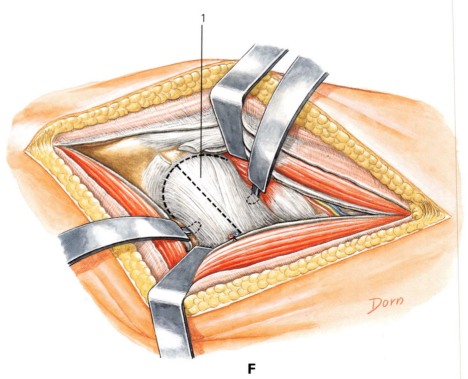

F

1 hip joint capsule

Hip

G A cross-section through the hip joint shows the approach to the joint.

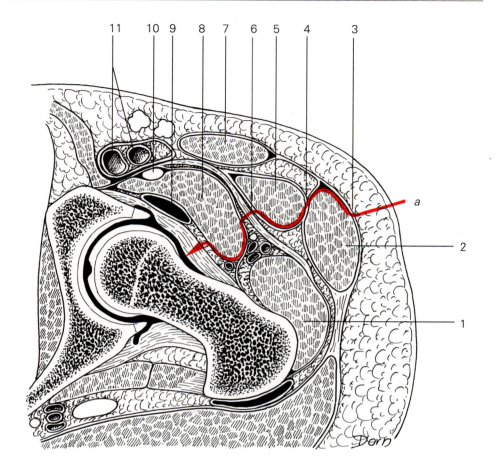

G

1 gluteus medius
2 tensor fasciae latae
3 incision of the fascia of tensor fasciae latae
4 incision of the fascia of rectus femoris
5 rectus femoris
6 incision through the deep fascial sheet
7 sartorius
8 psoas
9 iliopectineal bursa
10 femoral nerve
11 femoral vessels
a surgical approach

Closure

Closure is extremely easy — a 'self-closure' incision is used. It may be possible to reattach the hip capsule and the fascia of tensor fasciae latae is sutured with interrupted sutures, as are the subcutaneous fat and skin.

Extended anterior (Smith–Petersen) approach

Introduction

In comparison with the standard anterior approach the extended anterior approach allows a greater access to the superior aspect of the hip. Access to the iliac wing is variable and depends on the extent to which the muscles are freed from the external iliac fossa. It is possible to gain access to the upper border of the greater sciatic notch posteriorly.

The main disadvantage of this approach is the relatively high incidence of postoperative ectopic bone formation which may follow extensive elevation of muscle from the external iliac fossa. However, when this approach is used to perform a shelf operation — which does not include an arthrotomy of the hip joint — ectopic bone formation is exceptional.

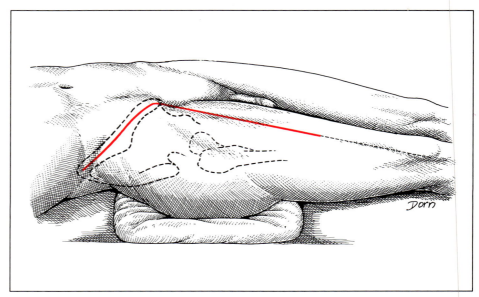

A

Indications

- Shelf operation for acetabular dysplasia.
- Hip arthroplasty.
- Acetabular reconstruction after loosening of total hip components.
- Hip arthrodesis, allowing the use of a muscle pedicle bone graft from the anterior part of the external iliac wing.
- Iliotrochanteric fusion to treat septic arthritis, or infected total hip arthroplasty.
- All operations that necessitate a wide exposure of the hip joint, to the iliac wing, can provide abundant material for cortico-cancellous bone graft.

Position of the patient

The patient lies supine on an ordinary table, and a suitable sandbag may be placed under the ipsilateral buttock. This approach is usually performed on the orthopaedic table.

The operative field is large, from at least the anterior three-quarters of the iliac crest and distally to the mid-thigh.

Incision

A The incision can be considered to consist of two limbs in continuity.

The first limb is placed over the iliac crest for a distance that depends on the access needed to the external iliac fossa, and ends at the anterior superior iliac spine.

From the anterior superior iliac spine the second limb, which is a straight incision, runs distally towards the outer border of the patella, exactly as described for the standard anterior approach. The length of this limb is approximately 20 cm but this depends on the required exposure of the femoral shaft.

Hip

Exposure

B Along the iliac crest the gluteal fascia is sharply incised and reflected from the lateral margin of the crest. An elevator is used to dissect tensor fasciae latae and the glutei subperiosteally which are reflected from the external iliac fossa. If the incision is extended posteriorly it is necessary to divide one or two neurovascular bundles which cross the iliac crest. From the anterior superior spine the fascia of tensor fasciae latae is incised longitudinally in line with the skin incision.

C The belly of tensor fasciae latae is freed from its fascial sheath along its medial border, to expose its origin from the iliac crest, which is incised adjacent to the bone. This allows a complete exposure of the external iliac fossa from the iliac crest to the superior aspect of the hip capsule, and as far posteriorly as necessary. Very close to the capsule lies the reflected head of rectus femoris, adjacent to the straight head. A forceps is introduced beneath the reflected head which is sharply divided and the tendon excised. When a shelf operation is performed the reflected head is left in place in order to delineate the upper border and roof of the trench into which the iliac graft will be introduced. The tendon is excised once the trench is completed.

The upper part of the capsule is exposed carefully with an elevator. Then the fascia covering rectus femoris is incised longitudinally. The muscle is retracted medially and proximally.

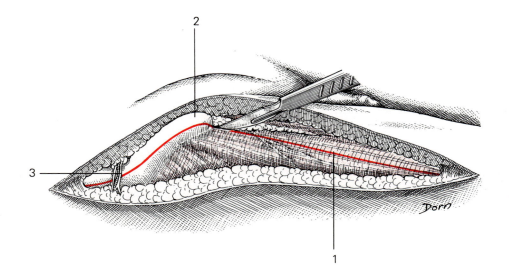

B

1 incision in the fascia of tensor fasciae latae
2 anterior superior iliac spine
3 lateral cutaneous branch of the hypogastric nerve (L1)

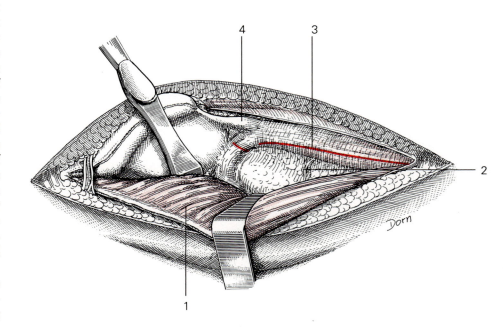

C

1 glutei and tensor fasciae latae, retracted
2 lateral circumflex femoral artery
3 incision in the deep fascia covering rectus femoris
4 anterior inferior iliac spine

D Following the same steps as described for the anterior approach the strong fascia deep to rectus femoris is incised (in line with the incision), beneath which the anterior circumflex vessels are identified and ligated.

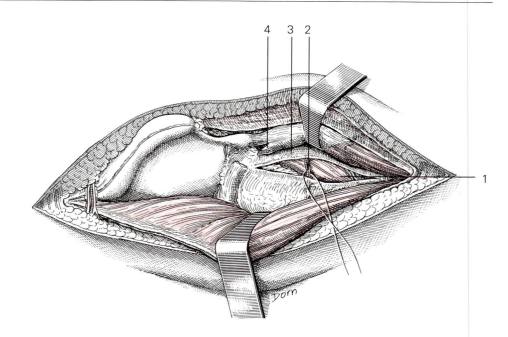

D

1 iliopsoas
2 ligation of the lateral circumflex artery
3 fascia beneath rectus femoris, incised
4 reflected head of rectus femoris, divided

E Once the vessels are ligated, a thin fascial sheet is seen covering that part of iliopsoas which is strongly attached to the anterior aspect of the hip capsule. This fascia is incised and psoas is elevated from the anterior capsule as far medially as the sheath of the iliopsoas tendon. The inferior border of the hip capsule is exposed by following the ilio-psoas tendon to its insertion into the lesser trochanter.

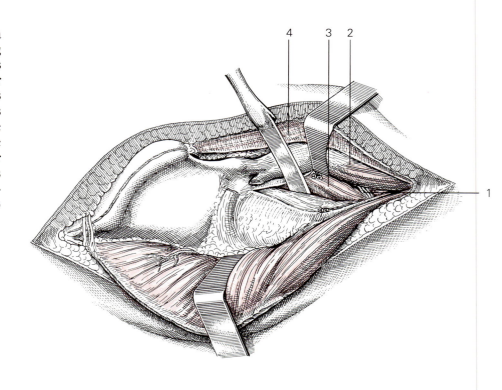

E

1 neurovascular bundle to vastus lateralis
2 rectus femoris, retracted
3 psoas, freed from the capsule
4 sartorius

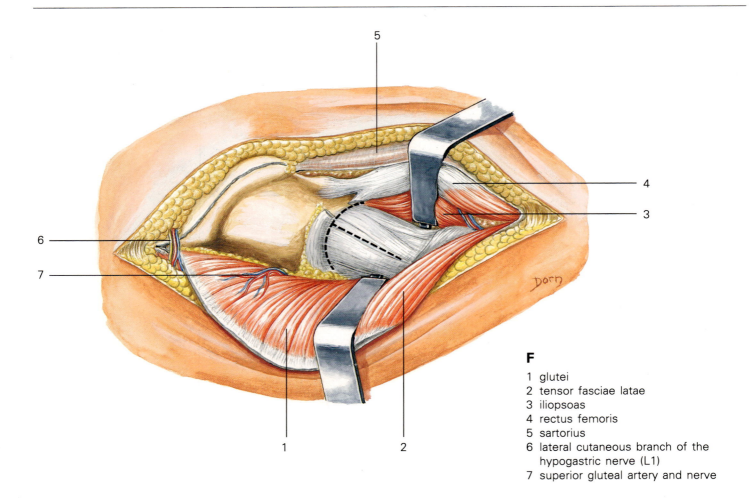

F

1 glutei
2 tensor fasciae latae
3 iliopsoas
4 rectus femoris
5 sartorius
6 lateral cutaneous branch of the hypogastric nerve (L1)
7 superior gluteal artery and nerve

F The exposure of the anterior aspect of the hip capsule is completed laterally with the elevator. An arthrotomy of the hip is performed as described in the anterior approach.

Closure

The capsule is sutured if possible. The gluteal fascia is reattached to the fascia of the abdominal muscles along the iliac crest with interrupted sutures. The fascia of tensor fasciae latae is closed in the same way, without trapping the branches of the lateral cutaneous nerve of thigh with the sutures. The subcutaneous tissues and skin are closed.

Possible extension

In some circumstances access to the internal iliac fossa may be necessary. First, the straight head of rectus femoris is divided close to the anterior inferior iliac spine. The tendon will be reattached at the end with a transosseous suture. This manoeuvre allows the exposure of the anterior wall of the acetabulum.

Secondly, the origins of the abdominal muscles are incised from the iliac crest and, in continuity, iliacus is elevated from the internal iliac fossa as far posteriorly as the sacroiliac joint and as far medially as the pelvic brim. It is essential to release sartorius and the inguinal ligament from the anterior superior iliac spine.

It is not possible to gain access beyond the posterior third of the pelvic brim and the iliopectineal eminence is reached with great difficulty.

Closure of such an extension necessitates the secure reattachment of the abdominal muscles and the gluteal fascia to the iliac crest with transosseous sutures.

Anterolateral (Watson-Jones) approach

Indications

- Internal fixation of femoral neck fractures, allowing control of the anterior aspect of the neck through a capsulotomy.
- Hip arthroplasty.

Position

The patient is positioned supine on an orthopaedic table, or on an ordinary table with a small sandbag beneath the ipsilateral buttock.

Incision

A The incision begins 2 cm distal and lateral to the anterior superior iliac spine, curves distally and posteriorly to the apex of the greater trochanter, and extends down over the greater trochanter to end 6–8 cm distal to the trochanteric line.

Exposure

B The deep fascia is incised over the greater trochanter and is continued distally in line with the skin incision. The incision is continued proximally along the posterior border of tensor fasciae latae which is palpable and often visible. The fascia lata with tensor fasciae latae is retracted anteriorly to expose the anterior border of gluteus medius. The plane between the two muscles is now developed by blunt dissection. Some blood vessels in this plane need to be coagulated. If the separation of the two muscles is continued too far anteriorly the branch of the superior gluteal nerve, which supplies tensor fasciae latae, is seen. It is unnecessary to dissect this far anteriorly.

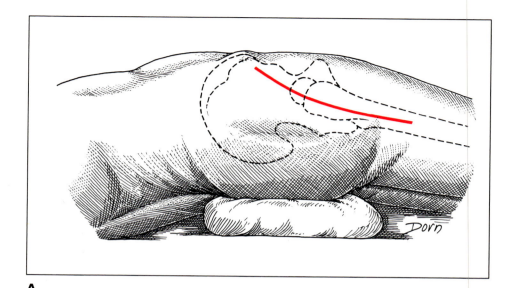

A

B
1 gluteus medius, covered by fascia
2 fascia lata (iliotibial tract)
3 tensor fasciae latae
4 superior gluteal nerve (deep to fascia)

Hip

C

1 reflection of vastus lateralis
2 tensor fasciae latae, retracted
3 glutei, retracted
a midline incision
b alternative incision along the
   trochanteric line

C Posterior retraction of gluteus medius, and anterior retraction of tensor fasciae latae exposes the fatty tissue covering the antero-superior aspect of the hip capsule. By rotating the femur laterally the capsule is stretched and its exposure facilitated.

Vastus lateralis may need to be reflected from the proximal femur distal to the greater trochanter. The muscle fibres may be split in the midline (*a*) and the muscle stripped from the bone anteriorly and posteriorly. Alternatively, the origin of the muscle can be incised along the trochanteric line, and the linea aspera and the proximal part reflected distally (*b*).

D A more complete exposure of the capsule is often needed. It is afforded by dividing the aponeurosis which inserts into the trochanteric line, and by elevating the attachments of iliopsoas from the anterior aspect of the hip capsule.

Along the superior acetabular lip the reflected head of rectus femoris can be excised without compromising function.

The hip capsule may be incised as usual by a 'T' incision, combining an incision along the anterior acetabular lip and a longitudinal incision along the line of the femoral neck. If the femur is rotated fully laterally, flexing and adducting it, the femoral head dislocates anteriorly.

D

1 origin of vastus lateralis, released
   and retracted distally
2 iliopsoas
3 tensor fasciae latae, retracted
4 reflected head of rectus femoris
5 straight head of rectus femoris

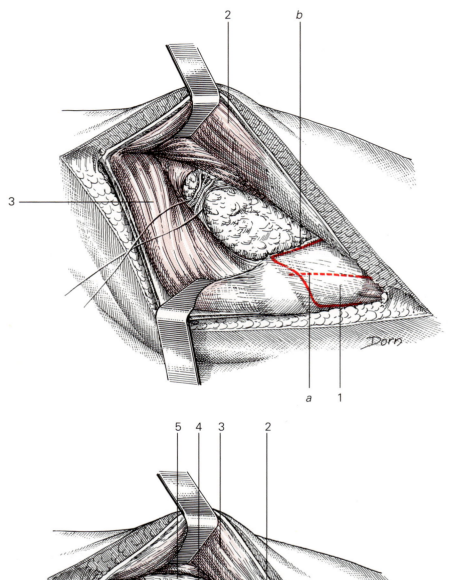

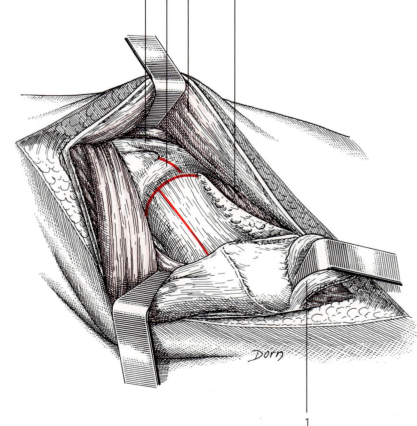

E The final exposure after retraction of the capsular flaps.

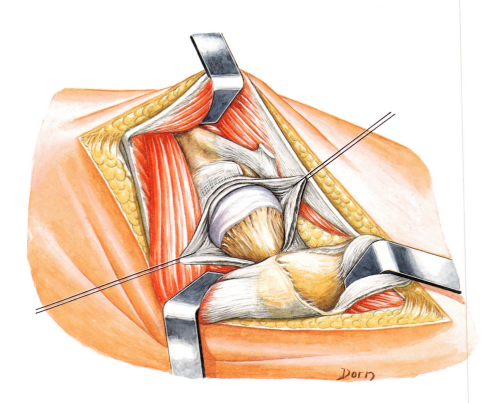

Extension

If it is necessary to expose the upper part of the femoral shaft the fibres of vastus lateralis may be split longitudinally (see *a* on **C**).

Alternatively, the origin of vastus lateralis from the trochanteric line is reflected distally (see *b* on **C**). A branch of the anterior circumflex artery adjacent to the bone must be diathermied. The hip capsule is attached to the medial aspect of the trochanteric line and thus the exposure of the anterior aspect of the hip can be increased.

The trochanteric insertion of gluteus medius can be partially divided to increase the exposure. Leaving a stump of tendon attached to the trochanter facilitates the repair.

Lateral (Gibson) approach

Introduction

Described by Kocher in 1904, this approach has been 'rediscovered' by Gibson (1950) with great success.

Indications

- Hip arthroplasty.
- Intertrochanteric osteotomy.
- Acetabular fractures of the posterior column involving either the posterior acetabulum or the posterior column.
- Removal of ectopic bone.

Position

The patient should either be prone on the orthopaedic table, or be strictly lateral on an ordinary table with the leg separately draped. Draping must extend anteriorly to the midportion of the inguinal ligament, superiorly to the costal margin, posteriorly one or two fingers' breadth medial to the posterior iliac spine, and inferiorly up to the mid-thigh.

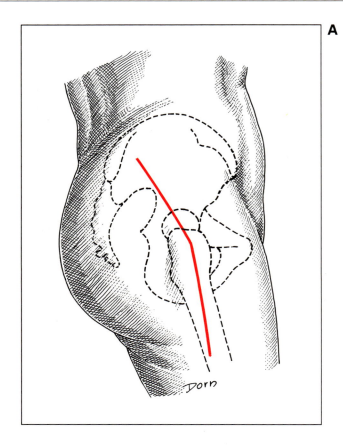

A

Incision

A The incision should be slightly angled and centred on the superior border of the greater trochanter. The upper limb of the incision runs towards a point on the iliac crest 6–8 cm anterior to the posterior superior iliac spine, but stops a few centimetres before the crest so that this limb of the incision overlies the anterior border of gluteus maximus. The lower limb extends distally following the long axis of the greater trochanter over 10–15 cm.

B

1 gluteus maximus
2 iliotibial tract, incised

B   The flaps of skin and subcutaneous fat are reflected by blunt dissection from the underlying deep fascia over a few centimetres. The fascia over gluteus medius is divided in the line of the skin incision along the anterior border of gluteus maximus. Distal to the greater trochanter the iliotibial tract is incised. Abduction of the thigh facilitates the division of the gluteal fascia along the sulcus at the anterior border of gluteus maximus. If necessary, the trochanteric bursa, which lies beneath the gluteal fascia, can be opened or excised.

C   Gluteus maximus is retracted posteriorly and the fascia lata retracted anteriorly to expose gluteus medius and posteriorly to expose the short external rotators. It is essential to identify and separate the posterior border of gluteus medius from piriformis by blunt dissection and to avoid injury to the vessels, some of which enter the joint, by working away from the greater trochanter. It is also essential to identify the sciatic nerve by following the line of the fibres of the short external rotators posteriorly. The nerve is always surrounded by adipose tissue.

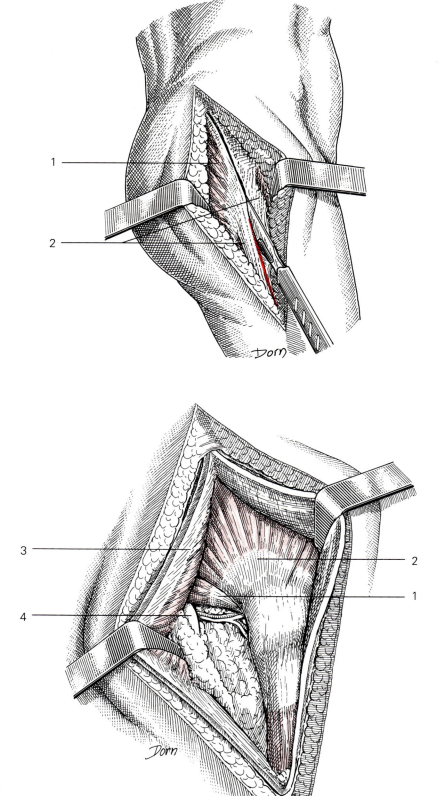

C

1 piriformis
2 gluteus medius
3 gluteus maximus, retracted
4 sciatic nerve

87

D There are two possible approaches to the joint:

- Divide the tendons of gluteus medius and gluteus minimus 0.5–1 cm away from their trochanteric insertions to facilitate their repair (*a*), and then dissect the muscles from the capsule by releasing their capsular insertions.
- Perform a trochanteric osteotomy. The trochanteric osteotomy can be performed with either a Gigli saw or an osteotome which is directed upwards and inwards from the base of the greater trochanter towards a forceps introduced between the capsule and the gluteal tendons adjacent to the trochanter. If the tendon of piriformis is retracted with the greater trochanter it is divided subsequently.

    The gluteal muscles are then dissected from the iliac wing as far proximally as necessary and held with one or two Steinmann pins inserted into the iliac wing.

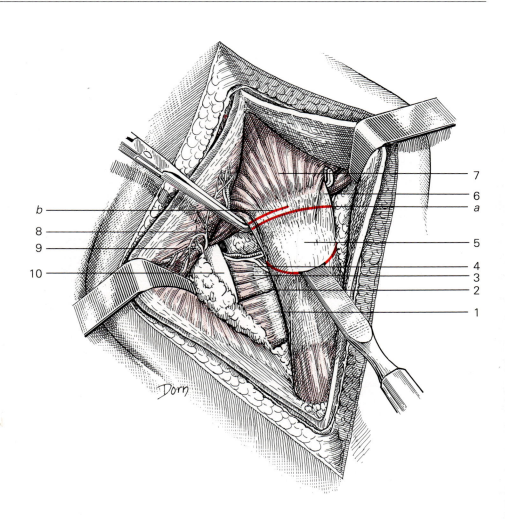

D

1 quadratus femoris
2 gemellus inferior
3 obturator internus
4 gemellus superior
5 greater trochanter
6 gluteus minimus
7 gluteus medius
8 piriformis
9 gluteus maximus

10 sciatic nerve
a complete division of tendons of gluteus medius, gluteus minimus and piriformis
b division of posterior half of tendons of gluteus medius and gluteus minimus with division of tendon of piriformis

E According to the surgical procedure, the approach to the hip capsule or the posterior column of the acetabulum can be enlarged by division of the short external rotators, which are held with stay sutures. The sciatic nerve has already been identified and posterior retraction of the short external rotators protects the nerve. The tendon of piriformis is divided.

Obturator internus and the gemelli are divided 2 or 3 cm from the trochanteric crest so as not to injure the posterior circumflex artery which supplies the head and neck of the femur. Retraction of obturator internus and the gemelli exposes the capsule and the posterior column. Following division of the short external rotators it is necessary to cauterize a transverse pedicle between the inferior gluteal and posterior circumflex vessels.

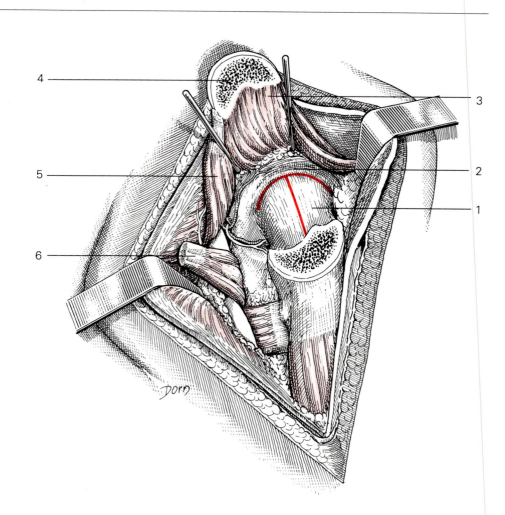

E

1 hip capsule
2 acetabular labrum
3 gluteus minimus and medius, retracted
4 greater trochanter, osteotomized
5 piriformis
6 obturator internus and gemelli

Hip

F The posterior capsule is fully exposed and can be opened by a 'T' incision. The capsule can be excised, and the hip dislocated posteriorly by flexion of hip and knee and adduction and internal rotation of the hip to about 90°.

Variation

If a less extensive access to the hip is required it is only necessary to divide the posterior part of the gluteal insertions into the greater trochanter (*b* on **D**) and to divide piriformis.

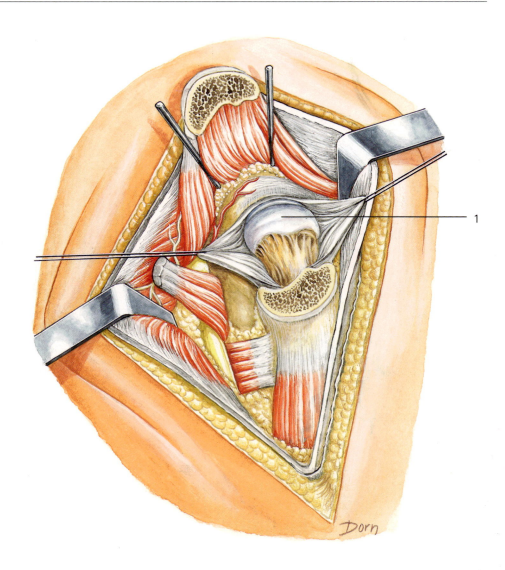

F

1 femoral head

Lateral transgluteal (Hardinge) approach

Indications

- Hip arthroplasty.
- Revision of hip arthroplasty or conversion of arthrodesis to total hip replacement.

Position

The patient lies supine with the greater trochanter lying over the edge of the table, thus freeing the buttock muscles from the table. The leg is draped separately.

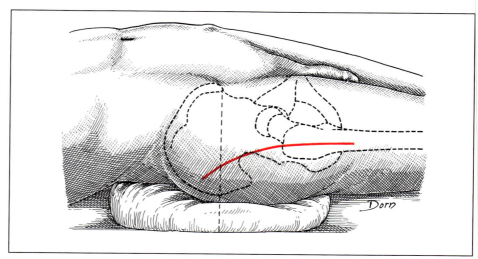

A

Incision

A The incision is curved and centred over the superior border of the greater trochanter; distally it proceeds parallel to the shaft of the femur along its anterior border for about 8–10 cm. Proximally it curves slightly posteriorly and ends at the vertical line dropped from the anterior superior iliac spine, but extends a little more proximally if the buttock is voluminous.

Exposure

B The gluteal fascia and the iliotibial tract are exposed by blunt dissection of the fat over a few centimetres on either side of the incision. The deep fascial incision begins over the long axis of the greater trochanter, or a little more anteriorly, and is continued distally in the midlateral line of the femur, and proximally in line with the skin incision.

The superficial fascia of gluteus maximus may also be divided in line with the direction of the muscle fibres which are then subsequently split over 5–8 cm.

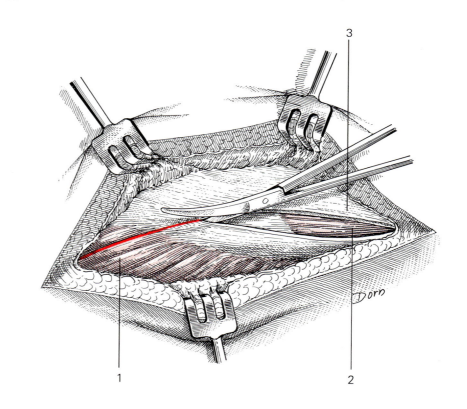

To expose the greater trochanter it may be necessary to divide the fibres of gluteus medius which arise from the deep surface of the gluteal fascia by blunt dissection, and to perform a partial or total excision of the trochanteric bursa. The insertion of gluteus medius into the proximal and lateral surface of the greater trochanter can now be clearly seen.

B
1 gluteus maximus
2 vastus lateralis
3 fascia lata (iliotibial tract)

Hip

C

1 gluteus maximus, split
2 vastus lateralis
3 transverse branch of the lateral circumflex artery, to be ligated
4 gluteus medius
5 course of the superior gluteal nerve

C Retractors are then positioned: one beneath the deep fascia anteriorly at the level of the anterior border of gluteus medius, and the other posteriorly at the level of the tendinous insertion of gluteus maximus into the posterior aspect of the femur.

The tendinous insertion of gluteus medius is split in the direction of its fibres at the junction of the anterior and middle thirds. This split is carried proximally 4 cm from the apex of the greater trochanter.

The incision is continued down to the bone, first over the trochanter, curved slightly anteriorly, and continued distally through vastus lateralis along the anterolateral surface of the femur for about 5–6 cm. During this last step the transverse branch of the lateral circumflex artery must be divided and cauterized.

D The anterior part of the tendinous insertion of gluteus medius is dissected from the trochanter, in continuity with the anterior part of vastus lateralis as a single layer, using a knife, the diathermy or (for some surgeons) a sharp chisel which then elevates the muscle with a slither of bone.

By flexing and adducting the hip the combined muscle mass that has just been detached is displaced forward. The tendon of gluteus minimus is now seen and divided from its insertion into the anterior aspect of the greater trochanter.

The capsule of the hip joint then comes into view.

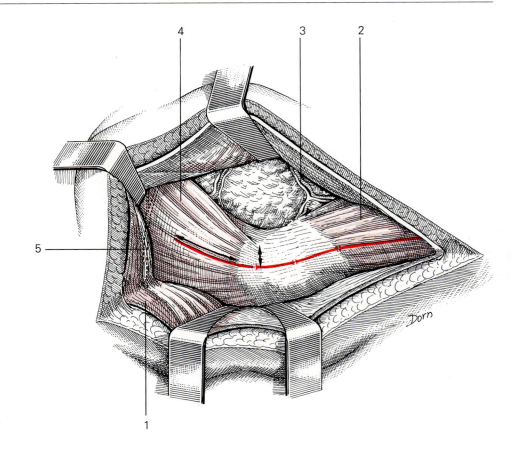

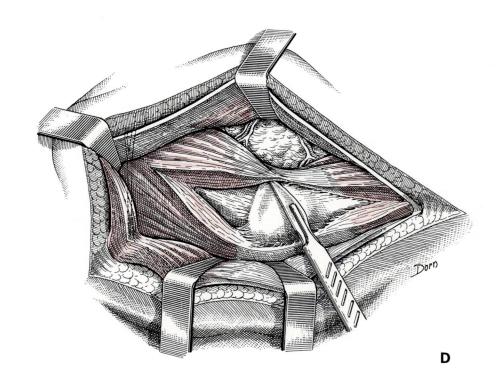

D

E The hip capsule is progressively freed, and finally incised circumferentially along the acetabular rim, after excision of the reflected head of rectus femoris; an additional longitudinal incision of the capsule allows the two capsular flaps to be reflected and the hip joint to be exposed.

F Further adduction of the thigh brings the femoral head into view and, on full adduction combined with increasing lateral rotation, the head will dislocate.

Closure

Gluteus minimus is reattached to its insertion. Gluteus medius is closed with a series of interrupted sutures, as is vastus lateralis. The deep fascia and the iliotibial tract are closed similarly. Two or three suction drains are inserted.

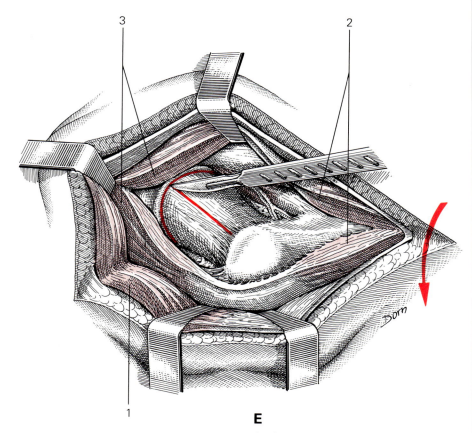

E

1 gluteus maximus, split
2 vastus lateralis, split
3 gluteus medius, split

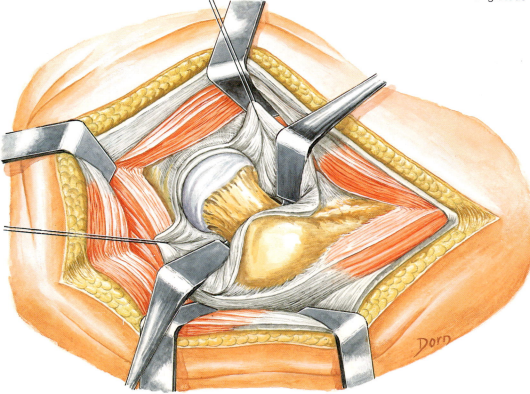

F

Posterolateral (Moore) approach

Introduction

The posterolateral approach is popular. However, it should be understood that it differs from the posterior approach to the acetabulum (see pages 36–42) only in the direction of the incision over the buttock. The incision is more acutely angled and thus the inferior part of gluteus maximus is split through its more horizontal fibres. This approach affords good access to the proximal femur but a more limited exposure of the acetabulum.

Indications

The approach allows exposure of the posterior aspect of the neck and the femoral head, and the lower half of the posterior column of the acetabulum. So it may be used for:

- Internal fixation of trochanteric fractures.
- Hip arthroplasty.

Position

The patient is placed on the unaffected side. Two supports securely maintain the lateral position, one (anterior) applied to the pubic symphysis and anterior superior iliac spine, the other (posterior) applied to the lumbosacral region.

Incision

A The incision is angled (or curved) centred over the posterior part of the superior border of the greater trochanter. The posterior limb extends proximally and medially to reach a point situated 8–10 cm below the posterior superior iliac spine, so its direction is parallel to the gluteus maximus fibres at that level. The inferior limb extends distally over 10–15 cm parallel with the femoral shaft.

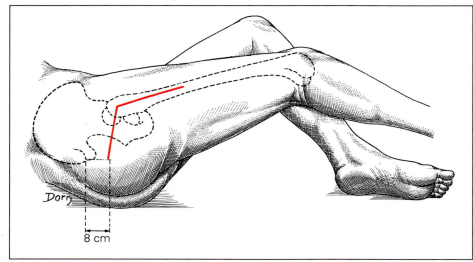

A

B

1 gluteus maximus
2 fascia lata (iliotibial tract)

B The deep fascia is exposed and divided in line with the skin incision; then, beginning at or below the greater trochanter, the fibres of gluteus maximus are separated by blunt dissection over 10–15 cm.

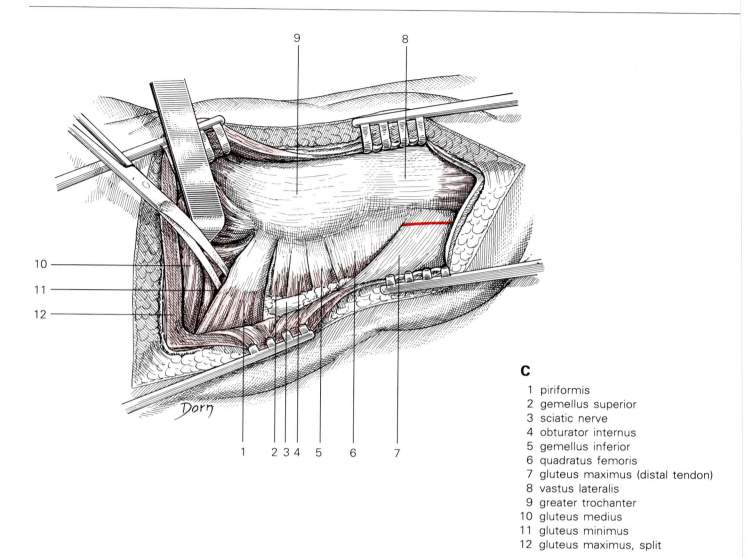

c

1 piriformis
2 gemellus superior
3 sciatic nerve
4 obturator internus
5 gemellus inferior
6 quadratus femoris
7 gluteus maximus (distal tendon)
8 vastus lateralis
9 greater trochanter
10 gluteus medius
11 gluteus minimus
12 gluteus maximus, split

C Retraction of the proximal part of gluteus maximus exposes the greater trochanter, and the overlying trochanteric bursa is either incised or partially excised.

Retraction of the posterior fibres of gluteus maximus posteriorly exposes the short external rotators of the hip. If it is necessary to enlarge the exposure, the tendinous insertion of gluteus maximus into the linea aspera can be divided in whole or in part a few millimetres from the bone, leaving a tendinous cuff to facilitate repair at the end of the procedure.

The short external rotators insert into the greater trochanter and proximal femur. They are,

from proximal to distal: piriformis, gemellus superior, obturator internus, gemellus inferior and quadratus femoris.

The fatty tissue should be dissected from their posterior surface; the horizontal direction of their fibres is then seen. The blunt dissection should be continued medially in order to identify the sciatic nerve that lies surrounded by adipose tissue. It is essential to identify the nerve. Stay sutures should be placed in these muscles 1 cm from their insertion. When these muscles are folded back following their division they will protect the sciatic nerve. The stay sutures facilitate their

reattachment at the end of the procedure.

The short external rotators are then divided. Piriformis is cut through its tendon lateral to the stay suture. Obturator internus and the gemelli may be divided adjacent to the trochanter (dotted line on **D**) if the head and neck are to be sacrificed, as in hip arthroplasty. If this is not the case, divide them 2 cm from their trochanteric insertion lateral to the stay suture in order to preserve the posterior circumflex artery. A horizontal anastomosis between the posterior circumflex artery and the inferior gluteal artery must always be divided.

D Elevation and retraction of the short external rotators expose the posterior part of the capsule and the posterior surface of the acetabulum. Internal rotation of the hip facilitates identification and division of the rotators because it stretches them.

Quadratus femoris may also be divided in its midportion or elevated from the femur to increase the exposure.

E The posterior part of the joint capsule is now well displayed, and is incised along the axis of the femoral neck. According to the procedure and access required, the capsule can also be incised along the posterior acetabular margin, so that two capsular flaps can be reflected. When inserting a total hip replacement, the capsule can be excised.

To dislocate the hip posteriorly it suffices to flex the thigh and knee to 90° and rotate the thigh internally.

D

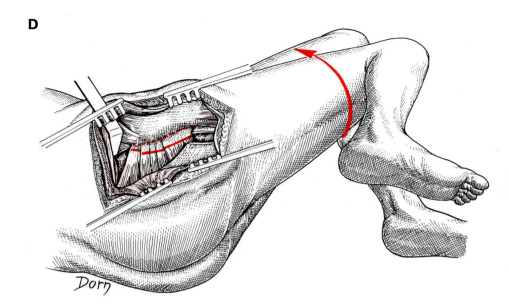

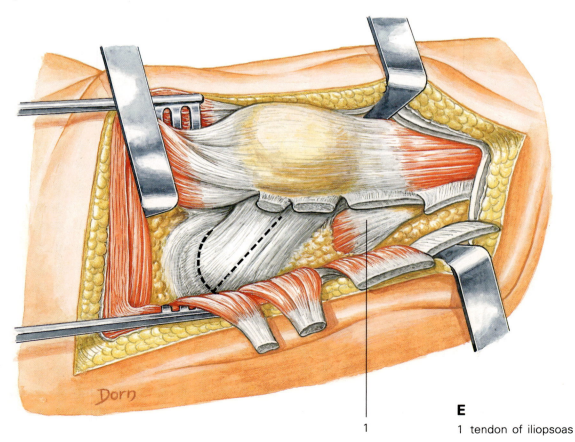

E

1   1 tendon of iliopsoas

F The femoral head is exposed.

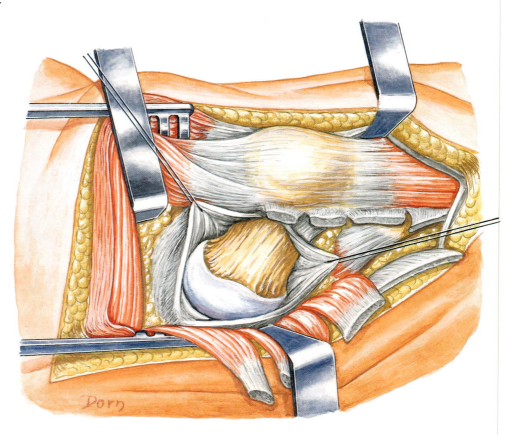

Medial (Ludloff) approach

Introduction

The medial approach was first developed to permit surgery on a congenitally dislocated hip with the hip flexed, abducted and externally rotated.

Indications

- Operative treatment of particular congenital hip dislocations.
- Approach to the inferior part of the hip joint to remove loose bodies.
- Tumours adjacent to the lesser trochanter.

Position

The patient lies supine on an ordinary table with the leg separately and fully draped. The hip is positioned in flexion, abduction and external rotation.

Incision

A The incision is longitudinal on the medial aspect of the thigh; it begins about 3 cm distal to the pubic tubercle, over the interval between gracilis and adductor longus, and is about 15–20 cm long.

Exposure

B The superficial fascia is incised in line with the skin incision. The plane between adductor longus and brevis anteriorly, and gracilis and adductor magnus posteriorly, is developed.

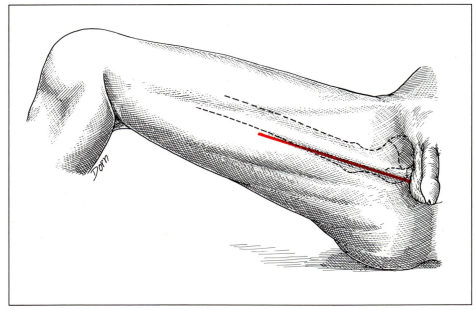

A

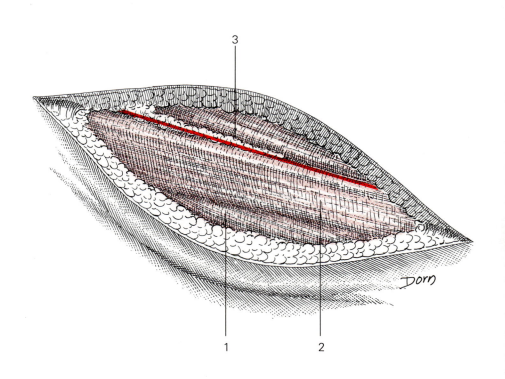

B

1 adductor magnus
2 gracilis
3 adductor longus

C In developing this plane the posterior branch of the obturator nerve and the neurovascular bundle to gracilis are exposed and protected.

D After retraction of adductor longus and brevis anteriorly, and adductor magnus and gracilis posteriorly, the lesser trochanter is exposed in the depths of the wound and the tendon of iliopsoas identified as it inserts into the lesser trochanter. Above it, the inferior part of the hip capsule is exposed and can be incised longitudinally, its inferior femoral attachments being freed by sharp dissection.

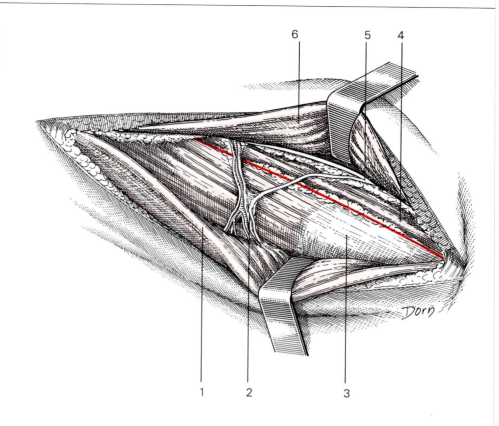

C

1 gracilis
2 nerve and vessels to gracilis
3 adductor magnus
4 adductor brevis
5 anterior division of obturator nerve
6 adductor longus

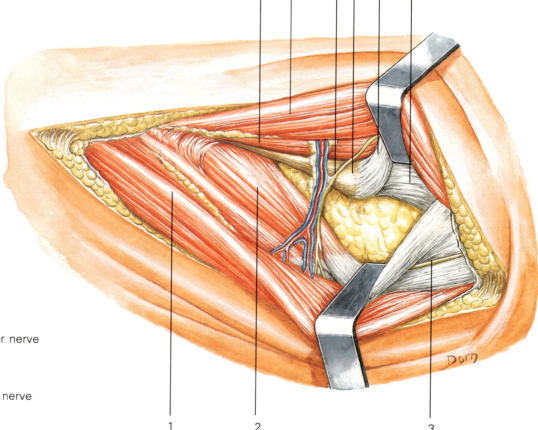

D

1 gracilis
2 adductor magnus
3 posterior division of obturator nerve
4 hip joint capsule
5 tendon of iliopsoas
6 lesser trochanter
7 anterior division of obturator nerve
8 adductor longus
9 adductor brevis

99

3

Femur

Femur

Introduction

The femur is one of the most frequently injured bones. It may also be the site of neoplasms or infection. The surgical approaches to the femur should, when possible, be safe, easy and bloodless, and should not lead to impairment of knee function. For these reasons, the approaches which split the muscles, for example the true lateral approach to the proximal third through the belly of vastus lateralis, should be avoided because haemostasis can be difficult to achieve. In addition, the approaches which split the quadriceps, for example, the anterolateral or anteromedial approaches, can lead to restricted knee flexion and are thus used for specific indications only. For the same reason, pins used for external fixation of fractures should not pass through the muscle bellies, in order to avoid adhesion formation.

Anatomical considerations

A Superficial muscles of the thigh

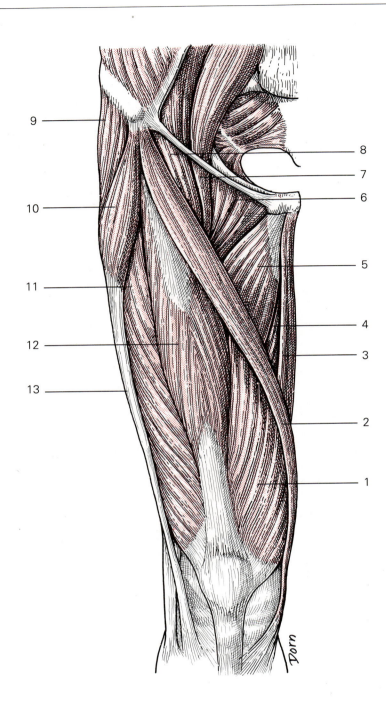

A

1 vastus medialis
2 sartorius
3 gracilis
4 adductor magnus
5 adductor longus
6 pectineus
7 psoas major

8 iliacus
9 gluteus medius
10 tensor fasciae latae
11 vastus lateralis
12 rectus femoris
13 iliotibial tract

**B Muscles of the thigh:
posterior aspect**

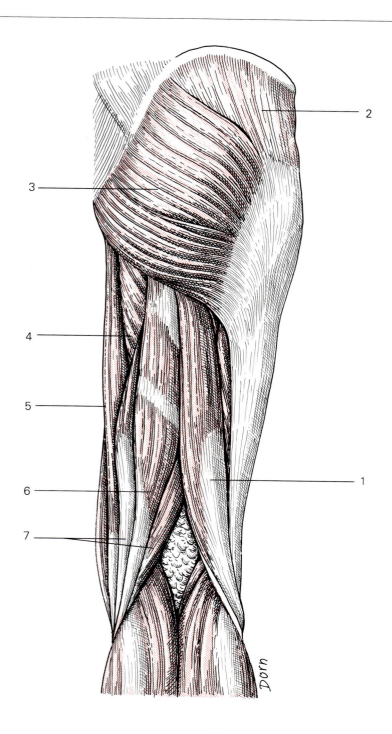

B

1 biceps femoris
2 gluteus medius
3 gluteus maximus
4 adductor magnus
5 gracilis
6 semitendinosus
7 semimembranosus

Femur

C Muscles of the thigh: lateral aspect

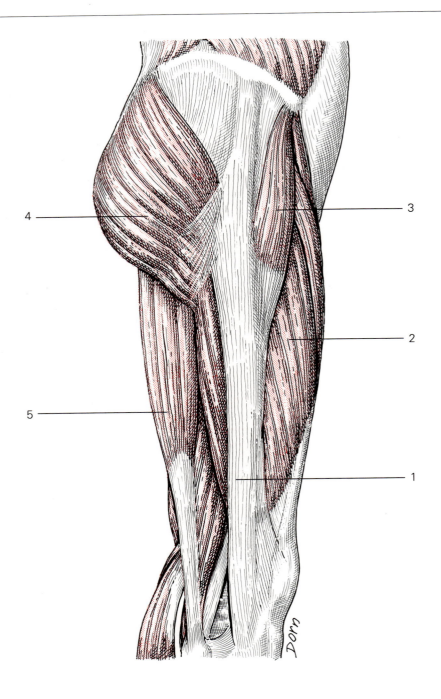

C
1 iliotibial tract
2 vastus lateralis
3 tensor fasciae latae
4 gluteus maximus
5 biceps femoris

D The thigh comprises three major muscle groups.

1 The adductors of the hip occupy the medial compartment of the thigh and are supplied by the obturator nerve. Adductor magnus is also supplied by the sciatic nerve.

2 The knee extensors comprise the anterior compartment and are supplied by the femoral nerve.

3 The knee flexors form the posterior compartment of the thigh and are supplied by the sciatic nerve.

The quadriceps are separated by an intermuscular septum from the hamstrings laterally and from the adductors medially. Compartment syndromes may occur in the thigh and require early surgical decompression.

The femoral artery changes position in relation to the femur: it is anterior to it in the upper third, medial in the middle third and posterior in the lower third. This spiral pathway influences the choice of surgical approach and also the placement of pins for traction and external fixators.

The perforating arteries arise from the profunda femoris and wind around the posterior femoral shaft before entering the anterior compartment by piercing the lateral intermuscular septum. These arteries carry a high risk of bleeding and must be carefully ligated.

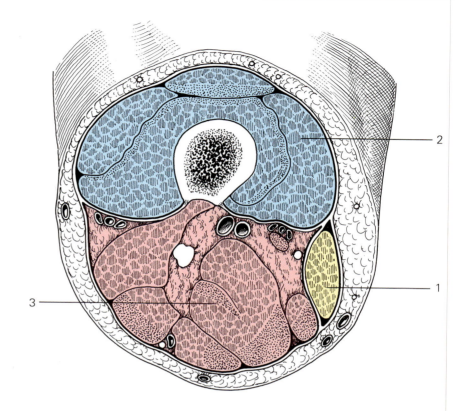

D
1 medial compartment (adductors)
2 anterior compartment (extensors)
3 posterior compartment (flexors)

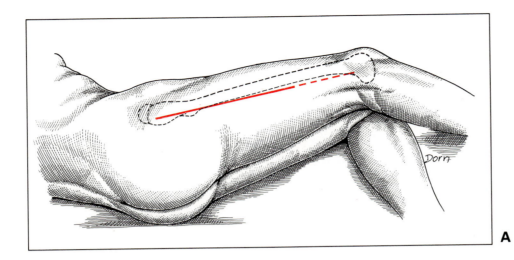

A

Proximal and middle third: posterolateral approach

Introduction

The plane between the lateral intermuscular septum and vastus lateralis is easy to define and, even if the muscle arises in part from the septum, the dissection is practically bloodless. However, the posterolateral approach extends to the linea aspera and, in order to expose the lateral aspect of the bone, the muscles need to be reflected anteriorly. The perforating arteries may need to be ligated. The key to the posterolateral approach to the proximal two-thirds is to detach the origin of vastus lateralis from the femur.

Indications

- Open reduction and internal fixation of intertrochanteric or subtrochanteric fractures.
- Intertrochanteric and subtrochanteric osteotomy.
- Open reduction or fixation of femoral shaft fractures.
- Biopsy and treatment of bone tumours.

Position of the patient

Patients with trochanteric or subtrochanteric fractures should be placed on an orthopaedic table in the supine position. For surgery of the femoral shaft, the patient should be placed on an orthopaedic table in the supine position or in the lateral position. Femoral shaft fractures can also be treated in a lateral position without an orthopaedic table. The posterolateral approach can be extended to the distal third of the femur.

Incision

A The limb being in a neutral position, the incision commences over the posterior border of the greater trochanter and is continued as far distally as necessary along a line drawn to the posterior margin of the lateral femoral condyle. A common mistake is to place the incision too anteriorly and thus for the approach to be impeded by the posterior border of the fascia lata.

B
1 vastus lateralis
2 fascia lata

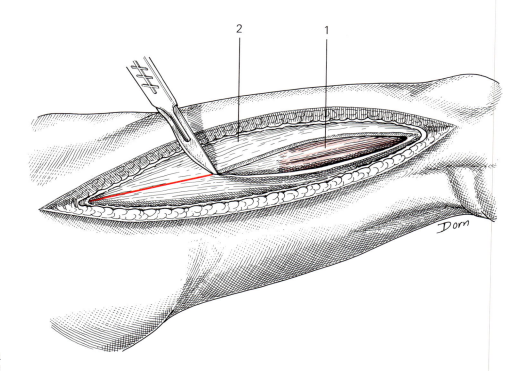

Exposure

B The fascia lata is incised in line with the skin incision and retracted, exposing the origin of vastus lateralis which is incised transversely leaving a tendinous portion attached to the bone. Haemostasis of the feeding artery is usually necessary over the anterior part of the muscle origin.

C The tendinous portion and the thin aponeurosis surrounding the muscles are incised along the femoral shaft close to the lateral intermuscular septum.

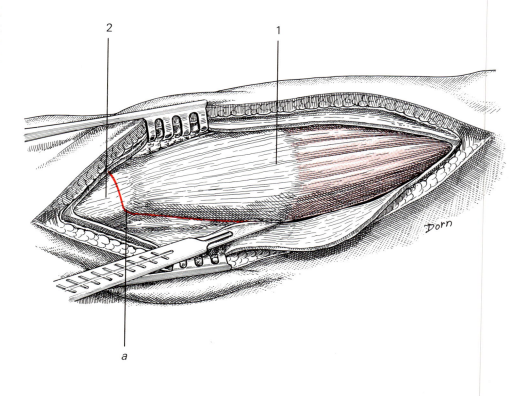

C

1 vastus lateralis
2 greater trochanter
a incision in tendon

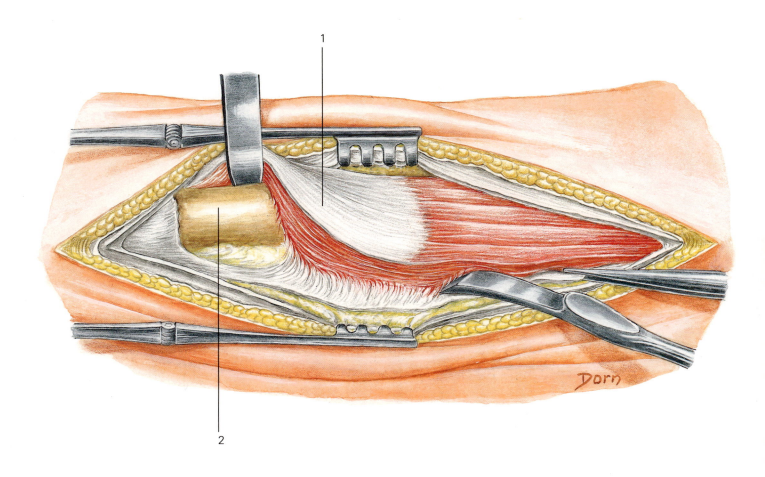

D   The muscle fibres are released from the lateral intermuscular septum from distal to proximal, and the muscle is progressively reflected anteriorly. A retractor is placed proximally and distally.

E   The perforating arteries are easily identified and ligated.

F   The exposure of the femur is carried out subperiosteally. The closure of the wound requires the proximal reattachment of vastus lateralis.

D
1   vastus lateralis, retracted
2   proximal femoral shaft (intertrochanteric region)

E

1 lateral intermuscular septum
2 perforating arteries

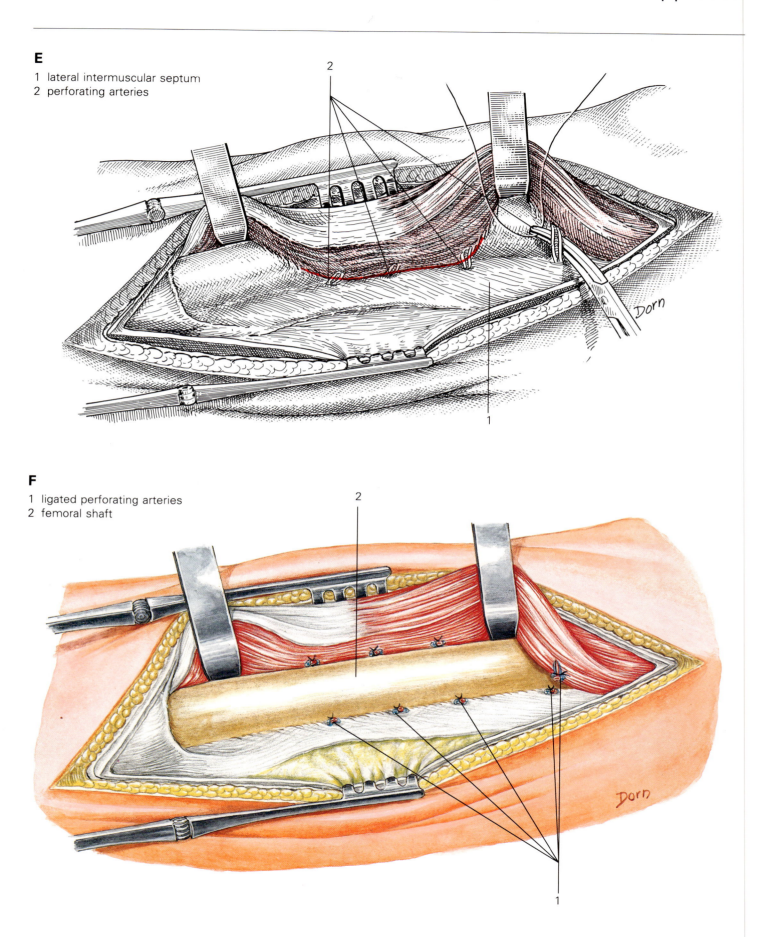

F

1 ligated perforating arteries
2 femoral shaft

Femur

G A cross-section through the mid-thigh shows the posterolateral approach to the femur.

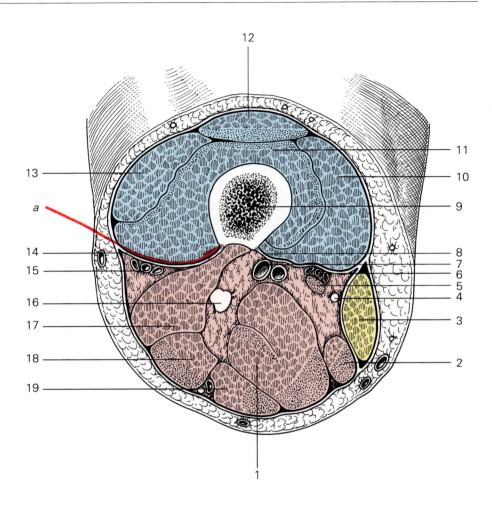

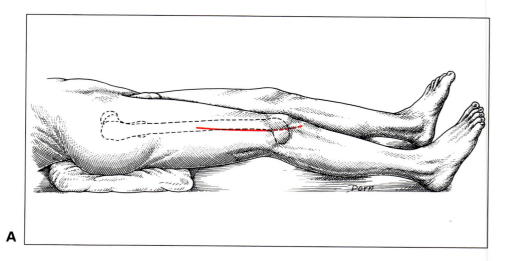

A

Distal third of the femur: lateral approach

Introduction

At the distal third of the thigh, the posterior border of vastus lateralis curves gently to join the extensor apparatus of the knee. It is easier to reflect the muscle in its distal third than in its proximal two-thirds. The lateral incision can be extended to expose the lateral aspect of the knee joint.

Indication

● Open reduction and internal fixation of distal metaphyseal fractures.

Position of the patient

The patient is in a lateral position or supine with a sandbag under the ipsilateral buttock.

Incision

A The incision commences at the level of the lateral aspect of the femoral condyle and extends proximally along the femoral shaft.

Femur

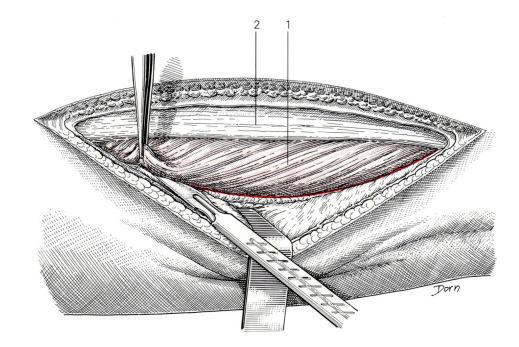

Exposure

B The fascia lata is incised in line with the skin incision and dissected from the underlying muscle. The posterior flap is retracted exposing the lateral border of vastus lateralis. The aponeurosis of the muscle is opened and the muscle fibres are released from the lateral septum in a distal to proximal direction.

C One or two perforating arteries may need to be ligated.

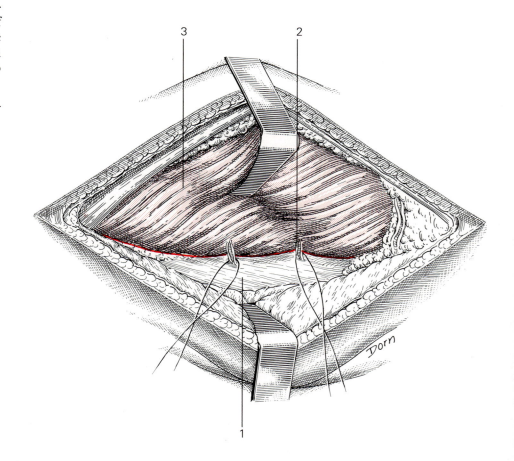

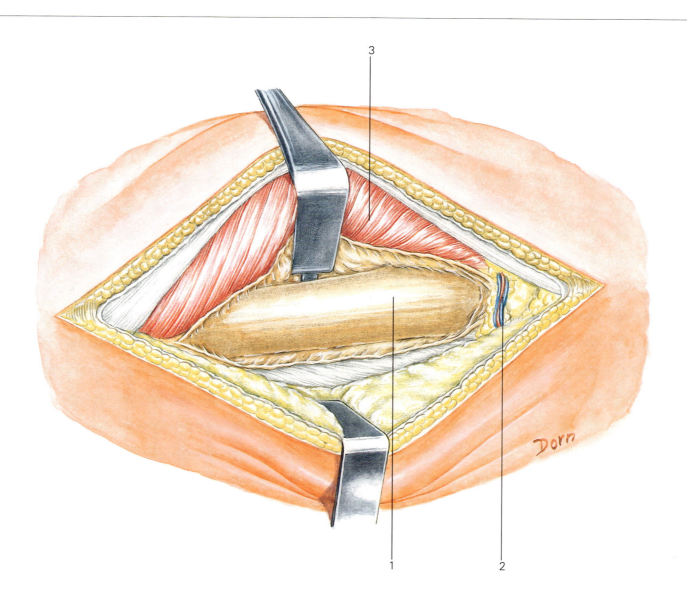

D The muscle is retracted anteriorly exposing the lateral aspect of the lower femur and the extra-articular portion of the lateral femoral condyle.

D

1 lateral femoral metaphysis
2 lateral superior genicular artery
3 vastus lateralis

Femur

E This approach can be extended as a lateral parapatellar approach to the knee.

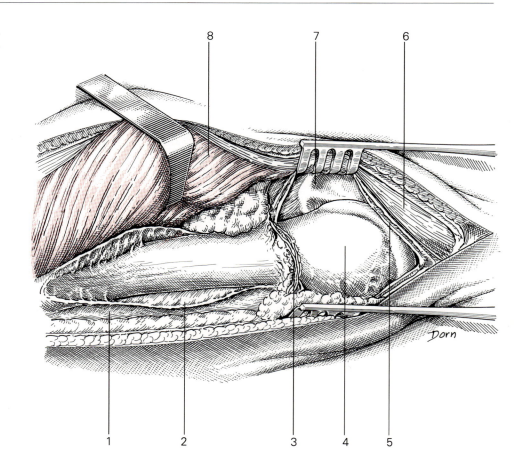

E

1 lateral intermuscular septum
2 periosteum
3 lateral superior genicular artery
4 lateral femoral condyle
5 lateral capsule of knee
6 lateral quadriceps expansion
7 patella
8 vastus lateralis

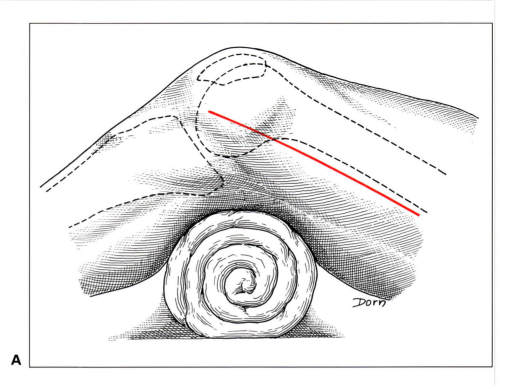

A

Distal quarter of the femur: medial approach

Introduction

The medial approach to the distal quarter of the femur, reflecting vastus medialis anteriorly, is not commonly used. However, it is simple and safe and is to be preferred to the anteromedial approach. It can be continued distally to expose the medial aspect of the knee joint.

Indications

- Resection of benign tumours of the femur.
- Supracondylar osteotomy.

Anatomy

In the distal third of the femur, the extensor compartment is separated from the flexor compartment by the medial intermuscular septum and bordered medially by the tendon of adductor magnus. The femoral vessels enter the popliteal space passing through the hiatus of the tendon of adductor magnus, although they are not usually seen in the medial approach to the lower femur. The articular and muscular branches of the descending genicular artery may need to be ligated; the saphenous nerve should be protected.

Position of the patient

The patient is supine, with the limb externally rotated.

Incision

A The incision is anterior to sartorius and begins distally midway between the posterior border of the medial femoral condyle and the patella. It extends proximally for about 10 cm.

Femur

B
1 deep fascia
2 vastus medialis

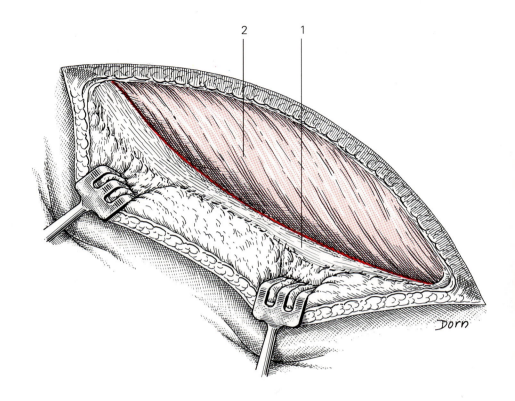

Exposure

B The fascia is opened in line with the skin incision. The aponeurotic sheet of vastus medialis is exposed and incised.

C The muscle fibres are released from the intermuscular septum in a distal to proximal direction. Perforating arteries and the muscular branch of the descending genicular artery should be ligated.

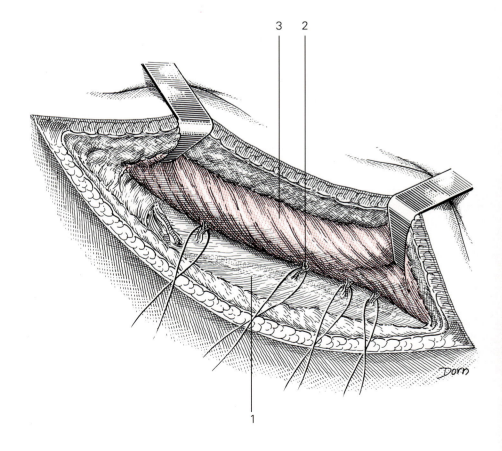

C
1 medial intermuscular septum
2 perforating artery
3 vastus medialis

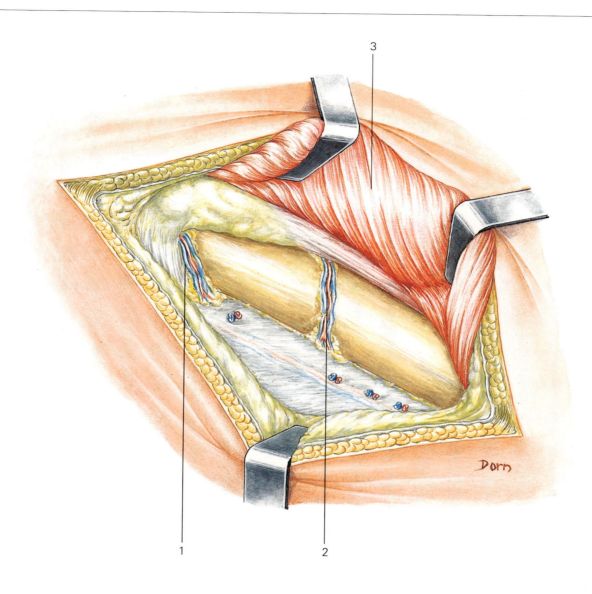

D The muscle is reflected anteriorly and the medial aspect of the femur is exposed subperiosteally. This approach can be extended to expose the medial aspect of the knee joint.

D

1 medial superior genicular artery
2 articular branch of descending genicular artery
3 vastus medialis

Femur

E A cross-section through the distal quarter of the thigh shows the medial approach.

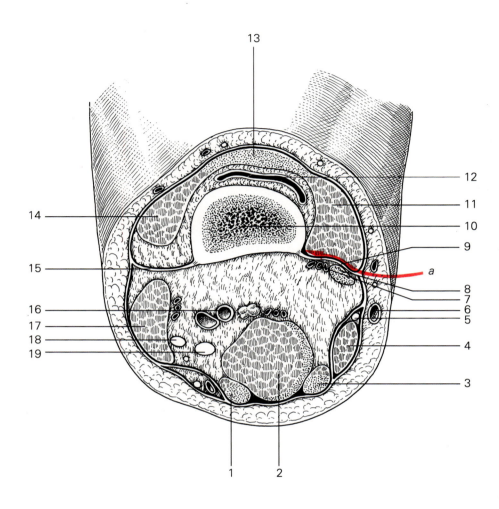

E

1 semitendinosus
2 semimembranosus
3 gracilis
4 sartorius
5 saphenous nerve
6 saphenous vein
7 descending genicular artery and veins
8 tendon of adductor magnus
9 medial intermuscular septum
10 femur
11 vastus medialis
12 suprapatellar pouch
13 quadriceps tendon
14 vastus lateralis
15 lateral intermuscular septum
16 popliteal artery and vein
17 biceps femoris
18 common peroneal nerve
19 tibial nerve
a medial approach

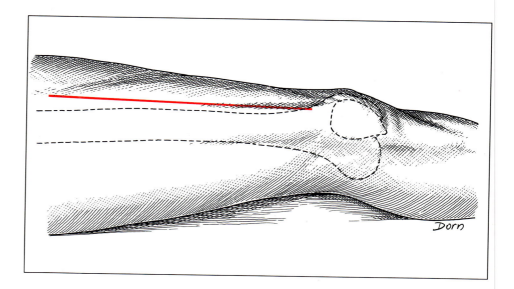

A

Distal two-thirds of the femur: anteromedial approach

Introduction

The anteromedial and the antero-lateral approaches to the distal two-thirds of the femur are similar. The former is rarely used for exposing only the distal femur and is not advocated for routine use, because it involves dissection between vastus medialis and rectus femoris and the splitting of vastus intermedius. This leads to adhesion formation and potentially to limitation of knee flexion. In practice, this approach should be considered as the proximal extension of the medial parapatellar approach to the knee.

Indications

- Excision of benign tumours.
- Insertion of a massive knee prosthesis as part of a proximal extension of a medial parapatellar approach to the knee.

Position of the patient

The patient is supine, with a sandbag under the ipsilateral buttock to maintain the limb in neutral rotation.

Incision

A The incision on the anteromedial aspect of the thigh runs along the lateral border of the contour of vastus medialis. If this muscle is wasted, the incision should be longitudinal commencing 1 cm above the superomedial angle of the patella.

Femur

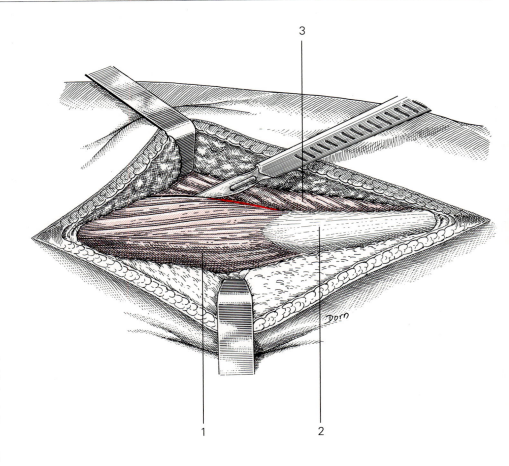

Exposure

B The deep fascia is incised in line with the skin incision and its two edges are reflected, exposing the interval between vastus medialis and rectus femoris. Retraction of the lateral skin flap exposes the quadriceps tendon.

C The plane is developed and the muscles retracted, exposing vastus intermedius. Distally, the incision is made in the quadriceps tendon close to its medial border, in order to preserve the muscle fibres of vastus medialis that insert into the tendon, and this facilitates the repair.

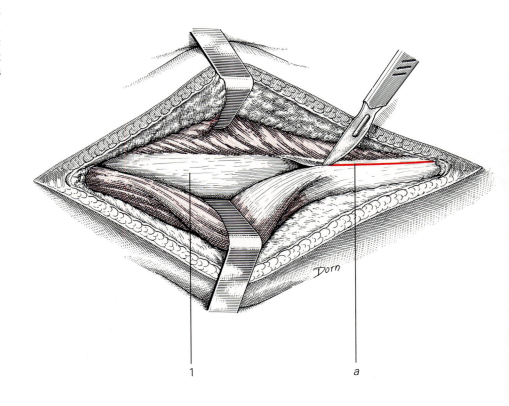

C

1 vastus intermedius
a incision through medial part of quadriceps tendon

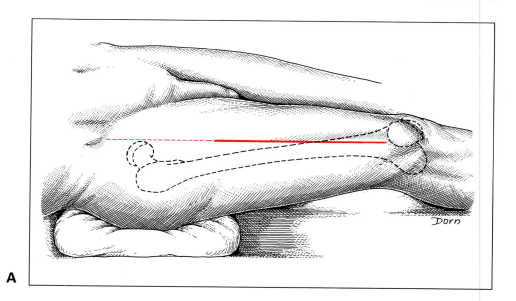

A

Femoral shaft: anterolateral approach

Introduction

The anterolateral approach is rarely used. It involves splitting vastus intermedius with the probable formation of adhesions between the muscles and the underlying femur.

Indications

This approach can be extended proximally and distally to expose the hip and knee joints. It is thus a good approach for a total replacement of the femur. It should not be used routinely for the internal fixation of fractures.

Anatomy

Two points should be emphasized:

- Vastus intermedius is entirely covered by the three other muscles of the extensor compartment: vastus lateralis, vastus medialis and rectus femoris. Between the superficial muscles and vastus intermedius, there is loose areolar gliding tissue.

- Vastus lateralis and rectus femoris are strongly attached to each other, but the plane of dissection is easily found in the middle third of the thigh. In the proximal third, this plane is crossed by the descending branch of the lateral femoral circumflex artery which runs deep to rectus femoris and enters vastus lateralis. One branch continues along the medial border of vastus lateralis to join the arterial anastomosis around the knee. These vessels may be ligated. The motor nerve of vastus lateralis accompanies the principal vessel and enters the muscle in its upper third. It should be preserved.

Indications

- Repair of the extensor apparatus of the knee.
- Exposure of the anterior aspect of the femur.
- Total replacement of the femur.

Position of the patient

The patient is supine, with a sandbag under the ipsilateral buttock to maintain the limb in neutral rotation.

Incision

A The incision is along a line drawn from the anterior superior iliac spine to the lateral border of the patella. The length and position of the skin incision are determined by the nature of the procedure.

Femur

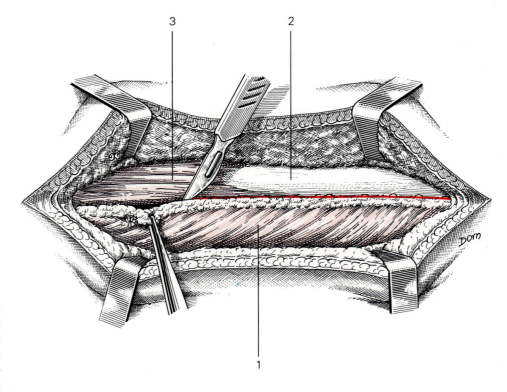

Exposure

B   The deep fascia is incised in line with the skin incision. The two fascial flaps are dissected from the underlying muscles. The junction of rectus femoris and vastus lateralis is exposed and can be identified by a line of fatty tissue in the middle third of the wound. The dissection is easy at this level and is extended distally by splitting the aponeurotic sheet that connects the two muscles.

C   Proximally, care should be taken to preserve the neurovascular bundle which crosses the operative field. Vastus lateralis and rectus femoris are retracted to expose vastus intermedius, which clothes the anterior two-thirds of the femoral shaft.

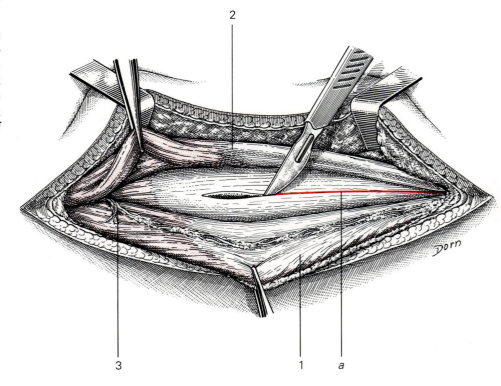

124

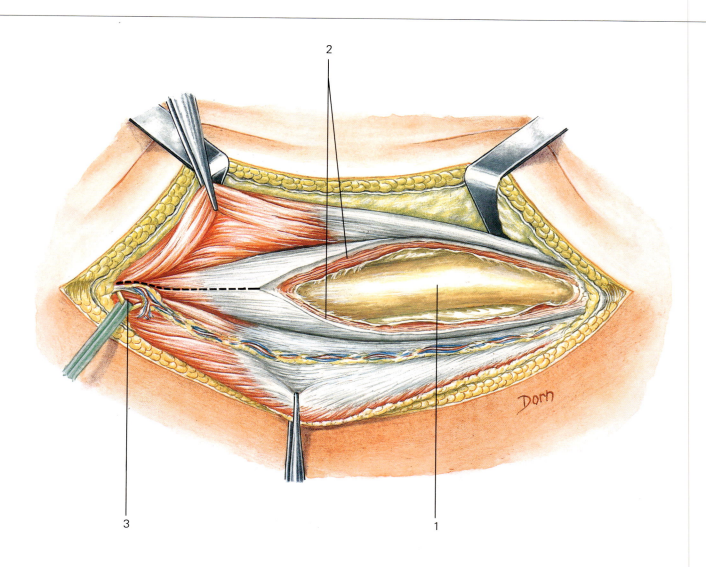

D The anterior surface of the femur is exposed by incising vastus intermedius and the periosteum.

D

1 femoral shaft
2 vastus intermedius and periosteum, split
3 proximal neurovascular pedicle to vastus lateralis

Femur

E A cross-section through the mid-thigh shows the anterolateral approach to the femur.

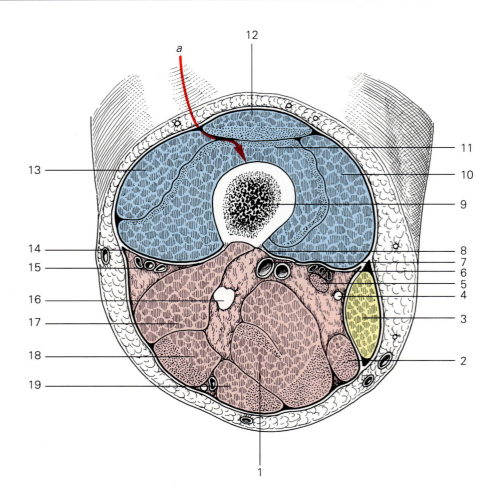

E

1 semimembranosus
2 gracilis
3 sartorius
4 saphenous nerve
5 tendon of adductor magnus
6 descending genicular artery and veins
7 femoral artery and vein
8 medial intermuscular septum
9 femur
10 vastus medialis
11 vastus intermedius
12 rectus femoris
13 vastus lateralis
14 lateral intermuscular septum
15 descending branch of lateral cir-cumflex femoral artery and veins
16 sciatic nerve
17 short head } biceps femoris
18 long head
19 semitendinosus
a anterolateral approach to femur

Femoral shaft: posterior approach

Introduction

The posterior approach to the femur is not used routinely. It is useful when the lateral approach can no longer be employed due to local skin problems. One of the indications is the treatment of non-union by bone grafting when other approaches are not available.

Anatomy

The key to the posterior approach is the relationship between the femur, biceps femoris and the sciatic nerve. Biceps femoris, the most superficial structure, crosses the line of the femoral shaft and the course of the sciatic nerve in the middle third of the thigh. In the upper part of the thigh, the sciatic nerve lies deep to biceps femoris and the correct intermuscular plane at this level is between biceps femoris and vastus lateralis. In the distal half, it is preferable to pass between biceps femoris and semimembranosus, the sciatic nerve being retracted laterally.

Position of the patient

The patient is prone.

Incision

A The skin incision is longitudinal and sited in the midline over the posterior aspect of the thigh. It commences just below the gluteal fold and ends at the apex of the popliteal fossa.

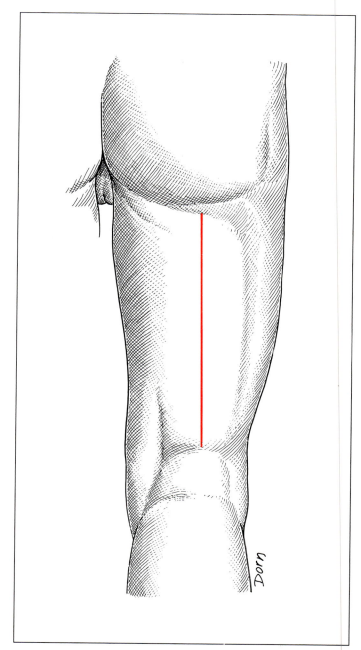

A

Femur

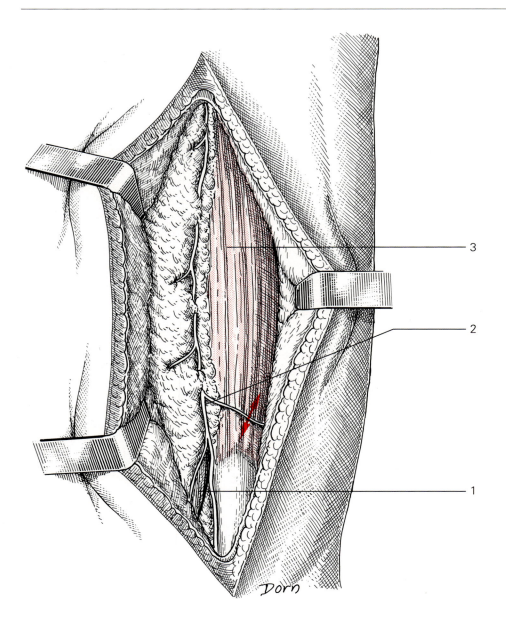

Dorn

B The deep fascia is incised in line with the skin incision. Care should be taken to avoid injury to the posterior femoral cutaneous nerve, which is deep to the fascia and lies in the groove between biceps femoris and semitendinosus.

B
1 semitendinosus
2 posterior femoral cutaneous nerve
3 biceps femoris

C The lateral skin flap is retracted laterally to identify the interval between biceps femoris and vastus lateralis.

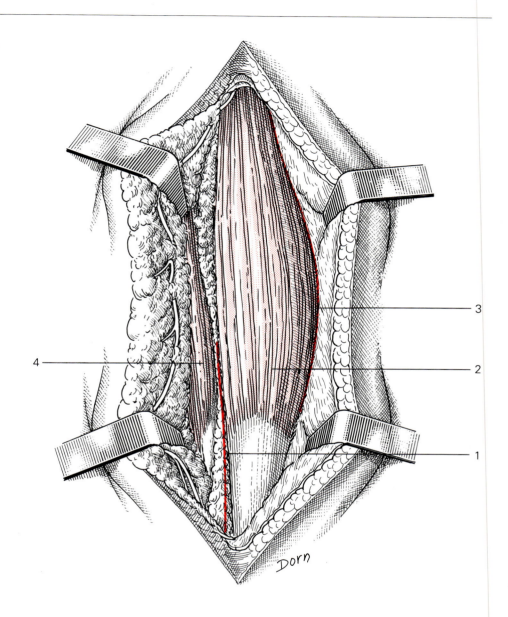

c

1 plane between biceps femoris and
  semitendinosus
2 biceps femoris
3 plane between biceps femoris and
  vastus lateralis
4 semitendinosus

Femur

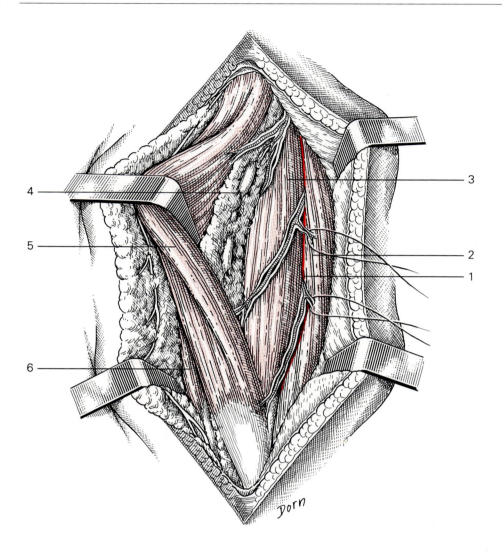

Dorn

D

1 plane of dissection
2 vastus lateralis
3 short head of biceps femoris
4 fatty tissue containing sciatic nerve
5 long head of biceps femoris,
  retracted
6 semitendinosus

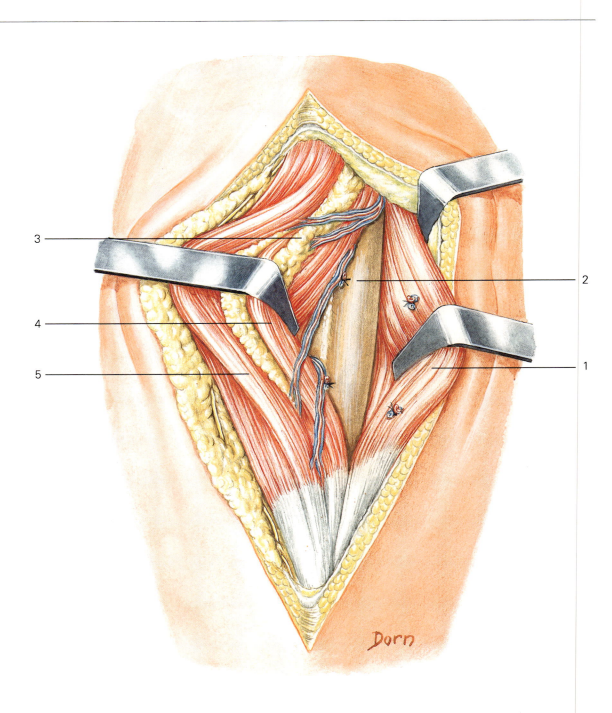

E The short head of biceps femoris is reflected from the femoral shaft and retracted firmly to the medial side to expose the linea aspera and the periosteum of the femur which can be incised. Care should be taken when retracting this muscle to protect the sciatic nerve, which lies in fatty tissue between the long and short heads of biceps femoris.

E

1 vastus lateralis
2 femoral shaft
3 fatty tissue containing sciatic nerve
4 short head ⎫ biceps femoris
5 long head ⎭

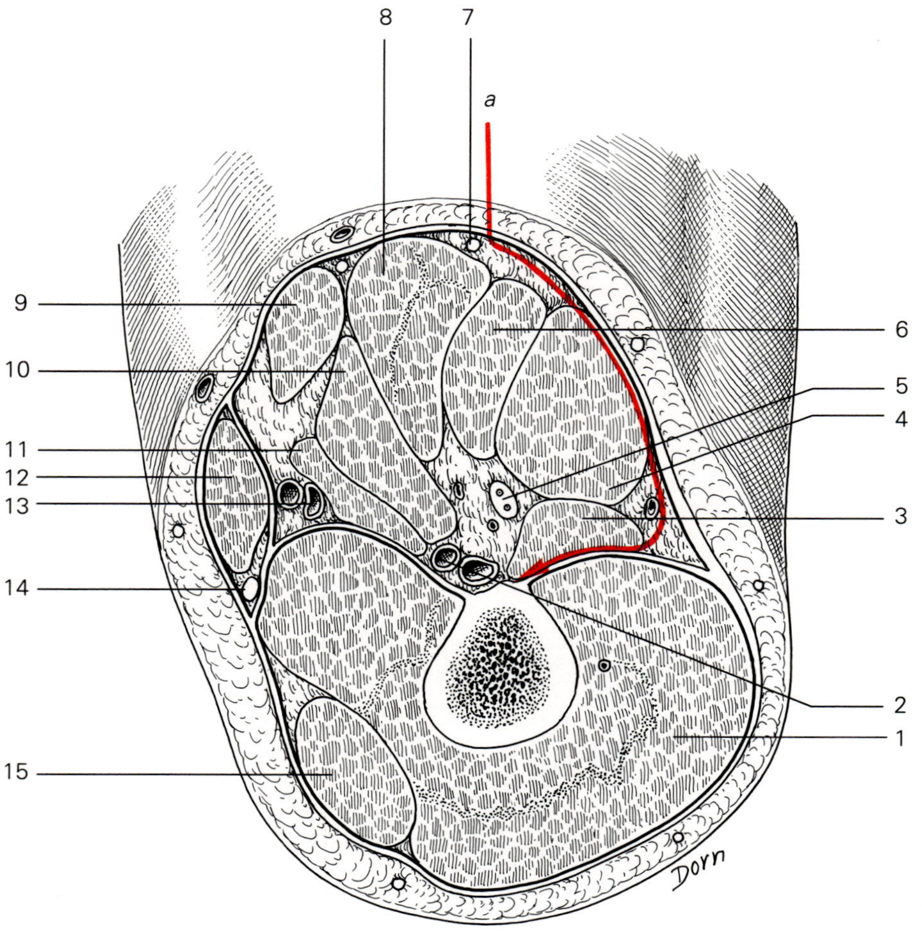

F A cross-section through the proximal third of the femur shows the posterior approach to the femur between biceps femoris and vastus lateralis. (The patient is prone.)

F

1 quadriceps (vastus lateralis)
2 profunda femoris artery and veins
3 short head } biceps femoris
4 long head } biceps femoris
5 sciatic nerve
6 semitendinosus
7 posterior femoral cutaneous nerve
8 semimembranosus
9 gracilis
10 adductor magnus
11 adductor longus
12 sartorius
13 femoral artery and vein
14 saphenous nerve
15 rectus femoris
a posterior approach to proximal third of femur

G If the distal femoral shaft is to be exposed, the dissection is medial to the long head of biceps femoris, between this muscle and semitendinosus and semimembranosus, exposing the sciatic nerve (see **C**).

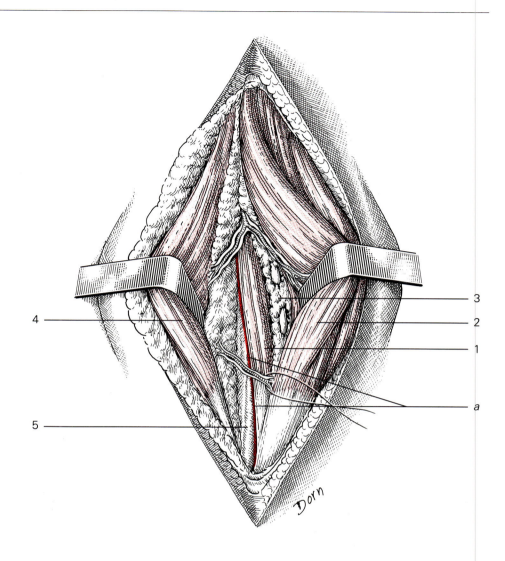

G

1 short head } biceps femoris
2 long head
3 sciatic nerve in fatty tissue
4 semitendinosus and
  semimembranosus
5 adductor magnus
a incision along linea aspera

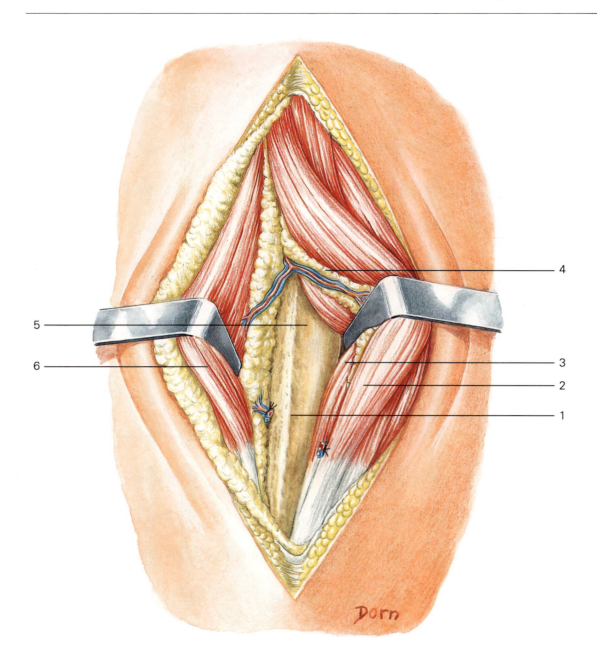

H

1 linea aspera
2 long head ⎫ biceps femoris,
3 short head ⎭ retracted laterally
4 sciatic nerve in fatty tissue
5 femoral shaft
6 semimembranosus and
   semitendinosus, retracted medially

H The long head of biceps femoris and the sciatic nerve are retracted laterally to gain free access to the linea aspera. The periosteum is incised and the femur exposed subperiosteally, stripping off adductor magnus medially, and the short head of biceps laterally. In some instances it may be necessary to divide the long head of biceps in order to obtain a wide exposure of the whole midshaft of the femur.

I A cross-section through the distal half of the femur shows the posterior approach to the femur between biceps femoris and semimembranosus. (The patient is prone.)

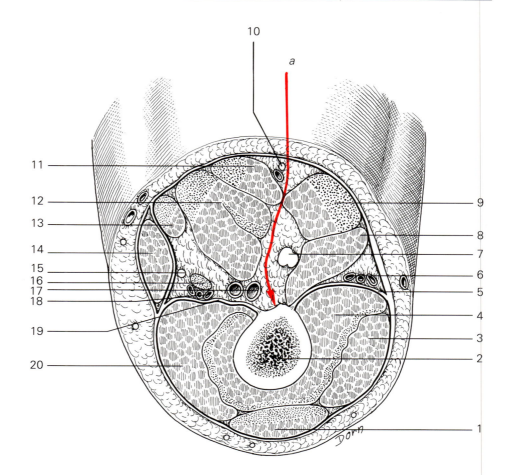

I

1 rectus femoris
2 femur
3 vastus lateralis
4 vastus intermedius
5 lateral intermuscular septum
6 descending branch of lateral
   circumflex femoral artery and veins
7 sciatic nerve
8 short head ⎫ biceps femoris
9 long head ⎭
10 posterior femoral cutaneous nerve
11 semitendinosus
12 semimembranosus
13 gracilis
14 sartorius
15 saphenous nerve
16 tendon of adductor magnus
17 femoral artery and vein
18 descending genicular artery
19 medial intermuscular septum
20 vastus medialis
a posterior approach to distal half of
   femur

4

Knee

Knee

Introduction

Whilst the overall anatomy of the knee, its muscles, tendons and ligaments, is relatively complex to facilitate the rolling, gliding motion of the knee, the arrangement of the soft tissues anteriorly allows ready access to the anterior compartments with minimal damage.

Approaches which involve division of the patella, quadriceps tendon or ligamentum patellae are best avoided. Approaches requiring extensive skin mobilization should be used with great caution in the arthritic and the elderly patient. The possibility of further surgery being required in the future should be borne in mind when planning skin incisions to avoid acute angled and distally based flaps. Transverse incisions across the knee should be avoided.

Anatomy

A The components of the quadriceps tendon form a fascial envelope for the patella; its retinacula and condensations form the proximal and distal patellofemoral ligaments. The iliotibial and semimembranosus fibres coalesce superficially over the insertion of the ligamentum patellae. These bands of fasciae would only be opened on extensive operative dissection.

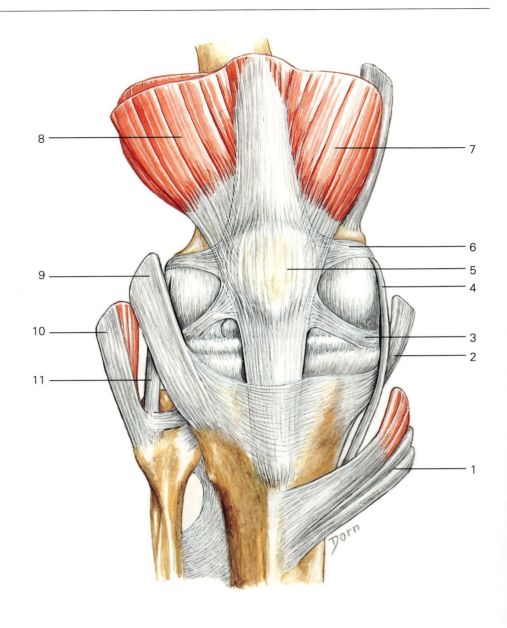

A

1 pes anserinus muscles
2 semimembranosus
3 patellomeniscal ligament
4 medial collateral ligament
5 patella
6 patellofemoral ligament
7 vastus medialis
8 vastus lateralis
9 iliotibial band
10 biceps femoris
11 lateral collateral ligament

B In surgical practice, the fascial layers of the anterior aspect of the knee joint are usually divided and repaired as one. The underlying infrapatellar fat pad contains the terminal anastomotic branches of the inferior genicular arteries which are best left undisturbed. The transverse ligament joins the anterior aspects of the menisci, overlying the insertion of the anterior cruciate ligament. The various approaches to the knee are demonstrated (*a-f*).

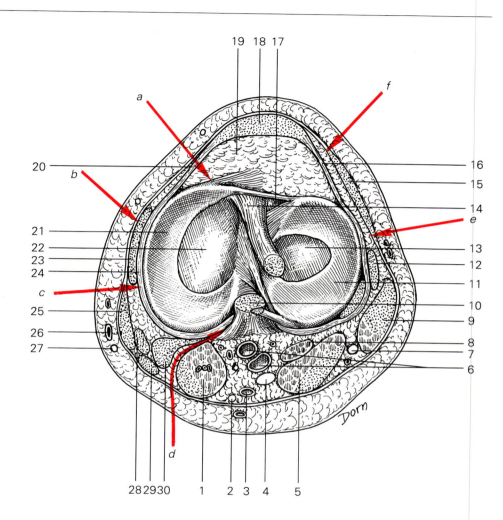

B

1 medial head of gastrocnemius
2 posterior cutaneous nerve of thigh
3 short saphenous vein
4 tibial nerve
5 lateral head of gastrocnemius
6 popliteal artery and vein
7 common peroneal nerve
8 plantaris
9 biceps femoris
10 posterior cruciate ligament
11 lateral meniscus
12 lateral collateral ligament
13 lateral tibial plateau
14 anterior cruciate ligament
15 lateral patellar retinaculum
16 lateral knee capsule
17 transverse ligament
18 ligamentum patellae

19 infrapatellar fat pad
20 medial patellar retinaculum
21 medial meniscus
22 medial tibial plateau
23 medial collateral ligament
24 medial knee capsule
25 sartorius
26 saphenous vein
27 saphenous nerve
28 semitendinosus
29 gracilis
30 semimembranosus
a anteromedial approach
b medial approach
c posteromedial approach
d posterior approach
e lateral approach
f anterolateral approach

Knee

C Although the cruciate ligament is covered by a vascular invagination of synovium, the anteromedial and posterolateral bundles of the ligament can usually be defined, the former being tight in flexion and the latter tight in extension. The posterior cruciate origin from the medial femoral condyle is covered by synovium.

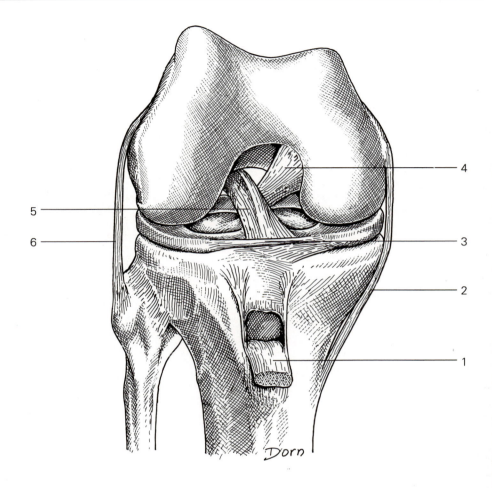

c

1 ligamentum patellae
2 medial collateral ligament
3 transverse ligament
4 posterior cruciate ligament
5 anterior cruciate ligament
6 lateral collateral ligament

D The fascial layers that close the medial aspect of the knee can be separated into three components. The superficial layer of patellar retinaculum invests sartorius to become continuous with the fascia over the medial head of gastrocnemius. The remaining pes anserinus muscles, gracilis and semitendinosus, lie deep to this. The anserinus group as a whole strengthens and overlies the medial collateral ligament.

The infrapatellar branches of the saphenous nerve are variable in number and position, but always pass forward subcutaneously across the anteromedial capsule to supply the skin over the lower pole of the patella, and are easily damaged by anteromedial incisions. The superior and inferior genicular arteries lie against the femoral and tibial condyles respectively.

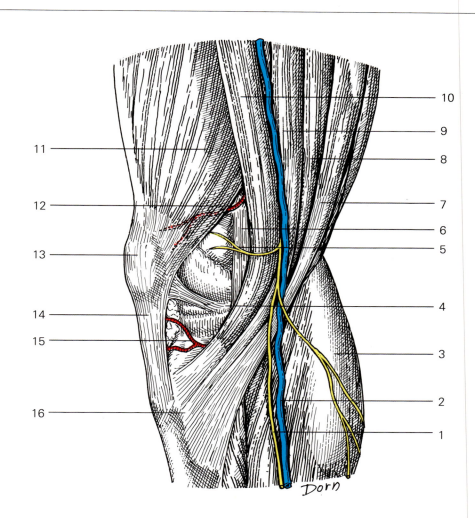

D
1 saphenous nerve
2 saphenous vein
3 medial head of gastrocnemius
4 medial meniscus
5 infrapatellar nerve
6 medial collateral ligament
7 semitendinosus
8 semimembranosus
9 gracilis
10 sartorius
11 vastus medialis
12 superior genicular artery
13 patella
14 ligamentum patellae
15 inferior genicular artery
16 pes anserinus insertion

Knee

E The deep layer of the medial structures comprises the medial collateral ligament which can be said to consist of two bundles. The more superficial anterior fibres pass obliquely from the femoral condyle to the tibia posterior to the pes anserinus insertion; the posterior oblique fibres insert into the tibia just below the articular surface, being firmly adherent to the medial meniscus. The third layer is the knee capsule itself which is continuous posteriorly with the fascia overlying the insertion of semimembranosus. An extension of the fibres of semimembranosus also passes deep to the collateral ligament to be inserted into the proximal tibia more anteriorly. The anterior fibres of the superficial medial collateral ligament resist forces in a valgus direction, being taut in extension. The posterior fibres and the posterior oblique fibres are said to be more important in resisting external rotation of the tibia on the femur, being reinforced in this role by the insertion of semimembranosus and the anterior cruciate ligament.

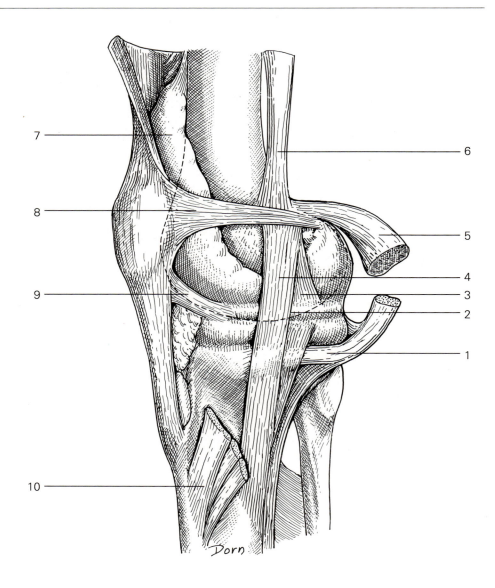

E

1 semimembranosus insertion
2 medial meniscus
3 posterior oblique fibres
4 medial collateral ligament
5 medial head of gastrocnemius
6 adductor magnus tendon
7 suprapatellar pouch
8 patellofemoral ligament
9 patellomeniscal ligament
10 pes anserinus insertion

F The fascia of the lateral aspect of the knee is less well differentiated into layers. A superficial layer is composed of the fascia of the iliotibial band joining the fascia over biceps femoris. The second layer commences anteriorly as the patellar retinaculum extending posteriorly, having received fibres from both the patellofemoral and patellomeniscal ligaments before joining the third layer, namely, the lateral joint capsule which anteriorly divides into two layers just posterior to the iliotibial band to envelop the lateral collateral ligament. The deeper layer is continuous with the lateral meniscus, forming the coronary ligaments for that structure. The lateral meniscus is, however, tethered less firmly than the medial meniscus. The hiatus for the popliteus tendon as it passes to the lateral tubercle of the femoral condyle further weakens the attachment of the meniscus. The superior genicular artery passes high over the femoral condyle proximal to the origin of the lateral collateral ligament. The inferior genicular artery passes deep to the ligament, close to the articular surface. The common peroneal nerve emerges from posterior to the biceps femoris tendon to wind round the fibular neck before dividing into its motor and sensory branches within the peroneal muscles.

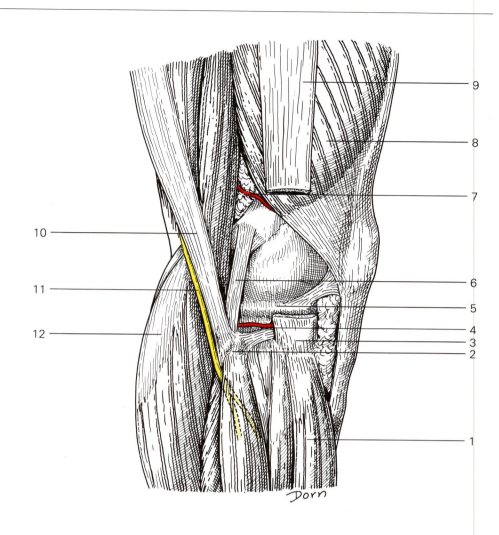

Dorn

F

1 tibialis anterior
2 head of fibula
3 Gerdy's tubercle
4 inferior genicular artery
5 lateral meniscus
6 lateral collateral ligament
7 superior genicular artery
8 vastus lateralis
9 iliotibial band (a section has been removed to show the lateral knee joint)
10 biceps femoris
11 common peroneal nerve
12 lateral head of gastrocnemius

Knee

G The lateral collateral ligament is the main restraint to varus rotation of the tibia on the femur in both extension and flexion. The role played by the iliotibial band, popliteus and biceps tendon decreases with increased flexion. The anterior tibial vessels reach the anterior compartment of the leg by passing between the neck of the fibula and the tibia, crossing the upper border of the interosseous membrane.

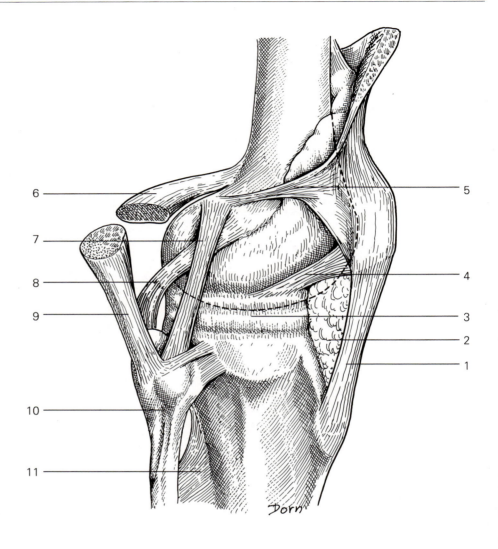

G

1 ligamentum patellae
2 infrapatellar fat pad
3 lateral meniscus
4 patellomeniscal ligament
5 patellofemoral ligament
6 lateral head of gastrocnemius
7 lateral collateral ligament
8 popliteus tendon
9 biceps femoris
10 neck of fibula
11 interosseous membrane

H The trapezoid shape of the popliteal fossa is formed proximally by the diverging hamstrings and distally by the converging heads of gastrocnemius. At a superficial level, the common peroneal nerve emerges from the medial border of biceps femoris gradually to move laterally around the neck of the fibula, giving several small cutaneous branches. The nerve is usually palpable during its excursion across the fossa.

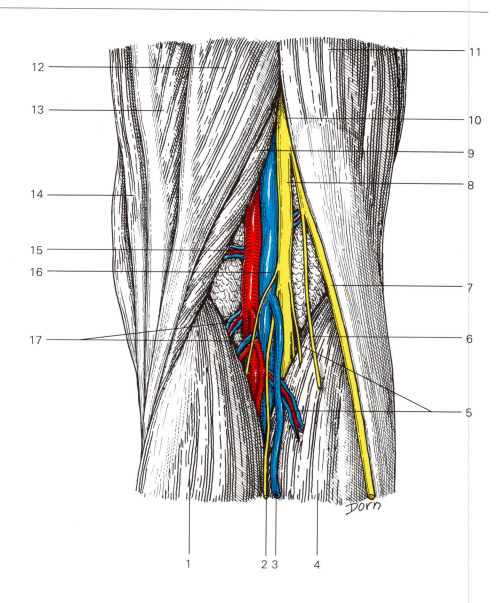

H

1 medial head of gastrocnemius
2 sural nerve
3 short saphenous vein
4 lateral head of gastrocnemius
5 neurovascular pedicle to lateral head of gastrocnemius
6 posterior cutaneous nerve of calf
7 common peroneal nerve
8 tibial nerve
9 semimembranosus

10 sciatic nerve
11 biceps femoris
12 semitendinosus
13 gracilis
14 sartorius
15 popliteal artery
16 popliteal vein
17 neurovascular pedicle to medial head of gastrocnemius

Knee

I The posterior capsule of the knee is weak in its medial portion at the site of entry of the median genicular vessels and at the arcuate arch of the popliteus tendon. Condensations of fascia from the semimembranosus insertion form the oblique popliteal ligament as it crosses the femoral condyle. This ligament crosses the posterior capsule obliquely and inserts close to the origin of plantaris and the lateral head of gastrocnemius. Bursae commonly lie under the medial head of gastrocnemius and under the semimembranosus insertion. The posterior ligamentous structures, popliteus, and to some extent the lateral collateral ligament, resist posterior movement of the tibia on the femur in early flexion. The posterior cruciate ligament is itself the main restraint as flexion increases.

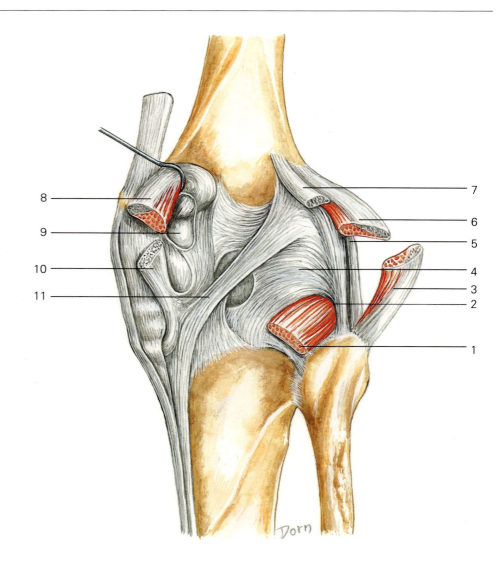

I

1 popliteus
2 popliteus hiatus
3 biceps femoris
4 arcuate ligament
5 lateral collateral ligament
6 lateral head of gastrocnemius
7 plantaris
8 medial head of gastrocnemius
9 bursa
10 semimembranosus
11 oblique ligament

Medial parapatellar approach

Introduction

The medial parapatellar approach is the most commonly used of the anterior approaches. If extended proximally and distally, wide exposure of both the medial and lateral joint compartments and the anterior cruciate ligament is possible. Lateral dislocation and eversion of the patella allows full access to the articular surface of the patella itself. This approach does not give a good exposure of the posterior compartments. However, it is suitable for the insertion of prosthetic joints and will allow the resection of the posterior cruciate ligament when indicated, depending on the prosthesis used.

A limited anterior approach is suitable for exploration of the anterior joint for removal of loose bodies, fat pad surgery and drilling of osteochondral fragments, arising most commonly from the lateral side of the medial femoral condyle. A more extensive exposure would be required either for the repair of the anterior cruciate ligament or when performing an anterior synovectomy.

A poor repair of the medial structures following any of these procedures will result in postoperative stretching of the medial quadriceps expansion, and subsequent lateral patellar subluxation or even dislocation. The approach may not infrequently result in damage to the infrapatellar branches of the saphenous nerve with a resultant neuroma formation. Reflection of large skin flaps, when performing the medial parapatellar approach, should be avoided in the elderly because the blood supply to the central portion of the incision is often poor. The rather fragile subcutaneous fat should be approximated with care, with preservation of the

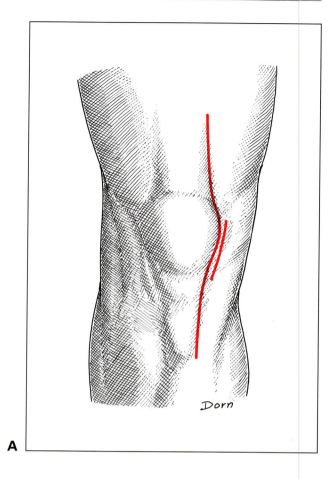

A

Dorn

blood supply to avoid fat necrosis. Similarly, continuous cutaneous suturing should be avoided.

Position of the patient

The patient is placed supine, with a small sandbag under the knee as necessary.

Incision

A The length of the incision is varied according to the exposure required. To provide a full exposure of the knee, it should commence 6–8 cm proximal to the patella over the medial aspect of the quadriceps and curve gently around the patellar margin to end medial to the lower border of the tibial tuberosity. The subcutaneous fat is divided similarly but with great care in the region of the saphenous nerve. Whenever possible, the infrapatellar branches are preserved. A more limited approach is adequate for performing a medial meniscectomy and is centred over the joint line itself.

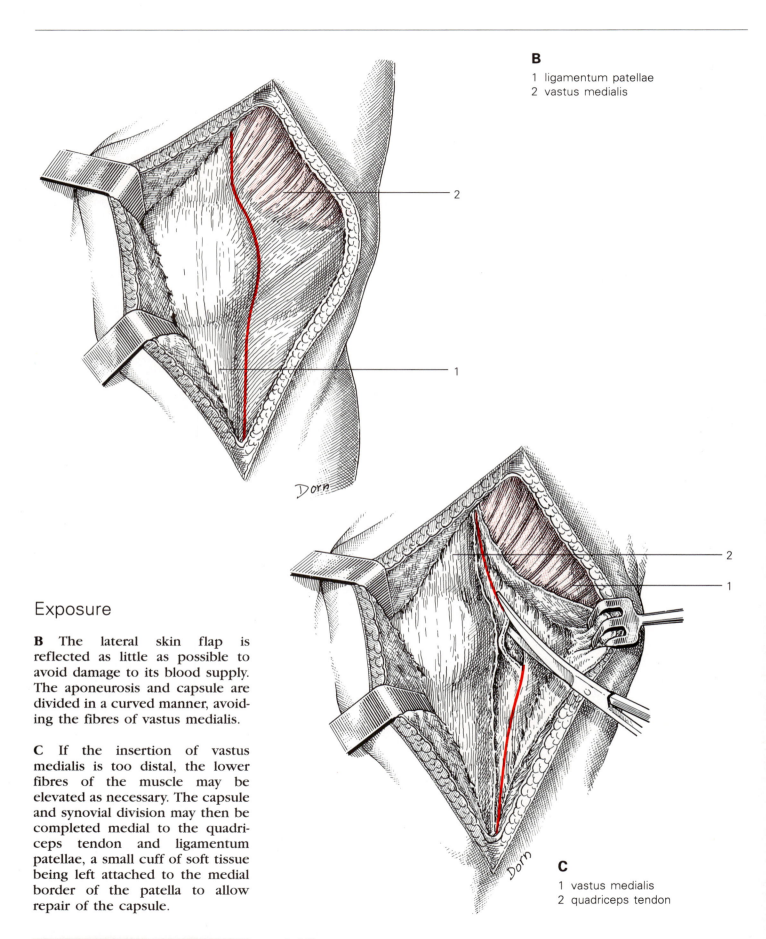

Exposure

B The lateral skin flap is reflected as little as possible to avoid damage to its blood supply. The aponeurosis and capsule are divided in a curved manner, avoiding the fibres of vastus medialis.

C If the insertion of vastus medialis is too distal, the lower fibres of the muscle may be elevated as necessary. The capsule and synovial division may then be completed medial to the quadriceps tendon and ligamentum patellae, a small cuff of soft tissue being left attached to the medial border of the patella to allow repair of the capsule.

C
1 vastus medialis
2 quadriceps tendon

D Lateral retraction with or without eversion or dislocation of the patella exposes the anterior joint. The exposure may be increased by subperiosteal elevation of the medial aspect of the ligamentum patellae, in continuity with the distal periosteal fibres, keeping the ligamentum patellae, the periosteum and overlying fascia as a complete continuous layer. The wound may be extended proximally along the lateral border of vastus medialis within the quadriceps tendon itself.

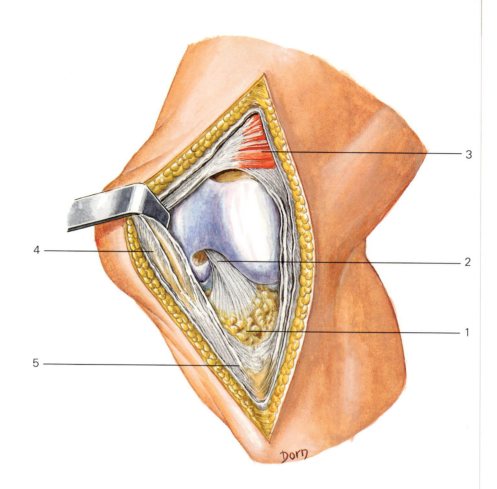

D

1 infrapatellar fat pad
2 anterior cruciate ligament
3 vastus medialis
4 retracted patella
5 ligamentum patellae, elevated from tuberosity

Knee

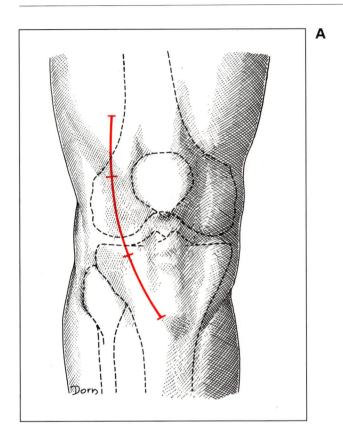

A

Lateral parapatellar approach

Indications

The lateral parapatellar approach gives a much more limited exposure of the anterior aspect of the knee. Its uses are therefore restricted to anterolateral joint exploration, particularly for meniscal problems, and removal of loose bodies or small intra-articular fractures.

Position of the patient

The patient is supine with the knee slightly flexed.

Incision

A The incision commences 2–3 cm proximal to the patella over vastus lateralis and is curved distally to end at the lower border of the tibial tuberosity. The middle third alone may be used for a lateral meniscectomy.

Exposure

B The incision is deepened through the subcutaneous fascia to expose vastus lateralis and the underlying lateral capsule and synovium. The capsule and synovium are divided. More extensive exploration of the lateral femoral condyle can be achieved by dividing longitudinally the lower fibres of vastus lateralis. The circumflex branches of the inferior genicular artery are commonly divided in the lower aspect of the wound and require cauterization.

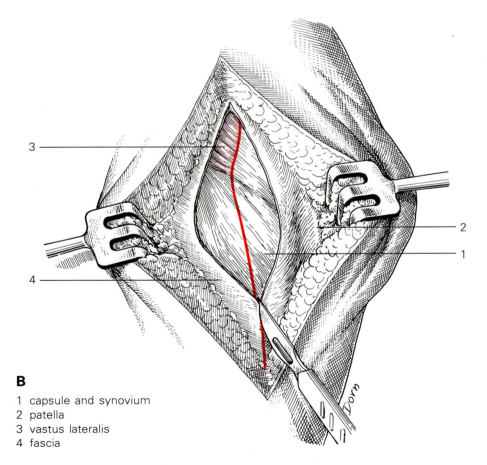

B

1 capsule and synovium
2 patella
3 vastus lateralis
4 fascia

C Medial retraction of the patella gives a limited exposure of the knee joint.

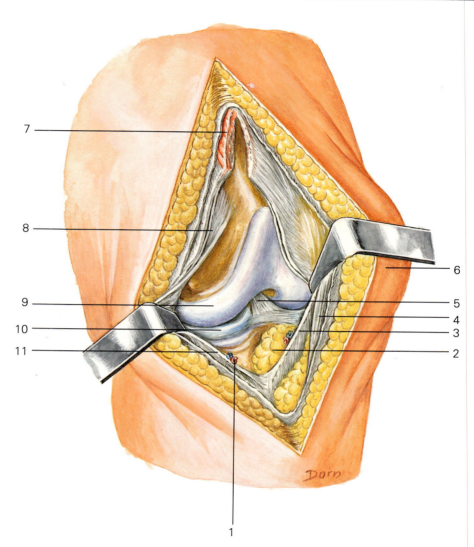

C

1 lateral genicular artery, ligated
2 infrapatellar fat pad
3 capsule
4 ligamentum patellae
5 anterior cruciate ligament
6 patella
7 vastus lateralis
8 synovium and capsule
9 lateral femoral condyle
10 lateral meniscus
11 capsule

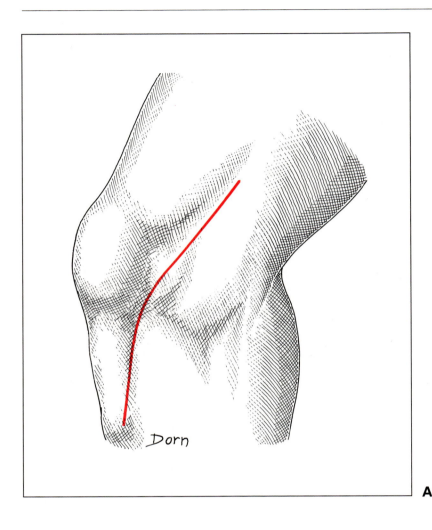

Dorn

A

Medial approach

Introduction

The medial approach to the knee gives a relatively limited exposure: it gives a poor exposure of the patella and an inadequate view of the lateral joint compartment. Wound healing is much better along this incision and a continuous subcuticular suture does not seem to compromise the blood supply to the skin flaps in this area.

Indications

- Repairs of the medial collateral ligament.
- Internal fixation of fractures of the medial tibial plateau or femoral condyle.

Position of the patient

The patient is placed supine with the hip externally rotated and the knee flexed to about 30°.

Incision

A The incision commences above the level of the medial femoral condyle curving gently downwards and forwards over the medial aspect of the knee joint, ending below the level of the tibial tuberosity. In a less extensive exposure, the infrapatellar branches of the saphenous nerve are easily preserved.

B

1 patella
2 vastus medialis

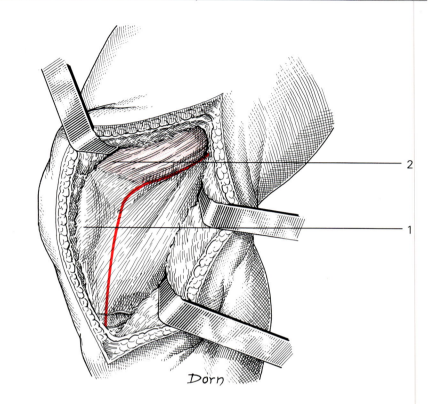

Exposure

B The incision is deepened to aponeurosis, where the border of vastus medialis can easily be defined. The incision of the aponeurosis and capsule commences medial to the muscle fibres and follows the curve of the muscle fibres to be extended distally in a straight line to end just medial to the tibial tuberosity. If the collateral ligament alone is to be exposed, then only the aponeurosis need be divided and retracted. The capsule can be left intact.

C The synovium can be opened in a longitudinal manner.

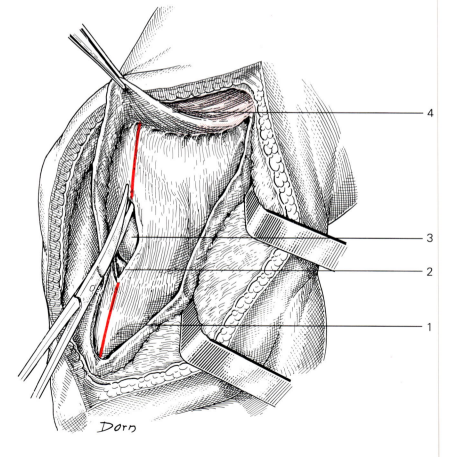

C

1 capsule
2 synovium
3 medial femoral condyle
4 vastus medialis

Knee

D   The patella is retracted anteriorly to expose the anteromedial joint compartment. The fat pad and the belly of vastus medialis require retraction. If access is restricted by the medial collateral ligament, its femoral origin may be elevated either subperiosteally or with a small block of bone. Immobilization in plaster for a period is then appropriate postoperatively.

D

1   medial femoral condyle
2   infrapatellar fat pad

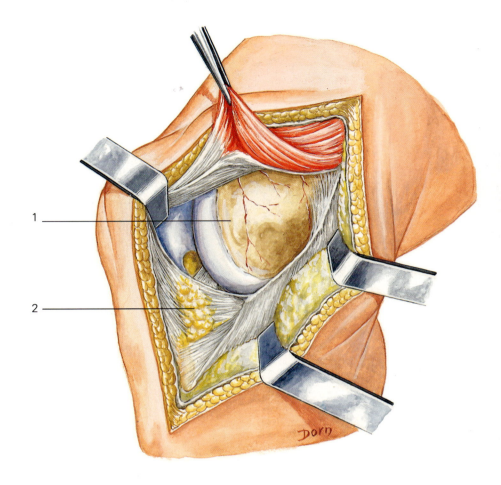

Posteromedial approach

Indication

The posteromedial approach may be used for the removal of loose bodies or a remnant of posterior horn of the medial meniscus. A more extensive exposure will be required for the repair of the posteromedial capsule. Extensive undermining of the skin can once again produce vascular compromise and delay wound healing. Visualization of the posterolateral joint compartment is inhibited by the cruciate ligaments and the overlying synovium.

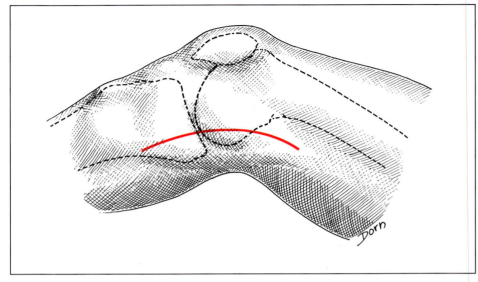

A

Position of the patient

The patient is placed supine with the hip externally rotated and flexed to 90°. The knee is flexed to approximately 30°.

Incision

A The incision curves from the level of the adductor tubercle of the femur to the posterior margin of the tibia, just distal to the tibial flare, but anterior to the border of sartorius.

Exposure

B The anterior margin of sartorius is defined, freed from the aponeurosis and retracted posteriorly, preserving the saphenous nerve. The underlying medial collateral ligament is thus exposed. The capsule is incised along the posterior oblique fibres of the collateral ligament.

B

1 semitendinosus
2 semimembranosus
3 gracilis
4 sartorius
5 medial head of gastrocnemius
6 medial collateral ligament
7 infrapatellar branch of saphenous nerve

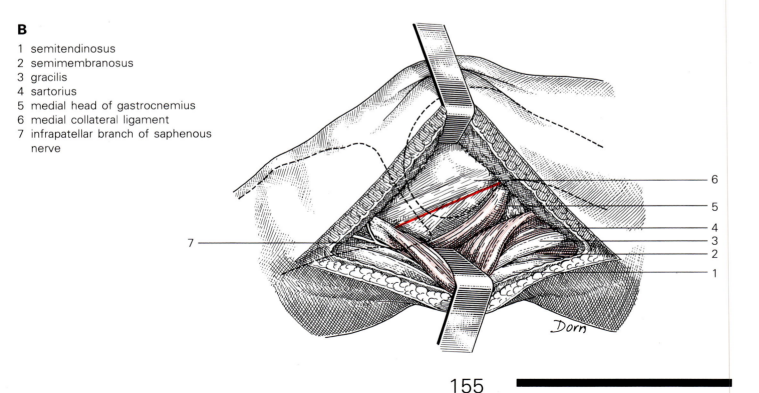

Knee

C The posteromedial joint compartment is entered by retracting the lax hamstrings posteriorly and the collateral ligament anteriorly with the capsule. The medial femoral condyle and the medial meniscus are thus exposed. The articular surface of the tibia is rarely seen clearly until the meniscus itself is mobilized. Careful closure of the wound is performed in layers with a continuous suture being appropriate for the synovium, and an interrupted suture for the capsule.

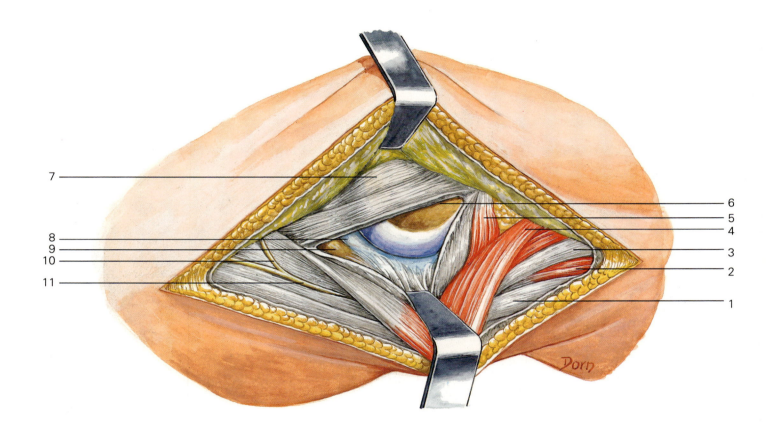

c

1 semitendinosus
2 semimembranosus
3 gracilis
4 sartorius
5 medial head of gastrocnemius
6 medial femoral condyle
7 capsule, opened
8 medial meniscus
9 tibia
10 infrapatellar branch of saphenous nerve
11 saphenous nerve

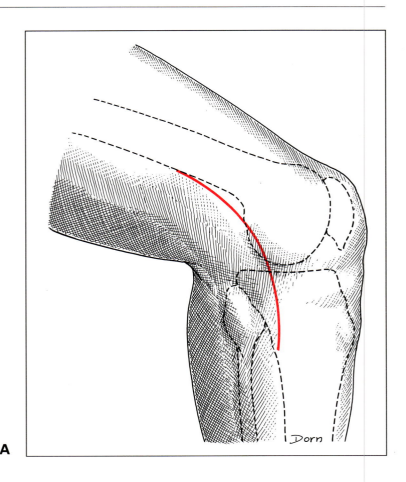

A

Lateral approach to the knee and proximal tibia

Introduction

This modified lateral approach can be made on either side of the iliotibial band. It allows a more extensive exposure of both the lateral femoral and tibial condyles, and the soft tissue of the lateral joint compartment.

Incising the capsule along the line of the joint itself will allow complete excision of a cyst of the lateral meniscus, but very careful reconstruction of the capsule is required at the end of the procedure. Extension of the lower end of the wound past the tibial flare, with incision of the deep fascia and elevation of the proximal tibialis anterior,

provides excellent exposure for a high valgus tibial osteotomy. However, the anterior tibial artery passes across the interosseous membrane close to the fibular neck and may be injured if retractors are placed between the tibia and fibula at this level, leading to vascular compromise of the anterior compartment. It is essential to insert a drain following a high tibial osteotomy to prevent an anterior compartment syndrome developing.

Indications

- Internal fixation of fractures of the lateral tibial plateau or lateral femoral condyle.
- Repairs of the lateral collateral ligament and posterolateral capsule.

Position of the patient

The patient is supine with a sandbag under the ipsilateral buttock and the knee flexed.

Incision

A The tendon of biceps femoris is palpated. A curved incision is made anterior to this tendon, above the level of the lateral femoral condyle, and is continued distally to end medial and anterior to the neck of the fibula. Subsequent dissection may then be either anterior or posterior to the iliotibial band.

157

B

1 iliotibial band

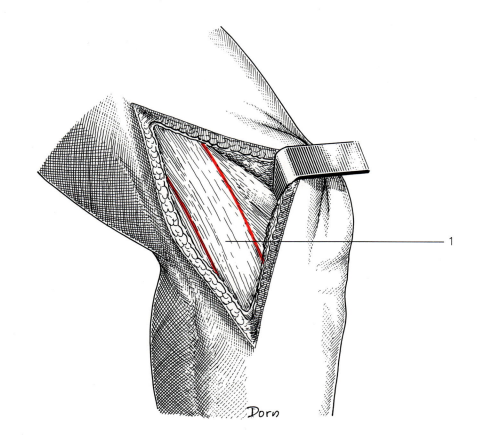

Exposure

B If the approach is posterior to the iliotibial band, access can be gained to the posterolateral capsule of the knee. The posterior border of the fascia lata is continuous with the lateral intermuscular septum and will need to be separated from it by longitudinal sharp dissection. The lateral intermuscular septum is then retracted posteriorly.

To expose the lateral collateral ligament, the approach will be made anterior to the iliotibial band which is then retracted posteriorly.

C The superior genicular artery is seen to pass across the lateral femoral condyle at the level of the origin of the lateral collateral ligament. The inferior genicular artery is seen to pass deep to this ligament distal to the knee joint. This artery is easily damaged in open operations on the lateral meniscus. The synovium should be incised well anterior to the lateral ligament. The incision may well involve division of the lower fibres of vastus lateralis.

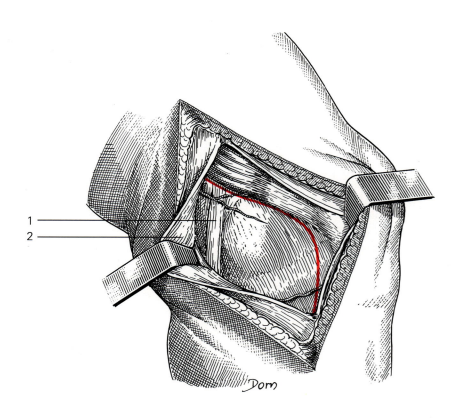

C

1 lateral collateral ligament
2 iliotibial band, retracted

D   The iliotibial band is retracted posteriorly. The anterior knee capsule, patella and infrapatellar fat pad are retracted anteriorly.

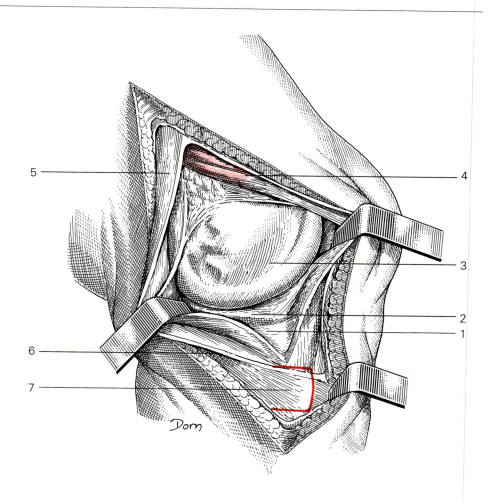

D

1 tibial plateau
2 lateral meniscus
3 lateral femoral condyle
4 vastus lateralis
5 fascia lata
6 iliotibial band
7 Gerdy's tubercle

Knee

E   If access is restricted by the tight iliotibial band, the fibres may be elevated in continuity with the periosteum or with a bone block raised from Gerdy's tubercle.

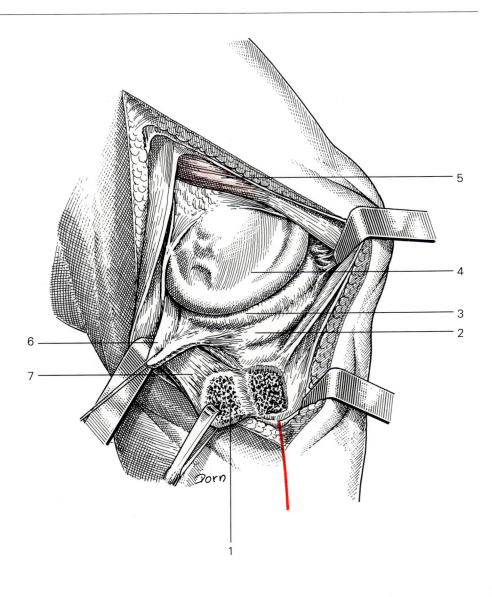

E

1 bone block, elevated
2 lateral tibial condyle
3 lateral meniscus
4 lateral femoral condyle
5 vastus lateralis
6 capsule
7 iliotibial band

F Elevation of the fibres of tibialis anterior from the lateral aspect of the tibia, with preservation of the anterior tibial vessels, will allow access to the lateral tibial condyle.

The fibular head and neck can be identified in this exposure and displayed subperiosteally by incising the anterior peroneal muscles and the periosteum longitudinally. Retractors can then be placed around the fibular head and a segment of head and neck can be resected as part of the operation of tibial osteotomy. Prior to this, the common peroneal nerve should be identified and safeguarded.

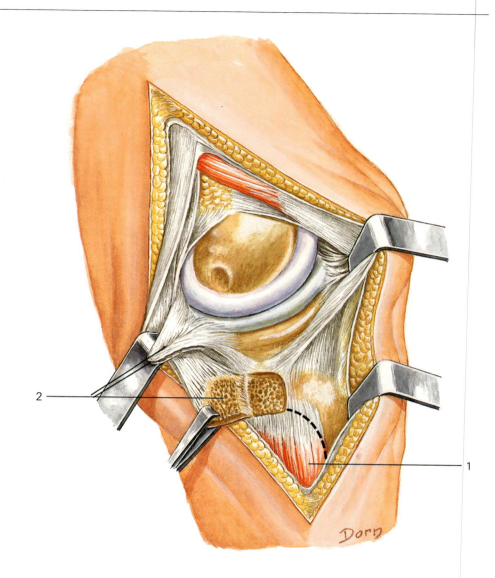

F

1 tibialis anterior
2 Gerdy's tubercle

Knee

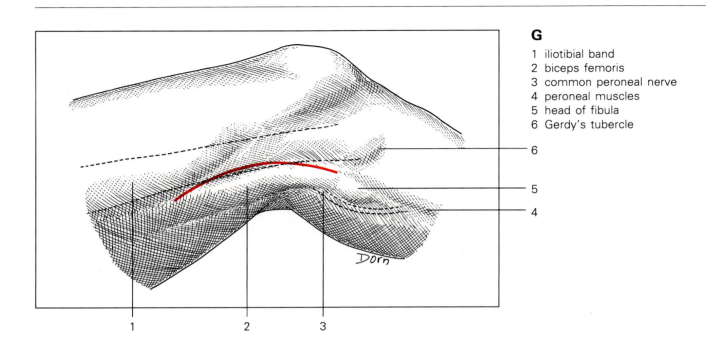

Dorn

G To expose the posterolateral capsule of the knee, an incision is made along the posterior border of the iliotibial band.

H The incision behind the iliotibial band is slightly more posterior and thus close to the common peroneal nerve. The position of this nerve is defined prior to incision of the deep fascia. The fascia is divided between the iliotibial band and biceps femoris, these structures then being retracted. The exposed underlying popliteal fat often contains friable vessels which require ligation. The lateral collateral ligament is defined. The capsule is identified posterior to the ligament and anterior to the lateral head of gastrocnemius which can easily be separated from the posterolateral knee capsule. A longitudinal incision is then made in the capsule.

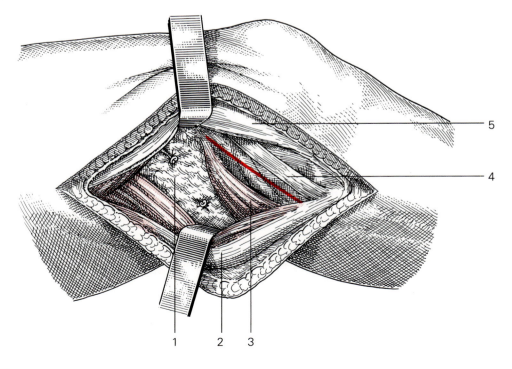

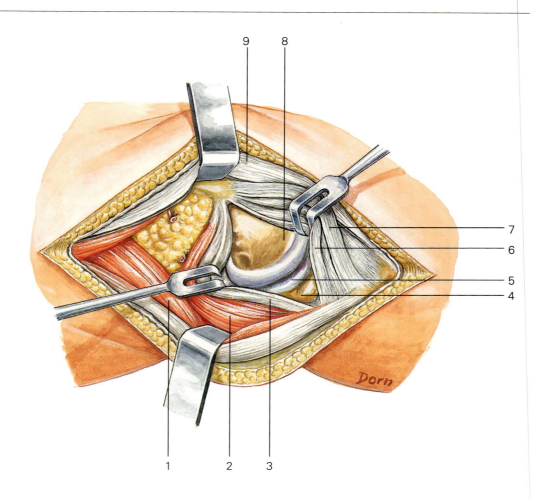

I The capsule is opened with care as the popliteus tendon lies immediately deep to the capsular incision. Posterior retraction of the lateral head of gastrocnemius and the capsule will reveal the posterolateral joint and lateral meniscus.

I

1 biceps femoris
2 lateral head of gastrocnemius
3 capsule, opened
4 lateral tibial condyle
5 lateral meniscus
6 capsule, opened
7 lateral collateral ligament, retracted
8 lateral femoral condyle
9 iliotibial band

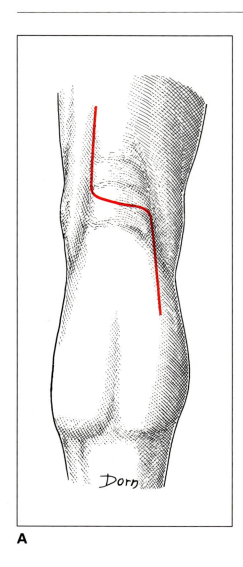

A

Posterior approach

Introduction

The posterior approach to the knee joint is indicated for surgery to the posterior cruciate ligament, particularly for suture of acute ruptures or reattachment of a distal evulsion with a bony fragment. The exposure is required also for excision of a Baker's cyst with reinforcement, repair of the posterior capsule, surgery to the nerves and vessels and correction of flexion contractures of the knee. A more limited approach is useful for removal of a semimembranosus bursa. Occasionally a posterior approach can be required for removal of loose bodies from the posterior compartment of the knee.

The posterior approach does, however, require quite extensive soft tissue dissection and, on occasions, division of the medial head of gastrocnemius which should be repaired at the end of the procedure, necessitating a period of immobilization post-operatively.

Preservation of the posterior sensory nerves is important, particularly the distal end of the posterior cutaneous nerve of the thigh and the sural nerve and its branches.

A lazy 'S' incision is made because this provides much greater access to the knee than a longitudinal incision, which may also give rise to a scar contracture over the popliteal fossa. Vascular compromise of the corner of the flaps following an angled incision is rarely seen.

Position of the patient

The patient is placed prone on pillows with the knees slightly flexed in a relaxed position.

Incision

A   A lazy 'S' incision is made commencing 10 cm proximal to the joint on the medial side and runs distally parallel to semimembranosus. At the level of the joint, it runs transversely before turning distally over the lateral head of gastrocnemius.

Exposure

B The sural nerve is visualized between the two heads of gastrocnemius and traced through the deep fascia to its origin from the tibial nerve. The popliteal aponeurosis is incised longitudinally.

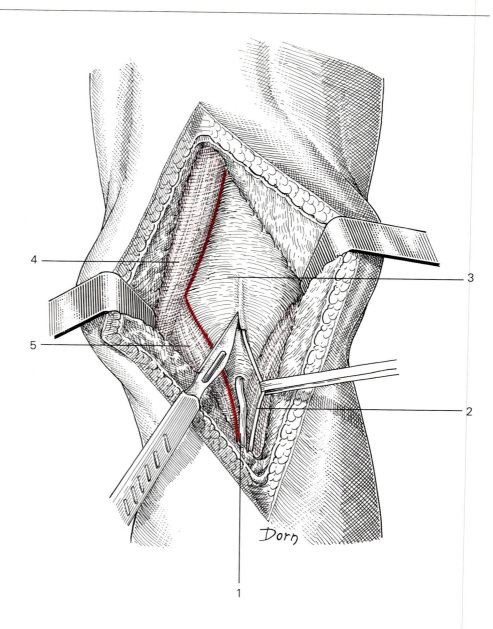

B

1 short saphenous vein
2 sural nerve
3 popliteal aponeurosis
4 semimembranosus
5 medial head of gastrocnemius

Knee

C   The tibial nerve, the common peroneal nerve and its branches are dissected free. The popliteal vessels are seen to lie medial to the nerve. The medial head of gastrocnemius is defined and its insertion visualized by medial retraction of semimembranosus. The medial head is then divided close to the femur and retracted laterally to protect the tibial nerve and popliteal vessels. The proximal neurovascular pedicle to the medial head of gastrocnemius must be protected.

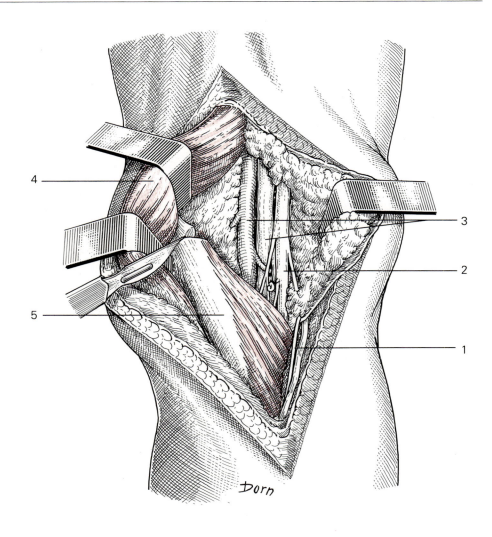

C

1 sural nerve
2 tibial nerve
3 popliteal artery and vein
4 semimembranosus
5 medial head of gastrocnemius

D The floor of the popliteal fossa is thus exposed, demonstrating the insertion of semimembranosus, its fascial extension and oblique ligament. The superior and middle genicular arteries are visualized and may require ligation.

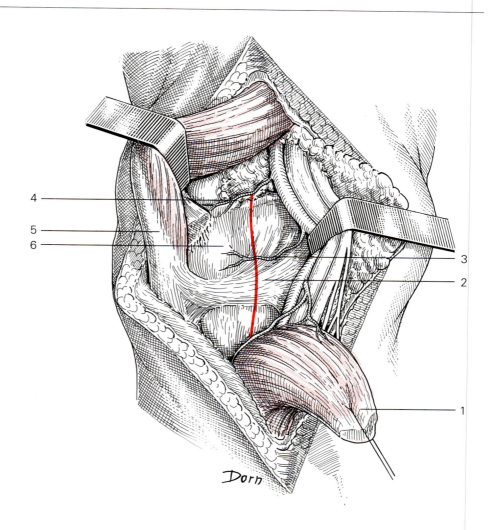

Dorn

D

1 medial head of gastrocnemius
2 oblique ligament
3 middle genicular artery
4 superior genicular artery
5 semimembranosus insertion
6 posterior knee capsule

Knee

E The posterior capsule is opened by a longitudinal midline incision and stay sutures are placed in the oblique ligament. The underlying posterior cruciate insertion into the tibia is exposed.

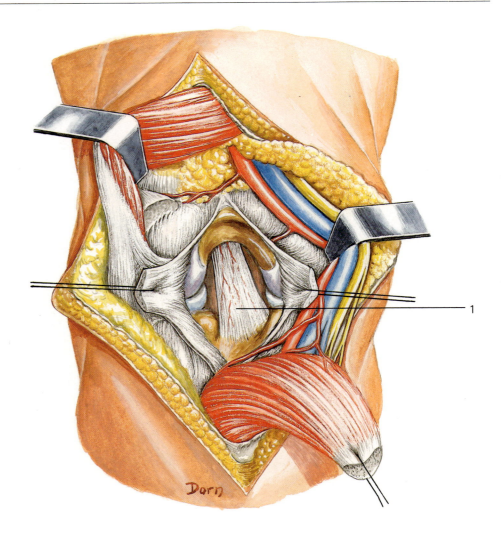

E

1 posterior cruciate ligament

5

Tibia and fibula

Tibia and fibula

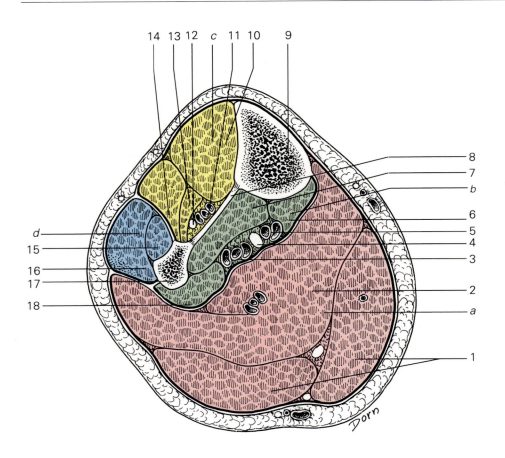

A

A
1. medial and lateral heads of gastrocnemius
2. soleus
3. peroneal artery and veins
4. tibial nerve
5. posterior tibial artery and veins
6. flexor digitorum longus
7. tibialis posterior
8. interosseous membrane
9. tibia
10. tibialis anterior
11. anterior tibial artery and veins
12. deep peroneal nerve
13. extensor hallucis longus
14. extensor digitorum longus
15. peroneus brevis
16. peroneus longus
17. fibula
18. flexor hallucis longus
   - a superficial
   - b deep } posterior compartment
   - c anterior compartment
   - d lateral compartment

Introduction

Surgical approaches to the tibia and fibula are commonly performed, especially in the field of trauma. Whatever the pathology, the siting of skin incisions is of vital importance because the postoperative complications are dominated by skin necrosis, resulting in soft tissue defects. The vascular anatomy of the skin and the principles of skin incisions should be clearly understood to limit the risk of skin necrosis. The creation of 'strap flaps', by placing an operative incision parallel to an area of traumatized skin or even a traumatic wound, must be avoided.

The anteromedial surface of the tibia is subcutaneous and thus eas-

ily exposed, but there are serious risks as the blood supply to the skin is highly vulnerable particularly following trauma. Local cutaneous flaps carry an even greater risk and should only be used by an expert to cover exposed bone following acute injury.

The posterior approaches to the tibia are more difficult, but carry much less risk of skin necrosis and wound failure. Even if postoperative skin necrosis were to result, the bone itself would not be exposed and the muscle offers a well-vascularized bed for a skin graft. Anterior and posterior approaches can be combined, but the incisions must be placed opposite to one another on the circumference of the leg and be separated by 180°.

Surgical access to the fibula is relatively easy except if the bone is to be excised in its entirety, because the peroneal vessels must then be dissected. For exposure of the proximal and middle thirds, the common and superficial peroneal nerves must be protected.

Anatomy

Four separate muscle compartments exist in the leg. The concept is of paramount importance during surgical procedures and following trauma, because compartment syndromes occur not infrequently in the leg and require urgent surgical decompression.

The anterior compartment contains the anterior tibial artery and its venae comitantes and the extensor muscles of the foot and ankle, namely tibialis anterior, extensor hallucis longus, extensor digitorum longus and peroneus tertius. The muscles are supplied by the deep peroneal nerve which runs in the anterior compartment and provides sensation over the dorsal aspect of the web space between the great toe and the index toe.

The lateral compartment contains the evertors of the foot and ankle, namely peroneus brevis and longus, which are supplied by the superficial peroneal nerve. There is no major artery within this compartment.

The posterior compartment is divided into two subcompartments by a fascial layer that runs in the coronal plane. The superficial posterior compartment contains the superficial flexor muscles, namely soleus, gastrocnemius and plantaris. The sural nerve, which is purely sensory, lies in the proximal third of this compartment. The deep posterior compartment contains the deep flexor muscles, namely tibialis posterior, flexor digitorum longus and flexor hallucis longus. In addition, the tibial nerve which supplies all these muscles, the posterior tibial artery and the peroneal artery lie within this compartment.

A A cross-section through the middle of the leg demonstrates the topography of the compartments.

B Muscles of the anterior aspect of the leg

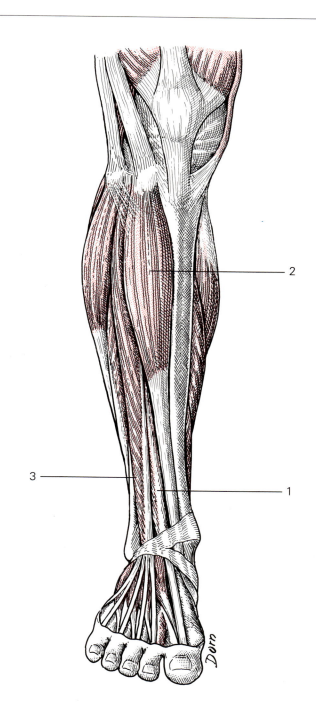

B

1 extensor hallucis longus
2 tibialis anterior
3 extensor digitorum longus

Tibia and fibula

C   Muscles of the posterior aspect of the leg

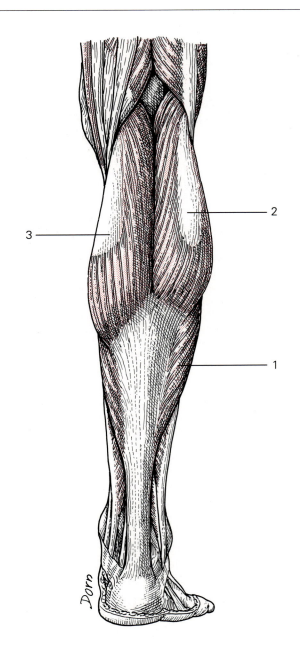

C

1 soleus
2 lateral head
3 medial head
} of gastrocnemius

D   Muscles of the lateral aspect of the leg

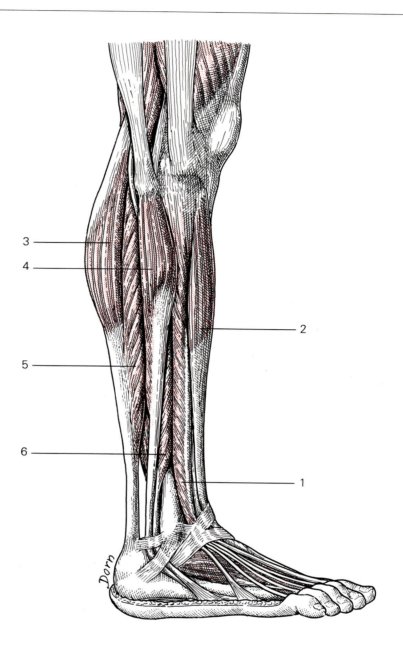

D

1 extensor digitorum longus
2 tibialis anterior
3 gastrocnemius
4 peroneus longus
5 soleus
6 peroneus brevis

E   Muscles of the medial aspect of the leg

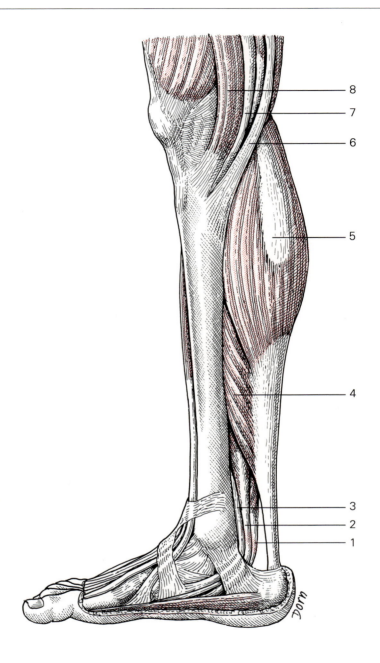

E

1 flexor hallucis longus
2 flexor digitorum longus
3 tibialis posterior
4 soleus
5 medial head of gastrocnemius
6 semitendinosus
7 gracilis
8 sartorius

Superficial veins and nerves

There are two major superficial veins in the leg: the short and long saphenous veins. The short saphenous vein follows the course of the sural nerve and may be ligated without impairing the venous return. The long saphenous vein runs along the postero-medial border of the tibia and crosses the bone in its distal quarter. It is very much at risk during the anterior approach to the tibia. The long saphenous vein should be preserved if at all possible, because it may be required for reconstructive vascular procedures.

The course of the superficial sensory nerves should be studied in order to avoid the development of painful neuromas or sensory loss. The saphenous nerve follows the long saphenous vein and is at risk during the medial approach to the tibia. The sural nerve is subject to damage in the distal third of the leg during the posterolateral approach to the tibia. The lateral sural nerve in the upper part of the leg and the superficial peroneal nerve in the distal part can be damaged during lateral exposures of the fibula.

See pages 272–4 for veins and 326–38 for nerves.

The blood supply of the skin and surgical approaches

The blood supply of the skin of the shin is of great importance because it affects the choice of surgical exposure and allows the possibility of raising various fasciocutaneous flaps. The skin of the leg is supplied by three main groups of vessels:

1 The fasciocutaneous vessels, which run along the intermuscular septa or interstitial spaces, and arise from the three main deep vessels of the leg, are arranged in three vertical rows. The medial row arises from the posterior tibial artery and emerges between the deep and superficial posterior compartments. The anterolateral row emerges between tibialis anterior and extensor hallucis longus, or between tibialis anterior and the lateral aspect of the tibia. The posterolateral row arises from the peroneal artery and emerges between the lateral and posterior compartments.
2 The second group of vessels comprises the arteries arising from the muscles which supply an area of skin overlying the particular muscle.
3 The third group comprises the cutaneous arteries which arise from the vessels that accompany the superficial nerves.

All three groups of vessels form anastomoses from which both suprafascial and subcutaneous vascular networks develop. The surgical implications derived from this knowledge are clear: skin incisions should avoid superficial nerves and the longitudinal rows of fasciocutaneous vessels. Extensive mobilization of skin flaps must include the underlying fascia to preserve the suprafascial vascular network.

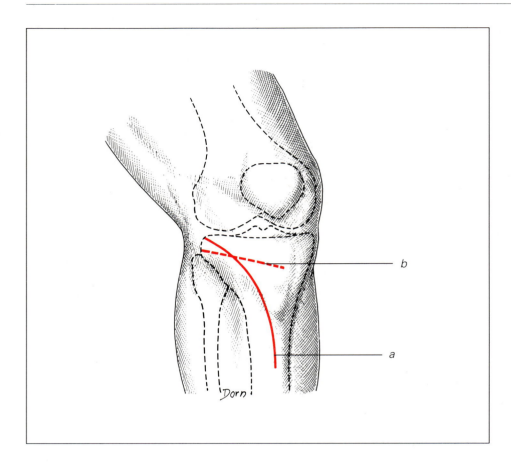

A

a incision
b transverse oblique incision

Proximal third of the tibia: anterolateral approach

Indications

- Reduction of fractures of the lateral tibial condyle.
- Tibial osteotomy.

Position of the patient

Reduction of fractures

The patient is in a lateral position which allows the space between the lateral meniscus and the tibial margin to be opened.

Tibial osteotomy

The patient is supine, with a sand-bag under the ipsilateral buttock. The whole limb is included in the operative field so as to appreciate the alignment of the limb clearly.

Incision

A A curved incision begins at the level of Gerdy's tubercle and descends along the lateral condyle to reach the tibial crest. It can be extended distally as necessary. An alternative incision is a skin crease 'transverse' incision, commencing posterior and proximal to the fibular head and extending to the midline, midway between the inferior pole of the patella and the tibial tubercle. This latter incision is suitable for tibial osteotomy but not for fracture fixation.

B

1 tibial tubercle
2 tibialis anterior
3 ligamentum patellae
4 tibial crest

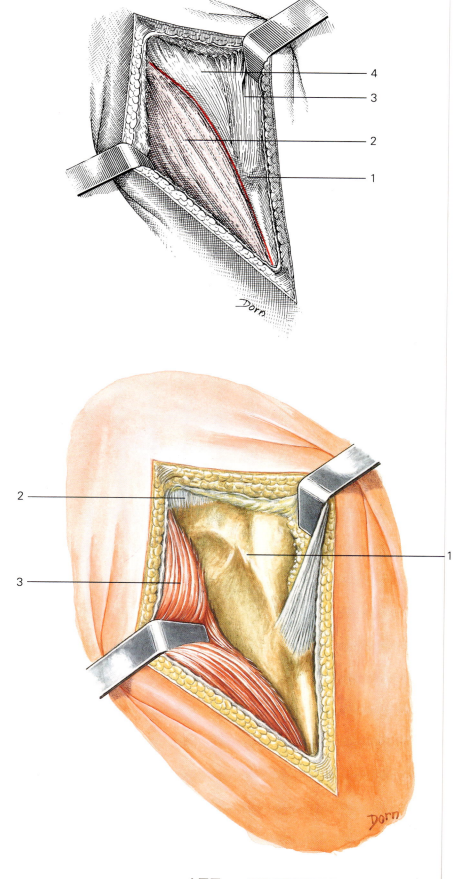

Exposure

B The skin margins are mobilized and retracted. An incision is made through the aponeurosis and periosteum along the tibial condyle and the tibial crest.

C Tibialis anterior is released subperiosteally and reflected, exposing the anterior and lateral surface of the condyle and the adjacent portion of the shaft of the tibia. Proximally, the insertion of fascia lata can be released from Gerdy's tubercle. The joint cavity can be opened by a horizontal incision in the synovial membrane beneath the meniscus. When closing the incision, the aponeurosis should not be reattached to avoid a compartment syndrome. In children, when undertaking a tibial osteotomy, a subcutaneous fasciotomy must be performed as far as the distal third of the leg.

C

1 proximal tibia
2 fascia lata, inserting into Gerdy's tubercle
3 tibialis anterior, retracted

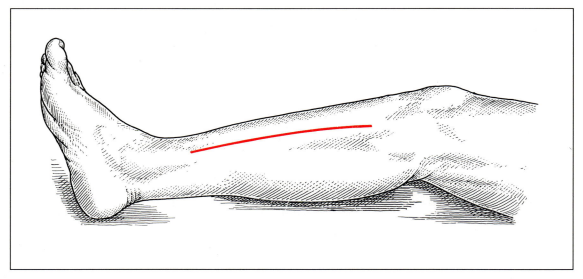

A

Midshaft of the tibia: anteromedial approach

Indications

- Open reduction of fractures of the tibia for tibial plating; the anterolateral approach is sometimes preferred to avoid the plate lying immediately deep to skin.
- Bone resection.
- Tibial osteotomy.

Position of the patient

The patient is supine and the limb externally rotated.

Incision

A A curved incision is made over the medial aspect of the tibia.

Exposure

B The saphenous nerve and the long saphenous vein must be protected in the lower part of the incision. The skin margins should not be mobilized from the underlying aponeurosis and muscles.

C The periosteum is incised along the midline of its medial surface, in continuity with the skin and subcutaneous tissues. The tibia is exposed subperiosteally.

Any desired segment of the tibia may be exposed. In the proximal third, the dissection is carried across the tendon insertions of sartorius, gracilis and semitendinosus, which are reflected together to gain access to the tibial metaphysis. In the distal third of the tibia, care should be taken in incising the skin because of its relatively poor blood supply. The advantage of the curved incision is to avoid tension on the skin edges. The incision should be longer than the area of tibia to be exposed.

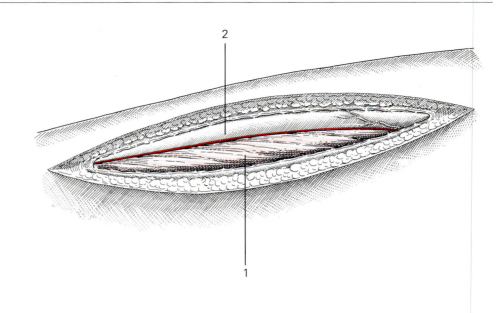

B
1 soleus
2 tibial shaft

C
1 tibial shaft

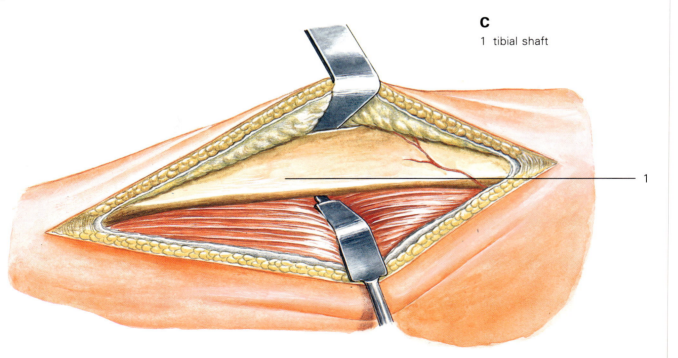

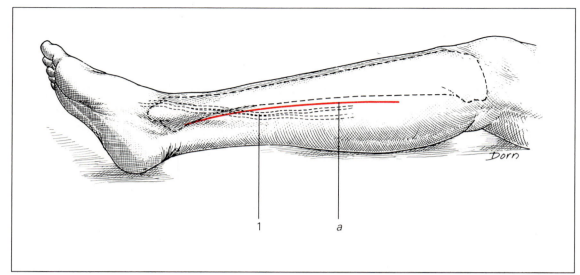

A
1 saphenous vein and
  nerve
a incision

Midshaft of the tibia: posteromedial approach

Indication

- Bone grafting of a fracture non-union.

Position of the patient

The patient is supine, the lower limb being externally rotated.

Incision

A The incision follows the posteromedial border of the tibia.

Exposure

B The skin margins are gently retracted to identify the posteromedial border of the tibia. The fascia is incised and the periosteum divided directly over the posteromedial border of the tibia.

C The posterior surface of the bone is exposed subperiosteally. The anteromedial surface is not exposed in its entirety. The deep flexor muscles are separated from the tibia, being attached to the periosteum.

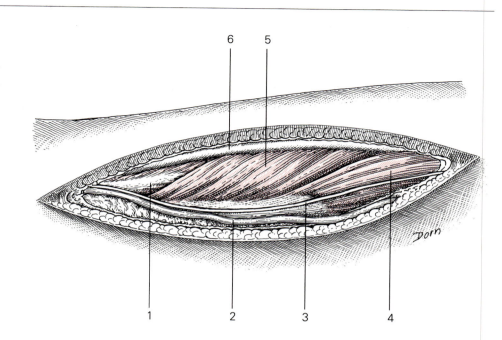

B

1 flexor digitorum longus
2 saphenous vein
3 saphenous nerve
4 gastrocnemius
5 soleus
6 tibia

C

1 tibial shaft

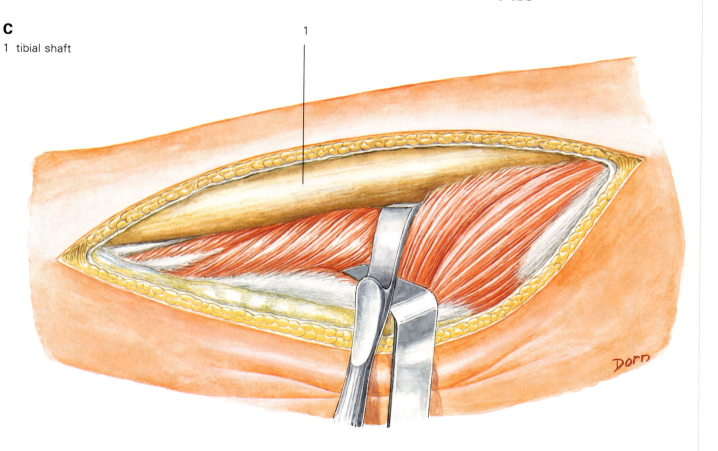

Tibia and fibula

D A cross-section through the mid-leg shows the posteromedial approach.

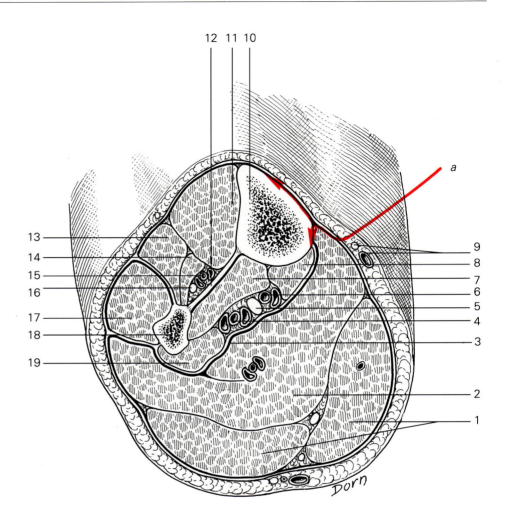

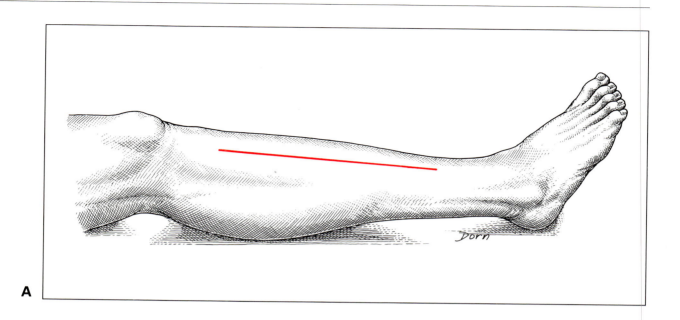

A

Midshaft of the tibia: anterolateral approach

Introduction

The anterolateral approach to the midshaft may be preferred when the skin on the medial aspect is of doubtful viability. It is also of value if the tibia is to be plated, because the plate can then be placed on the lateral aspect of the bone and covered by muscle.

Indication

- Open reduction and internal fixation of fractures of the tibia.

Position of the patient

The patient is supine, with a sandbag under the buttock of the affected leg.

Incision

A A straight longitudinal incision of the desired length is made 1 cm lateral to the anterior tibial crest.

Tibia and fibula

Exposure

B   The fascia and the periosteum are incised on the tibial crest and stripped from the anteromedial surface of the tibia.

C   Laterally, the periosteum, in continuity with tibialis anterior, is separated from the anterolateral surface of the tibia.

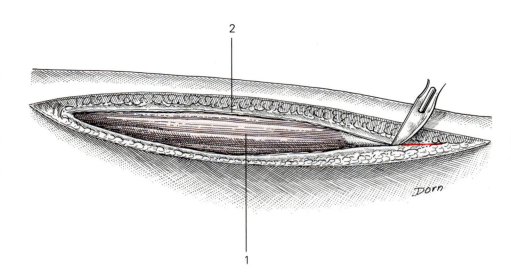

B

1 tibialis anterior
2 tibial crest

C

1 tibial shaft

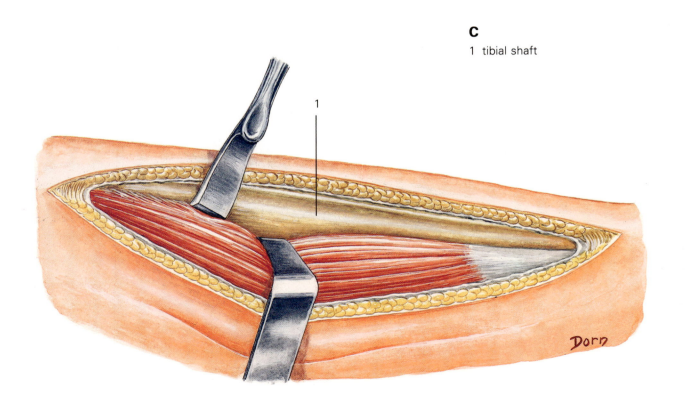

D A cross-section through the mid-leg shows the anterolateral approach.

At the end of the procedure, the fascia should not be closed in order to avoid the development of a compartment syndrome.

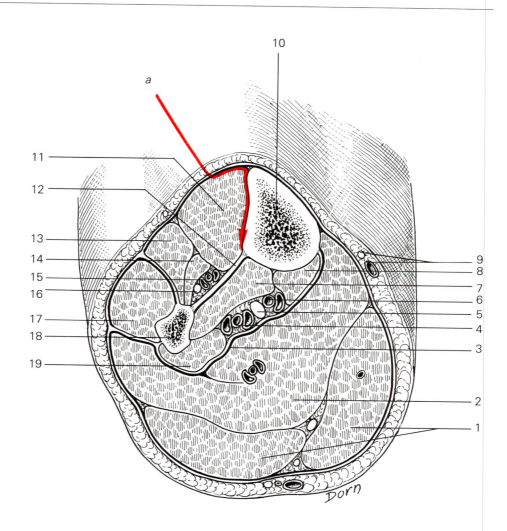

D

1 medial and lateral heads of gastrocnemius
2 soleus
3 fascia between deep and superficial posterior compartments
4 peroneal artery and veins
5 tibial nerve
6 posterior tibial artery and veins
7 tibialis posterior
8 flexor digitorum longus
9 saphenous nerve and vein
10 tibia
11 tibialis anterior
12 interosseous membrane
13 extensor digitorum longus
14 extensor hallucis longus
15 anterior tibial artery and veins
16 deep peroneal nerve
17 peronei
18 fibula
19 flexor hallucis longus
a anterolateral approach to the tibia

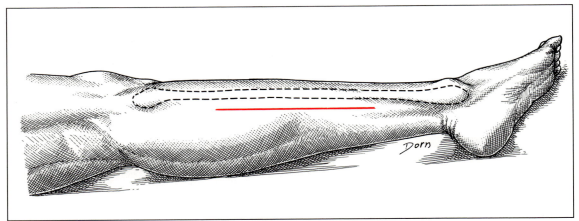

A

Tibia and fibula: posterolateral approach

Introduction

The posterolateral approach to the tibia and fibula is of considerable surgical importance, because the skin is usually healthy and undamaged. The dissection is difficult and carries the risk of damage to the posterior tibial and peroneal arteries and their venae comitantes. Nonetheless, two main points facilitate the dissection:

1 The first is to identify the plane between soleus in the superficial posterior compartment and the peroneal muscles in the lateral compartment.

2 The second point which is of value when considering the deep dissection is to release the deep flexor muscles sequentially from the fibula subperiosteally, from the interosseous membrane and finally from the posterior surface of the tibia. The neurovascular bundles are retracted medially and posteriorly without exposing them. If the posterior tibial artery and its venae comitantes are encountered, considerable venous oozing can occur.

Indications

- Treatment of non-union by an intertibiofibular graft.
- Access to the tibia when the anterior approach is impossible, usually due to unhealthy skin.

Position of the patient

The patient is prone or lying on his or her non-affected side.

Incision

A A straight longitudinal incision is made overlying the lateral border of gastrocnemius. The lateral sural nerve should be protected in the proximal third of the leg.

B

1 soleus
2 flexor hallucis longus
3 peronei

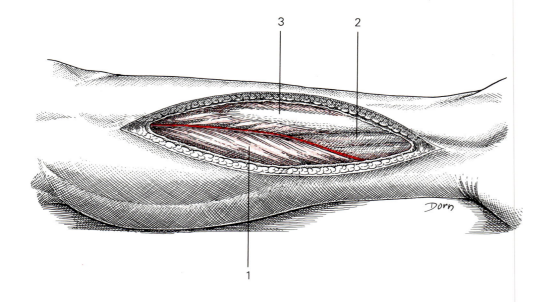

Exposure

B The fascia is incised in line with the skin and the plane between the peronei and soleus is defined by the septum separating the two compartments. Soleus is released from the septum and the fibula. In the proximal part of the incision, muscular branches of the peroneal artery, supplying peroneus brevis, may be ligated.

C Soleus and gastrocnemius are retracted medially and posteriorly to reveal, in the depth of the incision, the posterior crest of the fibula. The periosteum of the fibular crest is incised and flexor hallucis longus is progressively released from the bone.

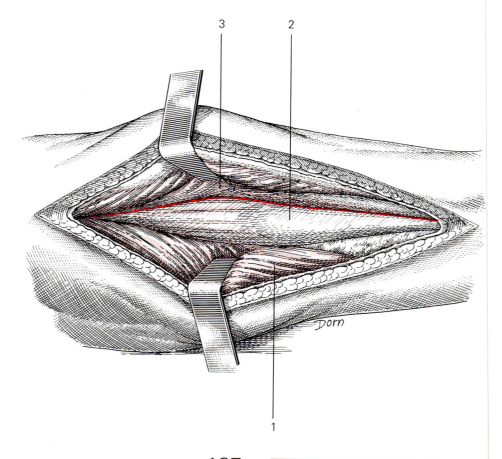

C

1 gastrocnemius and soleus
2 flexor hallucis longus
3 peronei

Tibia and fibula

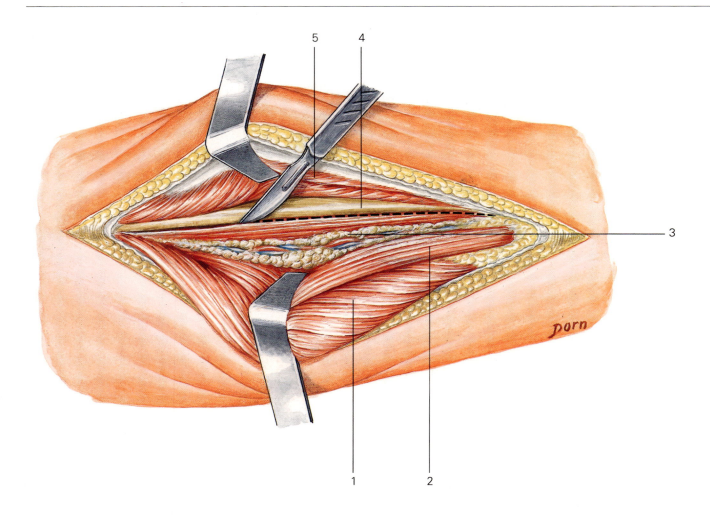

D As flexor hallucis longus is retracted medially, the peroneal artery and vein are exposed. The dissection should hug the surface of the fibula, detaching tibialis posterior, to expose the interosseous membrane.

D
1 soleus
2 flexor hallucis longus
3 peroneal artery and veins
4 lateral fibula
5 peronei

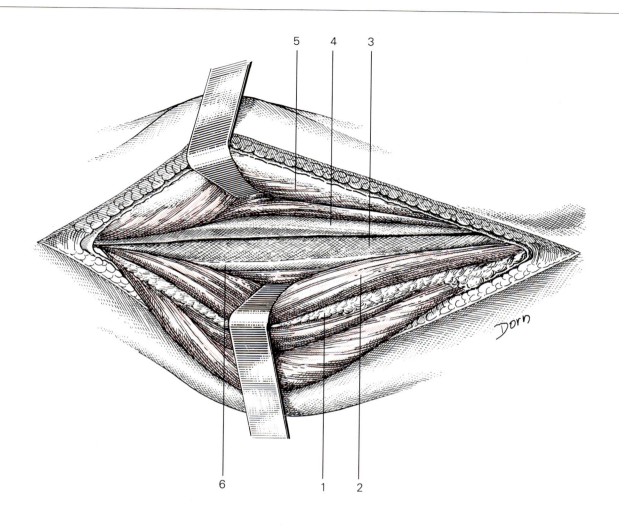

E Tibialis posterior is progressively detached from the membrane and, with flexor hallucis longus, is retracted medially and posteriorly, thus protecting the peroneal and tibial vessels and the tibial nerve. The dissection continues adjacent to the posterior surface of the interosseous membrane as far as the lateral border of the tibia, where the periosteum is divided and stripped from the posterior surface of the bone in order to expose it.

E
1 peroneal vessels
2 tibialis posterior
3 interosseous membrane
4 lateral fibula
5 peronei
6 lateral border of the tibia

Tibia and fibula

F A cross-section through the mid-leg shows the posterolateral approach.

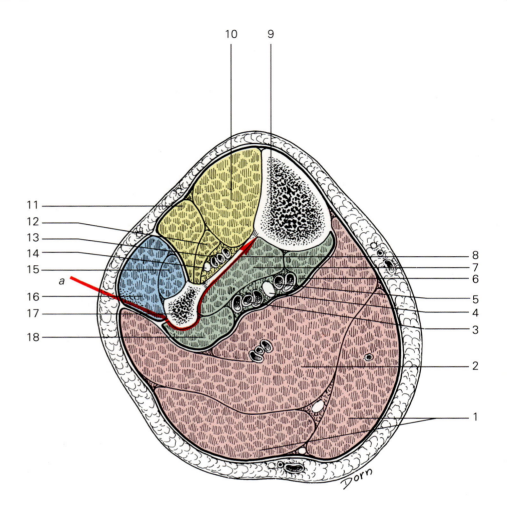

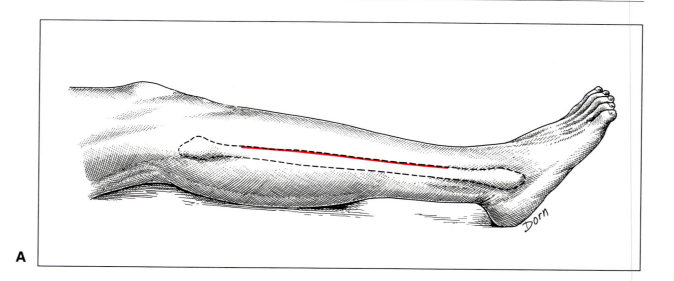

A

Lateral approach to the tibia: anterior to the fibula

Introduction

This approach is an alternative to the posterolateral approach described previously. It should only be performed when the anterior tibial vessels have previously been destroyed. It does not give good access to the tibia and the route is between the lateral and anterior compartments. It carries the risk of damage to the anterior tibial vessels and the deep peroneal nerve which lie on the interosseous membrane.

Indication

- Intertibiofibular graft.

Incision

A A straight longitudinal incision is made anterior to the fibular crest.

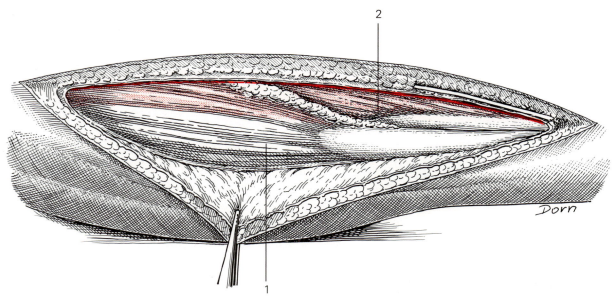

Exposure

B The skin is gently retracted to reveal the septum between the anterior and lateral compartments. The fibula is reached between extensor digitorum longus and the peronei.

C All the muscles are released from the fibula subperiosteally and from the anterior surface of the interosseous membrane. Care should be taken to protect the anterior tibial vessels and deep peroneal nerve which lie on the interosseous membrane.

B

1 peroneus longus
2 peroneus brevis

C

1 peronei
2 fibula
3 septum between anterior and lateral compartments

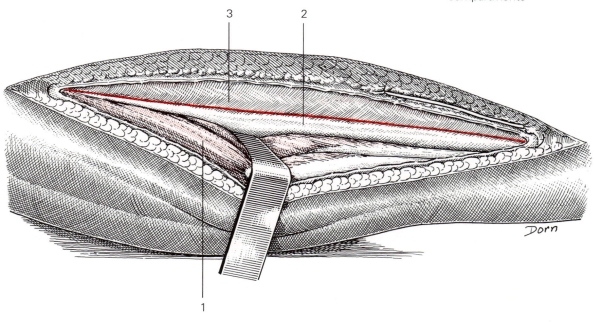

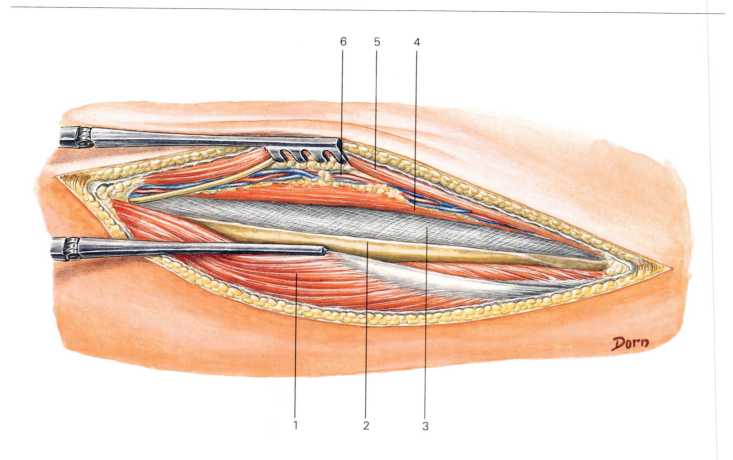

D Tibialis anterior is partially released from the lateral aspect of the tibia. The muscles are retracted anteriorly and medially, exposing the medial aspect of the fibula, the interosseous membrane and the lateral border of the tibia. When an intertibiofibular graft is planned, the membrane should be excised.

D
1 peronei
2 fibula
3 anterior surface of interosseous membrane
4 tibialis anterior
5 extensor digitorum longus
6 deep peroneal nerve and anterior tibial artery and vein

Tibia and fibula

E A cross-section through the mid-leg shows the lateral approach to the tibia.

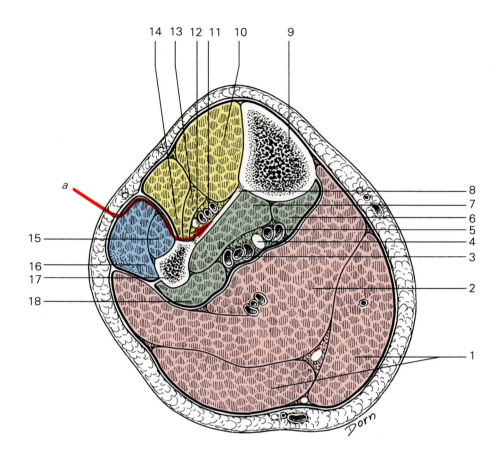

E

1 medial and lateral heads of gastrocnemius
2 soleus
3 peroneal artery and veins
4 tibial nerve
5 posterior tibial artery and veins
6 flexor digitorum longus
7 tibialis posterior
8 interosseous membrane
9 tibia
10 tibialis anterior
11 anterior tibial artery and veins
12 deep peroneal nerve
13 extensor hallucis longus
14 extensor digitorum longus
15 peroneus brevis
16 peroneus longus
17 fibula
18 flexor hallucis longus
a lateral approach to the tibia anterior to the fibula

Distal quarter of the tibia: posterolateral approach

Introduction

The posterolateral approach to the distal quarter of the tibia is the distal extension of the posterolateral approach to the tibia. The distal quarter of the tibia is relatively difficult to approach. The medial approach is not advocated because the skin is thin and the risk of necrosis high. The posterolateral approach provides good access to the posterior surface of the distal quarter of the tibia and allows reduction and internal fixation of the fractures.

Indications

- Open reduction and fixation of fractures of the posterior distal tibia.
- Open reduction of posterior intra-articular fractures of the tibia.

Position of the patient

The patient is prone or alternatively may be placed on the non-affected side.

Incision

A The longitudinal incision runs midway between the lateral border of the Achilles tendon and the posterior border of the fibula. It begins at the level of the tip of the lateral malleolus and can be extended proximally as far as necessary.

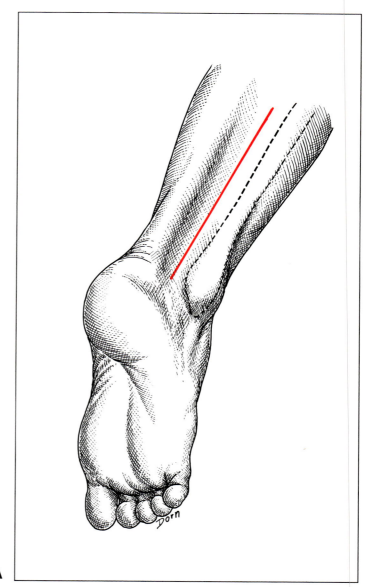

A

Tibia and fibula

B

1 short saphenous vein
2 sural nerve
a incision through peroneal
retinaculum

Exposure

B In the subcutaneous tissues,
care must be taken when isolating
and protecting the short saphenous vein and the sural nerve. In
the lower part of the incision, the
nerve and vein are anterior to it,
and they cross the wound. If the
incision is extended proximally, it
is sometimes necessary to mobilize a long segment of this neurovascular bundle in order to
retract it both medially and laterally. If the incision is lateral, the
neurovascular bundle is retracted
with the medial skin margin without exposing it, except in the
lower part of the incision. The fascia is incised in line with the skin
incision.

C The peroneal retinaculum is
incised, and the tendon of peroneus longus and the muscle belly
of peroneus brevis are retracted
laterally and anteriorly. Flexor hallucis longus is exposed and, in the
proximal part of the incision,
soleus is released from the fibula.
A longitudinal incision is made on
the fibula through the fibres of
flexor hallucis longus which is
released subperiosteally and
retracted medially and posteriorly.

C

1 sural nerve
2 peronei
3 fascia between lateral and posterior
compartments of the leg
4 short saphenous vein

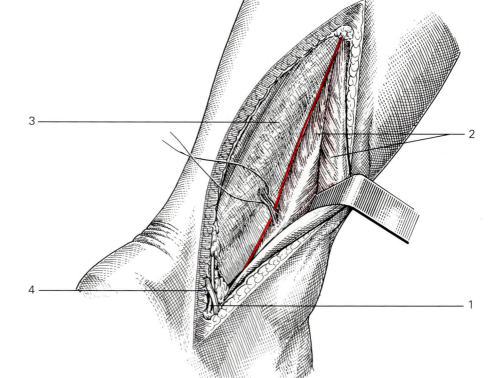

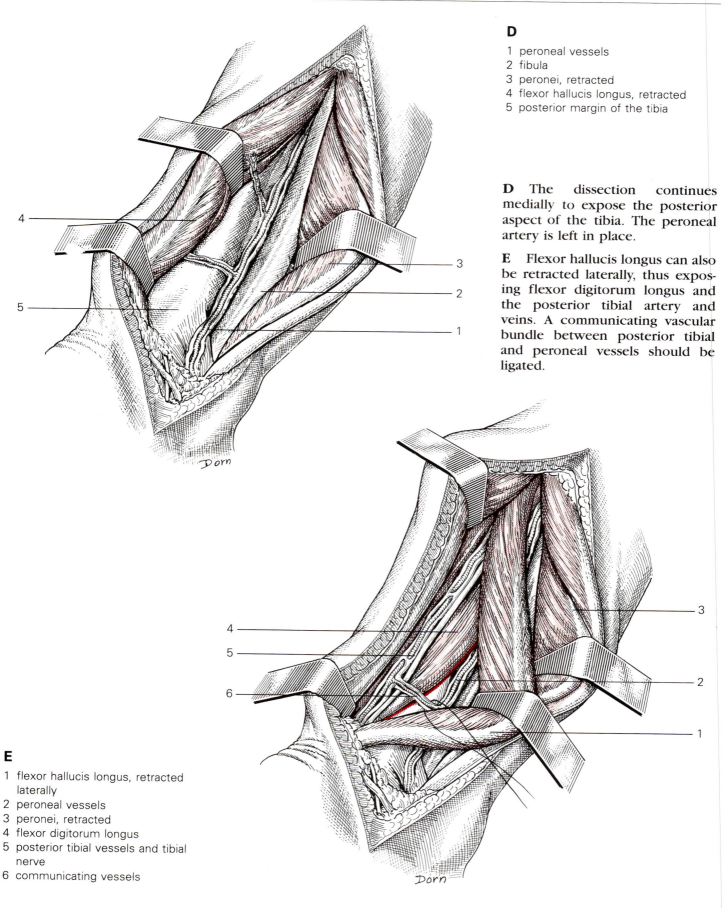

D
1 peroneal vessels
2 fibula
3 peronei, retracted
4 flexor hallucis longus, retracted
5 posterior margin of the tibia

D The dissection continues medially to expose the posterior aspect of the tibia. The peroneal artery is left in place.

E Flexor hallucis longus can also be retracted laterally, thus exposing flexor digitorum longus and the posterior tibial artery and veins. A communicating vascular bundle between posterior tibial and peroneal vessels should be ligated.

E
1 flexor hallucis longus, retracted laterally
2 peroneal vessels
3 peronei, retracted
4 flexor digitorum longus
5 posterior tibial vessels and tibial nerve
6 communicating vessels

Tibia and fibula

F

1 posterior margin of the tibia
2 flexor hallucis longus, retracted
3 peronei, retracted
4 flexor digitorum longus, retracted

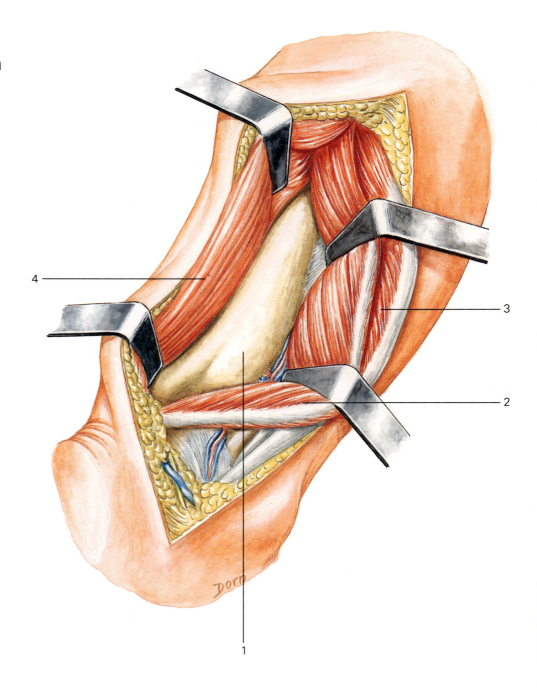

F Flexor hallucis longus is retracted laterally and protects the peroneal vessels while flexor digitorum longus is retracted medially and protects the posterior tibial vessels and the tibial nerve.

A

1 superficial peroneal
  nerve
a incision

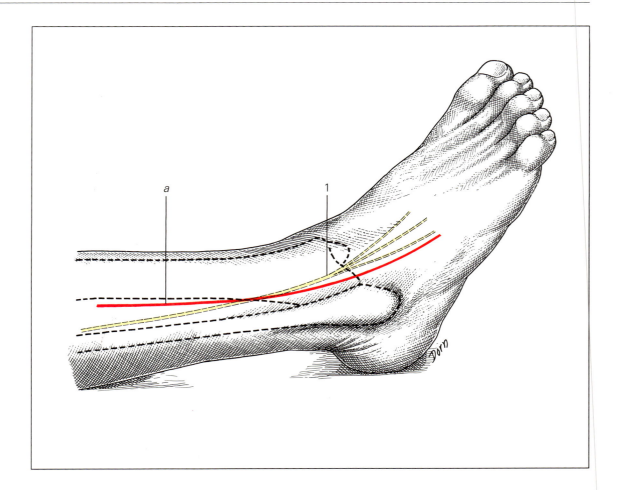

Distal quarter of the tibia: anterolateral approach

Introduction

The distal quarter of the tibia is subcutaneous on its medial aspect and would be exposed if the overlying skin were to undergo necrosis.

The anterolateral approach carries the same advantages as the posterolateral, because the skin is usually viable, being supplied by multiple vessels, and the bone is protected by the muscles of the anterior compartment. The anterolateral approach is easier than the posterolateral and is necessary when the intra-articular tibial fracture involves a large anterior fragment. The anterolateral approach does not necessitate the detachment of any muscle insertion from the tibia. Extensor digitorum longus and peroneus tertius arise from the fibula. The tendons of extensor hallucis longus and tibialis anterior have no bone attachment.

Indications

- Reduction and internal fixation of fractures of the distal tibia and fibula.

- Reduction of intra-articular fractures of the tibia.

Position of the patient

The patient is supine, with a sandbag under the buttock of the affected limb to maintain it in neutral rotation.

Incision

A The longitudinal incision lies anterior to the lateral border of the fibula.

Tibia and fibula

B

1 extensor digitorum longus
2 extensor retinaculum
3 superficial peroneal nerve

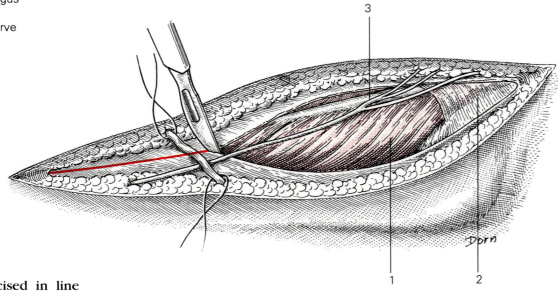

Exposure

B The fascia is incised in line with the skin incision. The anterior skin margin is retracted anteriorly, including the superficial peroneal nerve. Sometimes a branch to the lateral malleolus may have to be sacrificed.

C Extensor digitorum longus and peroneus tertius are released extraperiosteally from the anteromedial aspect of the fibula and from the interosseous membrane. The vascular anastomosis between the lateral malleolar artery and the perforating ramus of the peroneal artery is diathermied.

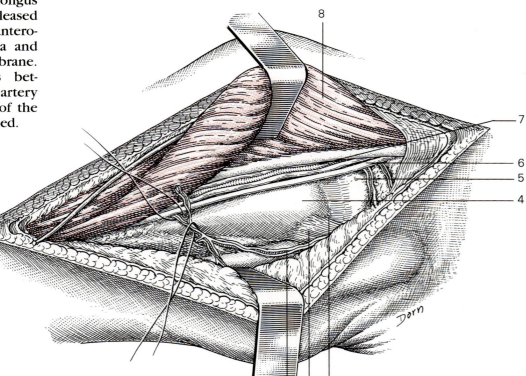

C

1 lateral malleolar artery
2 anterior distal tibiofibular syndesmosis
3 ankle joint
4 anterior distal tibia
5 talar dome
6 deep peroneal nerve
7 anterior tibial artery
8 extensor digitorum longus, retracted

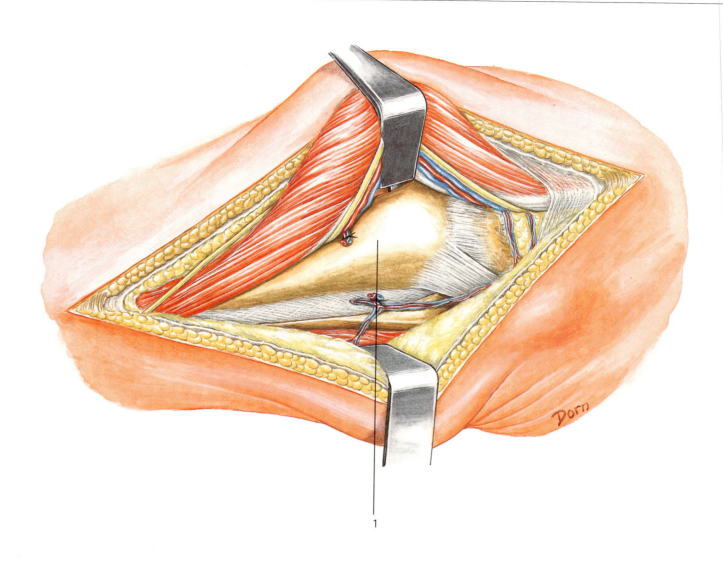

D All muscles of the anterior compartment with the anterior tibial vessels and the deep peroneal nerve are retracted medially and anteriorly, exposing the anterolateral aspect of the distal quarter of the tibia.

D

1 distal quarter of tibia

Tibia and fibula

E A cross-section through the distal quarter of the tibia and fibula shows the anterolateral approach.

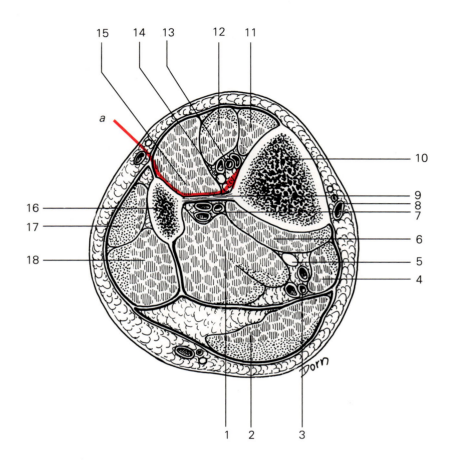

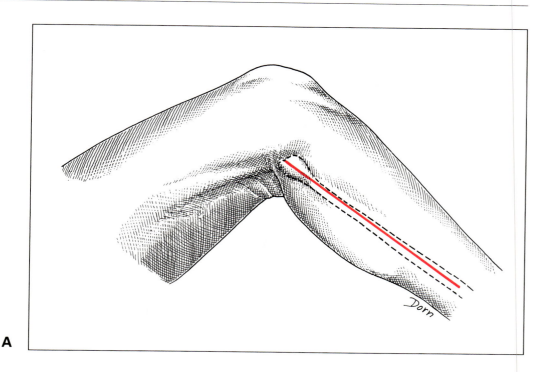

A

Proximal and middle third of the fibula: lateral approach and lateral extended approach to the distal third of the fibula

Introduction

The fibula is triangular in cross-section. A medial surface faces the tibia with the anterolateral and posterolateral surfaces being separated by the lateral fibular crest. The head and distal artery of the fibula are subcutaneous and easily palpable. The shaft is enclosed in muscle and only the crest can be palpated. Simultaneous access to the anterolateral and posterolateral surfaces can be carried out by separating the peronei in the lateral compartment from the muscles of the posterior compartment. Access to the anterolat-eral surface can be achieved by dissection between the anterior and lateral compartments, but the superficial peroneal nerve is at risk.

The approach to the proximal third and the middle third of the fibula is easier and safer between the lateral and posterior compartments, the superficial peroneal nerve being protected by the reflected peronei.

The common peroneal nerve is at risk as it winds around the neck of the fibula, where it is covered by the muscle fibres of peroneus longus. The distal third of the fibula is exposed by a lateral approach in which the tendons and muscle fibres of the peronei are retracted posteriorly.

Osteosynthesis, or the raising of a non-vascularized or vascularized graft, is carried out via the same exposure.

Indications

- Osteotomy of the fibula associated with tibial osteotomy.
- Excision of the fibula.
- Open reduction and internal fixation of fractures.
- The raising of a bone graft.

Position of the patient

The patient is supine, with a sandbag under the ipsilateral buttock. Alternatively, the patient may be placed on his or her non-affected side.

Incision

A A longitudinal incision is made just posterior to the crest of the fibula. It is continued proximally to the head of the fibula in line with the tendon of biceps femoris.

Tibia and fibula

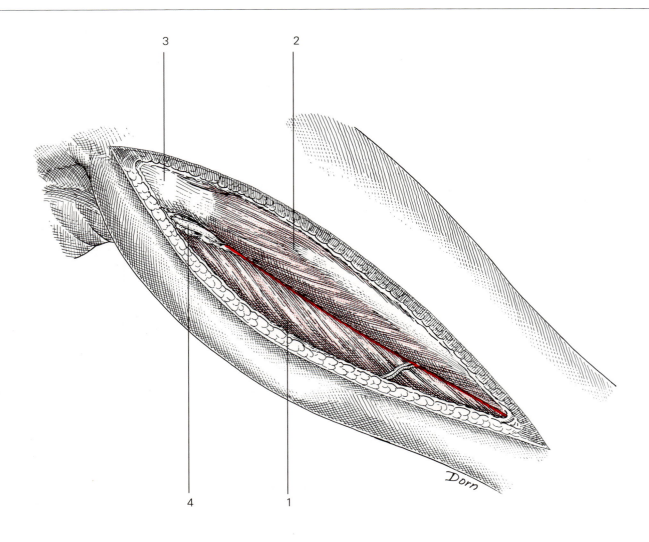

Exposure

B The first step is the identification of the common peroneal nerve (see pages 365-7). The skin is gently retracted and proximally the fascia is carefully incised. The common peroneal nerve is identified just posterior to the tendon of biceps femoris. It is isolated and dissected as far as the neck of the fibula, at which point the superficial fibres of peroneus longus are separated to expose the nerve. The nerve can be very gently drawn over the fibular head. Following this, the plane between the lateral and posterior compartments is identified by incising the fascia over the fibular crest.

B
1 gastrocnemius and soleus
2 peroneus longus
3 head of fibula
4 peroneal nerve

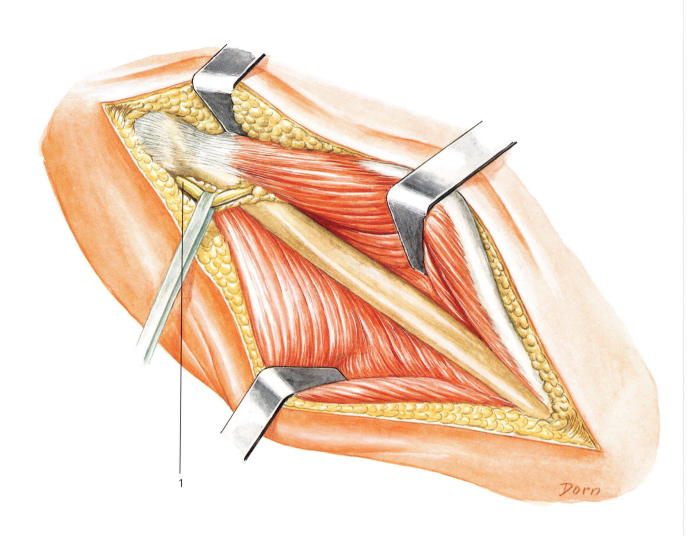

C Soleus (posteriorly) and the peronei (anteriorly) are released subperiosteally and retracted. In the middle third, flexor hallucis longus is detached from its insertion on the posterior aspect of the fibula.

C
1 peroneal nerve

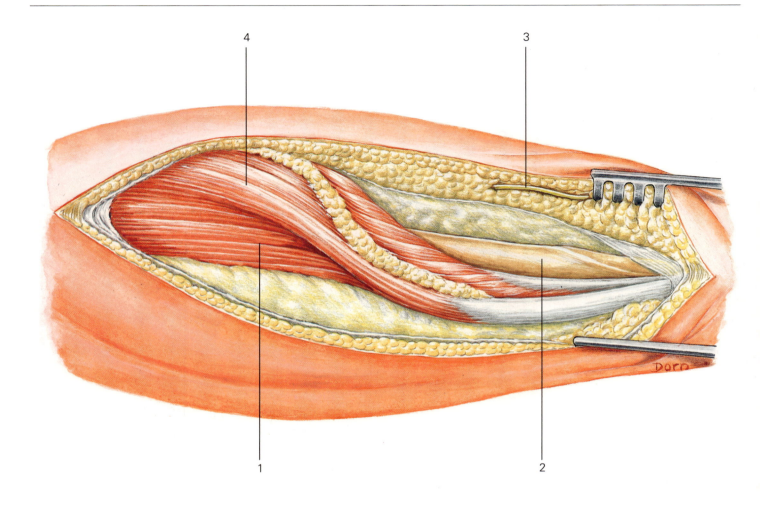

D Beyond the middle third, the peronei should be retracted posteriorly to expose the distal third of the bone.

D

1 peroneus longus
2 distal third of fibula
3 superficial peroneal nerve
4 peroneus brevis

E A cross-section shows the lateral approach to the fibula in the proximal two-thirds.

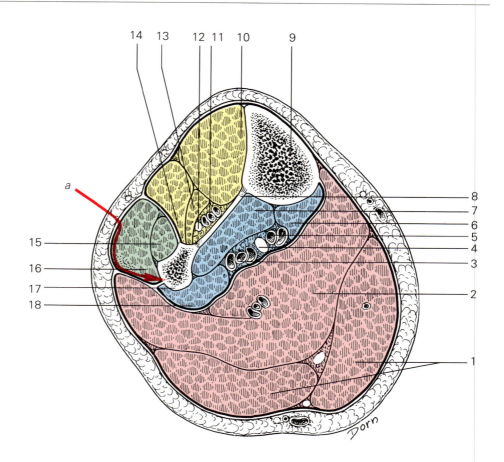

E

1 medial and lateral heads of gastrocnemius
2 soleus
3 peroneal artery and veins
4 tibial nerve
5 posterior tibial artery and veins
6 flexor digitorum longus
7 tibialis posterior
8 interosseous membrane
9 tibia
10 tibialis anterior
11 anterior tibial artery and veins
12 deep peroneal nerve
13 extensor hallucis longus
14 extensor digitorum longus
15 peroneus brevis
16 peroneus longus
17 fibula
18 flexor hallucis longus
a lateral approach to the fibula (proximal and middle third)

Tibia and fibula

F A cross-section shows the lateral approach to the fibula distal to the middle third.

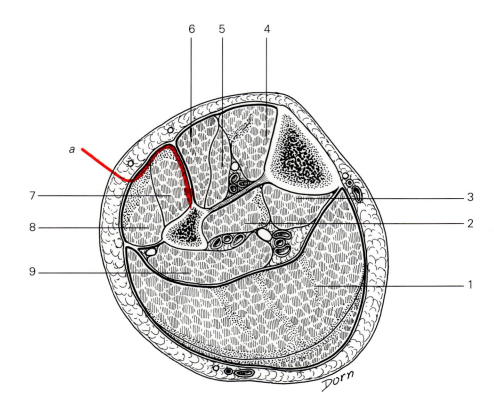

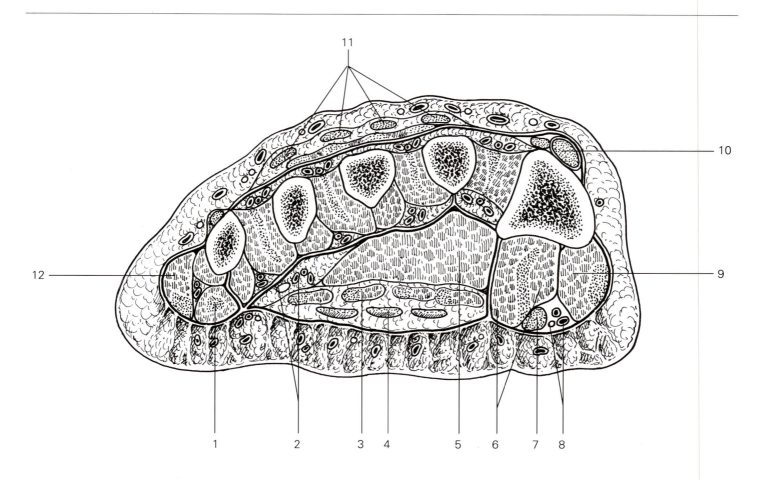

A,B Most foot surgery is performed from the dorsal surface and the sole is avoided unless there is a special reason such as the resection of a Morton's neuroma. Incisions on the sole heal well because the blood supply is excellent but access to the deep surface of the foot is not often needed. The muscles on the sole of the foot are traditionally grouped in four layers but the details of the layers do not have great clinical significance. Abductor hallucis, as pointed out by AK Henry, is 'the door to a vaulted cage that opens widely at the inner sole'. If the muscle belly is mobilized on its superior surface it can be turned towards the plantar surface and the cage can be opened. If the incision is extended proximally up the leg to expose the neurovascular bundle, one can then even expose the medial surface of the calcaneum which may sometimes be necessary for the open reduction of calcaneal fractures.

B

1 flexor digiti minimi brevis
2 lateral plantar nerve and artery
3 flexor digitorum longus tendon
4 flexor digitorum brevis tendon
5 adductor hallucis
6 medial and lateral heads of flexor hallucis brevis
7 flexor hallucis longus tendon
8 medial plantar artery and nerve
9 abductor hallucis
10 extensor hallucis longus tendon
11 extensor digitorum longus tendons
12 abductor digiti minimi

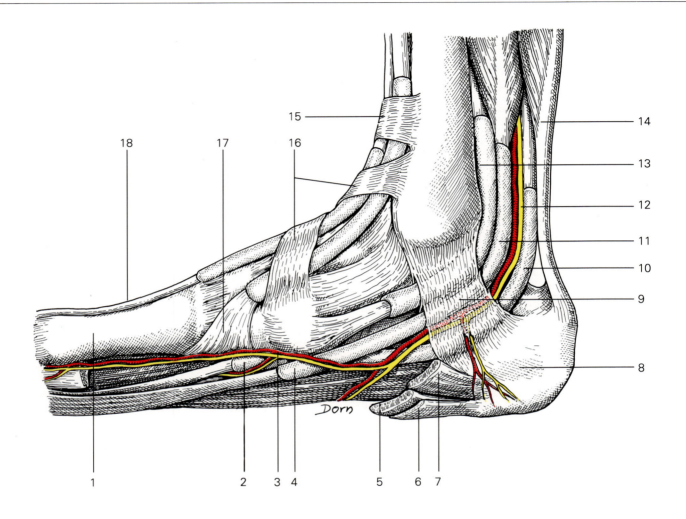

C The most important structures lie on the medial side of the ankle in the tarsal tunnel. This region is not truly comparable to the carpal tunnel in so far as tendons do not lie free but in fibro-osseous tunnels, that is, tibialis posterior, flexor digitorum longus and flexor hallucis longus. The flexor retinaculum is much thinner than the transverse carpal ligament at the wrist. The only structure which lies free is the neurovascular bundle and this should be carefully protected and isolated in a sling in all surgical approaches to the medial side of the ankle and foot.

C

1 first metatarsal
2 sheath of flexor hallucis longus tendon
3 medial plantar artery and nerve
4 sheath of flexor digitorum longus tendon
5 flexor digitorum brevis, cut
6 plantar aponeurosis, cut
7 abductor hallucis, cut
8 os calcis
9 flexor retinaculum
10 sheath of flexor hallucis longus tendon

11 sheath of flexor digitorum longus tendon
12 posterior tibial artery and tibial nerve
13 sheath of tibialis posterior tendon
14 Achilles tendon
15 superior extensor retinaculum
16 inferior extensor retinaculum
17 tibialis anterior tendon
18 extensor hallucis longus tendon

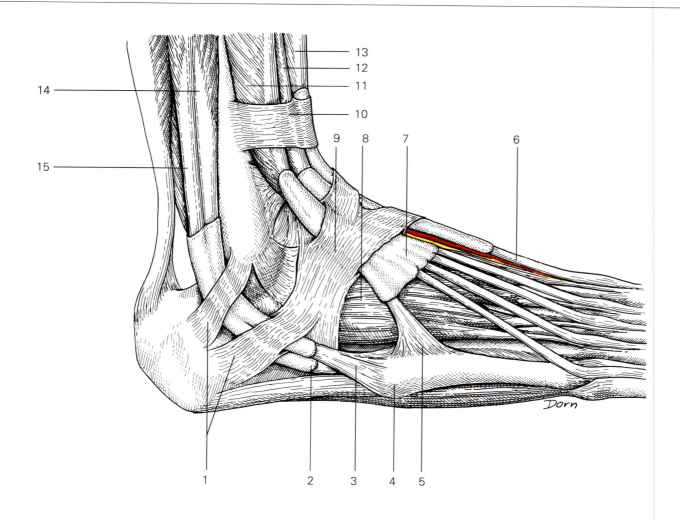

D   On the lateral side of the foot, extensor digitorum brevis is a key structure, because elevation of this muscle belly in a distal direction will give a clear exposure of the subtalar joints.

D

1 superior and inferior peroneal retinacula
2 peroneus longus tendon
3 peroneus brevis tendon
4 tuberosity of fifth metatarsal
5 peroneus tertius tendon
6 extensor hallucis longus tendon
7 sheath of extensor digitorum longus and peroneus tertius tendons
8 extensor digitorum brevis
9 inferior extensor retinaculum
10 superior extensor retinaculum
11 extensor digitorum longus
12 extensor hallucis longus
13 tibialis anterior
14 peroneus brevis
15 peroneus longus

Ankle and foot

E The skin on the dorsal aspects of the foot is thin and there is little subcutaneous fat. All the underlying structures are readily palpated through the thin skin covering.

E

1 extensor hallucis longus tendon
2 arcuate artery
3 dorsalis pedis artery and medial branch of deep peroneal nerve
4 synovial sheath of extensor hallucis longus tendon
5 synovial sheath of tibialis anterior tendon
6 superior extensor retinaculum
7 anterior tibial artery and deep peroneal nerve
8 tibialis anterior tendon
9 peroneus longus tendon
10 extensor digitorum longus
11 peroneus brevis
12 synovial sheath of extensor digitorum tendons
13 inferior extensor retinaculum
14 extensor digitorum brevis
15 peroneus tertius tendon
16 extensor digitorum longus tendons

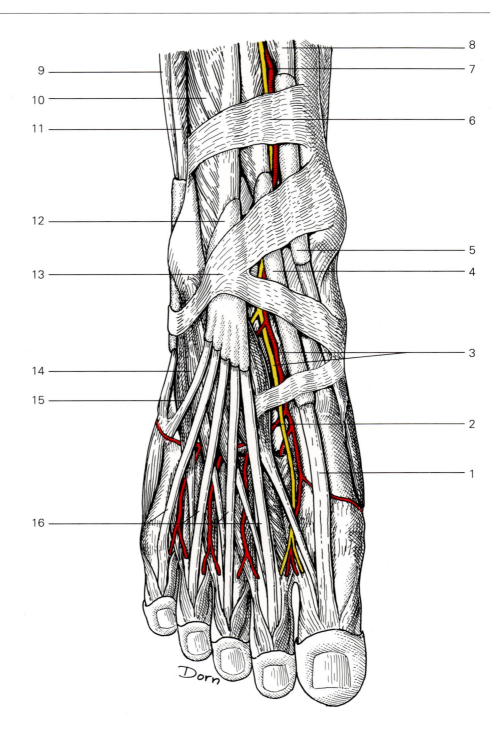

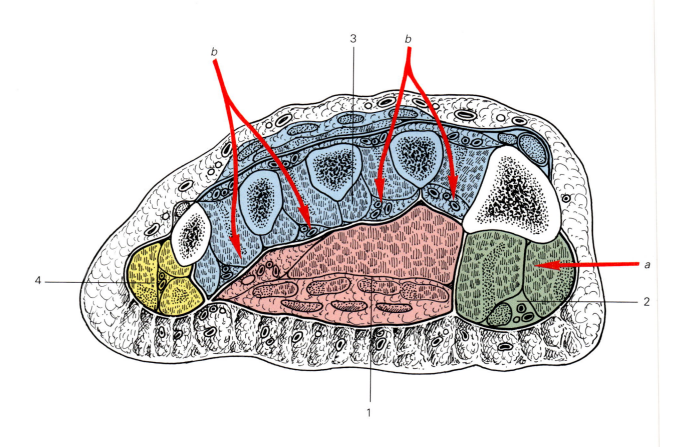

F Compartment syndromes of the foot have only recently been recognized and may result from crush injuries and require decompression. There are four compartments. The medial and lateral compartments contain the muscles running along their respective borders. A central compartment is bounded by the plantar aponeurosis inferiorly and the intermuscular septae medially and laterally. The interosseous compartment is bounded by the interosseous fascia and the metatarsals and contains the seven interossei. Decompression of the foot can be carried out through a single medial incision along the length of the inferior surface of the first metatarsal. The dorsal approach utilizes two longitudinal incisions along the length of the second and fourth metatarsals.

F
1 central compartment
2 medial compartment
3 interosseous compartment
4 lateral compartment
a medial incision
b dorsal incisions along the second and fourth metatarsals

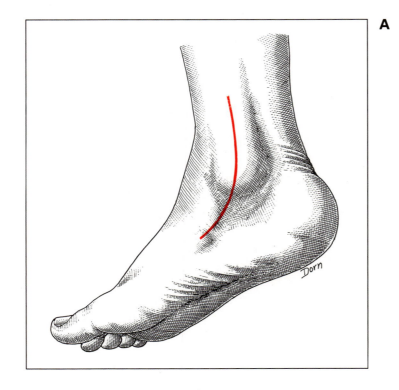

Anteromedial approach to the ankle

Indications

- Surgery to the medial malleolus following fracture.
- Exploration for osteochondritis dissecans of the talus.

Incision

A This starts about 5 cm proximal to the tip of the medial malleolus, passes across the joint and then curves posteriorly ending 1 or 2 cm below the medial malleolus.

Exposure

B The long saphenous nerve and vein which lie in the anterosuperior part of the wound must not be damaged. A longitudinal incision along the anterior margin of the deltoid ligament and retraction of the anterior capsule laterally will give access to the anteromedial portion of the ankle joint.

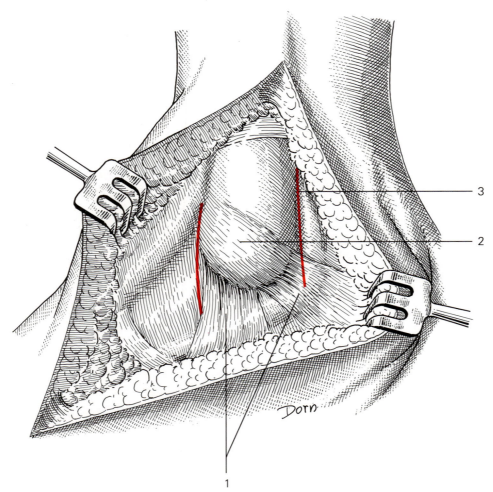

B

1 deltoid ligament
2 medial malleolus
3 posterior incision for mobilization of medial malleolus

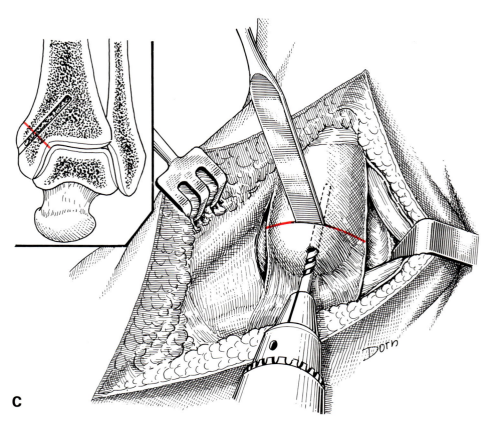

C

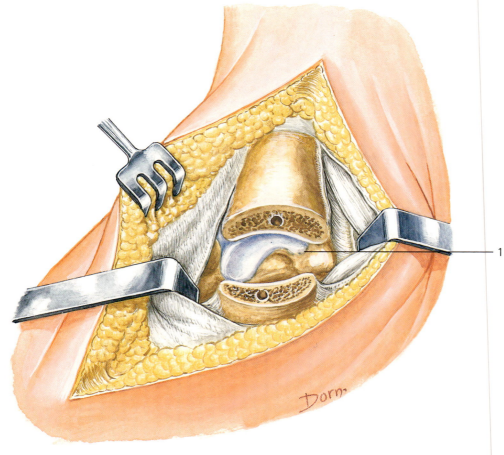

D

C For better access it may occasionally be necessary to carry out an osteotomy of the medial malleolus. This is best performed in an oblique line with a power saw. The attachment to the deltoid ligament must be carefully preserved. To make reattachment of this bony fragment easier, it is best to drill the hole for the lag screw before the osteotomy is performed.

D The medial malleolus is retracted inferiorly to expose the medial talar dome.

1 talus

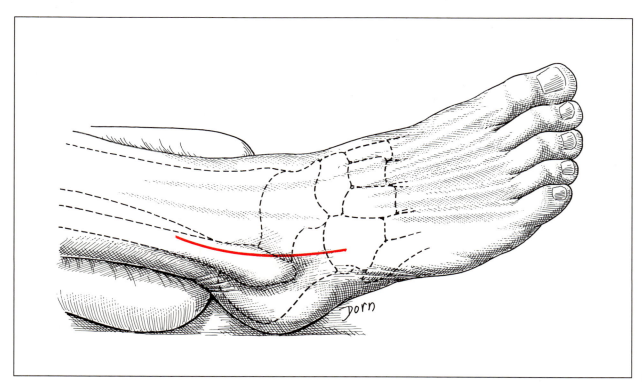

A

Anterolateral approach to the ankle

Indications

- Internal fixation of the lateral malleolus.
- Inspection of the anterior tibiofibular joint.
- Opening the lateral aspect of the ankle joint.
- Gaining access to the anterior and middle band of the lateral collateral ligament.

Position of the patient

The patient is supine with a sandbag under the buttock of the side to be operated upon.

Incision

A A slightly curved longitudinal incision about 10 cm long is made over the lateral malleolus and extended distally to pass across the ankle joint.

B

1 superior extensor retinaculum
2 superficial peroneal nerve

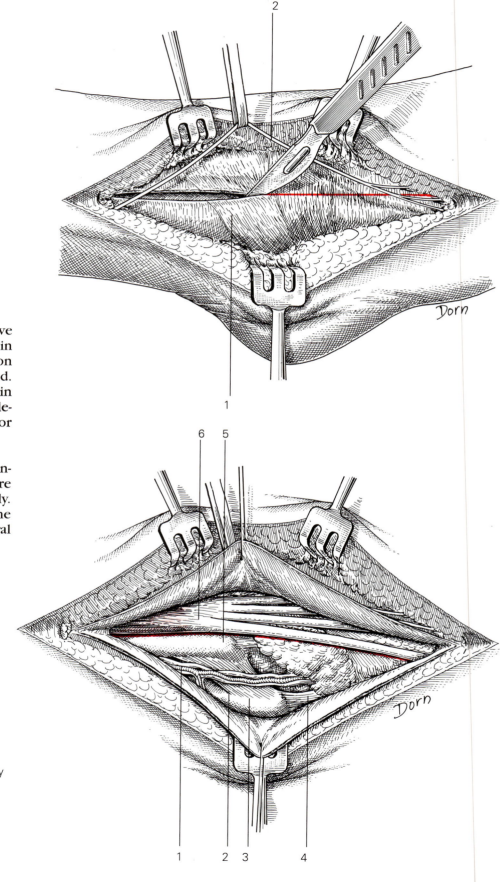

Exposure

B The superficial peroneal nerve lies in the subcutaneous tissues in the anterior part of the incision and must not be damaged. Dissection of the posterior skin flap will expose the lateral malleolus. The superior extensor retinaculum is incised.

C The lateral tendons of extensor digitorum longus are mobilized and retracted medially. The perforating branch of the peroneal artery lies to the lateral side of the ankle capsule.

C

1 perforating branch of peroneal artery
2 anterior tibiofibular ligament
3 lateral malleolus
4 calcaneofibular ligament
5 tibia
6 extensor digitorum longus muscle
  and tendons

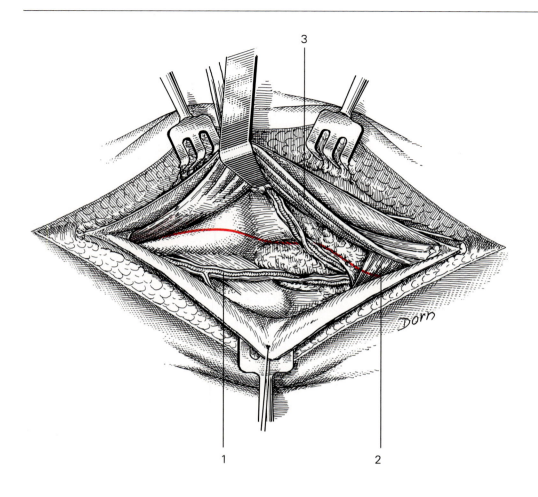

D The anterior capsule of the ankle can be clearly seen and, when incised in the line of the skin incision, it will give access to the anterolateral aspect of the talus and the inner side of the fibular malleolus.

D

1 perforating branch of peroneal artery
2 extensor digitorum brevis
3 extensor digitorum longus tendons, retracted

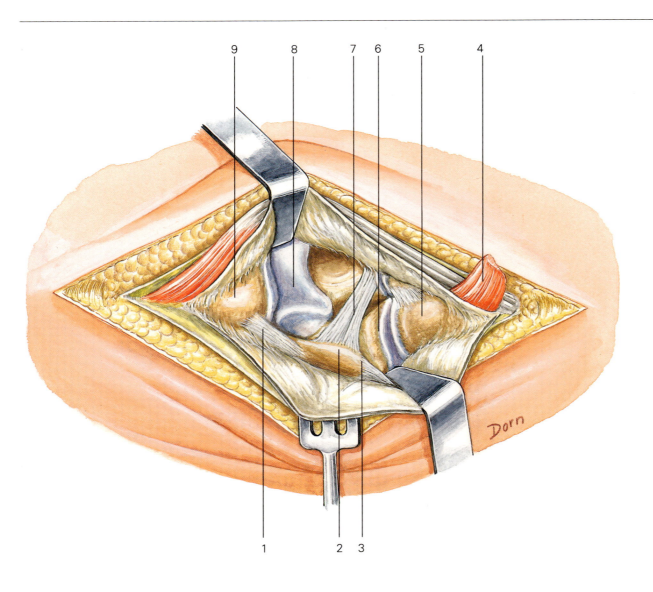

E To expose the calcaneofibular band of the lateral ligament of the ankle, the inferior peroneal retinaculum is incised and the peroneal tendons are retracted. Incision of the capsule allows exposure of the lateral aspect of the ankle joint. Where it is intended to carry out an ankle arthrodesis, osteotomy of the distal fibular shaft and a complete resection of the distal fibula will produce an excellent view of the lateral surface of the ankle joint (see pp. 237-9). The incision can be extended distally to the level of extensor digitorum brevis which can be mobilized from its origin on the calcaneum to reveal the subtalar and calcaneocuboid joints.

E

1 anterior tibiofibular ligament
2 lateral malleolus
3 calcaneofibular ligament
4 extensor digitorum brevis, released proximally and retracted
5 cuboid
6 calcaneum
7 anterior talofibular ligament
8 talar dome
9 tibia

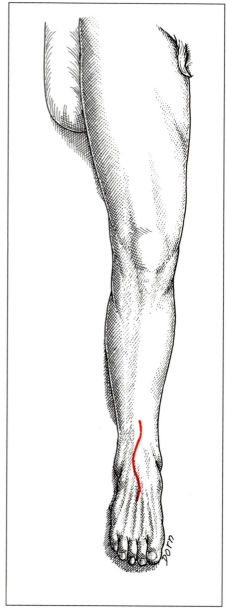

A

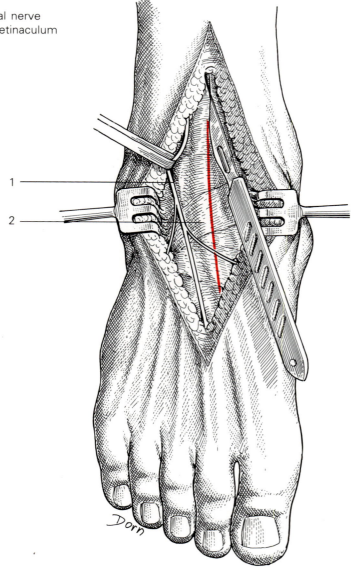

B
1 superficial peroneal nerve
2 inferior extensor retinaculum

Anterior approach to the ankle

Indications

- Ankle arthrodesis.
- Ankle arthroplasty.

Position of the patient

The patient lies supine.

Incision

A The incision is midway between the medial and lateral malleoli and extends from a point about 10 cm above the joint line to end 5 cm below it. As the incision passes across the front of the ankle joint, it is preferable to make it slightly curved above and below the joint, in the shape of a lazy 'S'.

Exposure

B The deep fascia is reinforced by the superior and inferior retinacula. Both retinacula are divided in the line of the skin incision. The superficial peroneal nerve is isolated and retracted.

C The tendons of extensor digitorum longus are retracted laterally to expose the deep peroneal nerve and the dorsalis pedis artery and veins. The anterior malleolar and lateral tarsal arteries are ligated and divided to allow the dorsalis pedis vessels to be mobilized and retracted medially with the deep peroneal nerve.

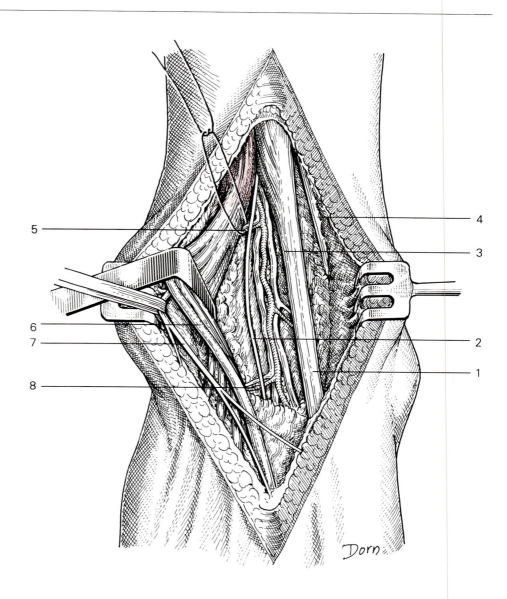

C

1 extensor hallucis longus tendon
2 deep peroneal nerve
3 dorsalis pedis artery
4 tibialis anterior
5 anterior malleolar artery
6 extensor digitorum longus tendons, retracted
7 superficial peroneal nerve
8 lateral tarsal artery

D,E The anterior ankle capsule is thus exposed and incised transversely to give a clear view of the anterior aspect of the tibiotalar joint.

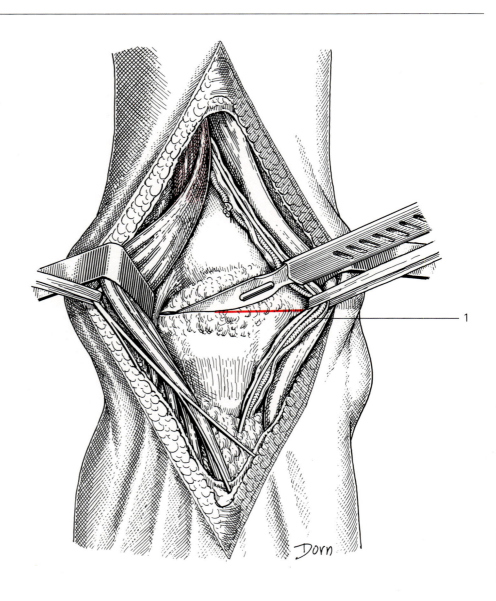

D

1 dorsalis pedis artery and deep peroneal nerve, retracted

E

1 anterior talar dome

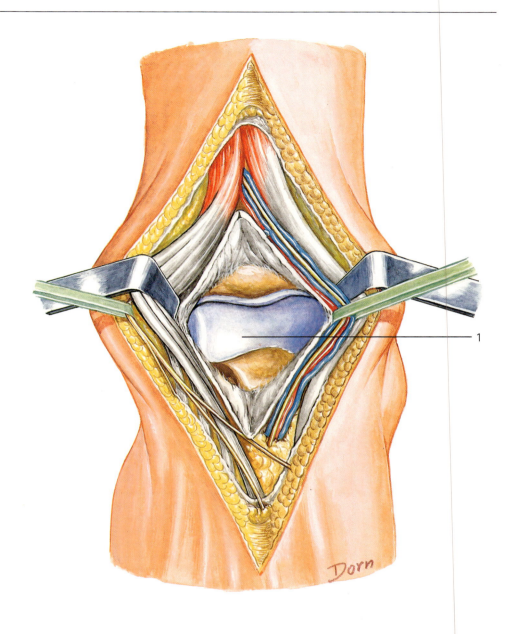

1

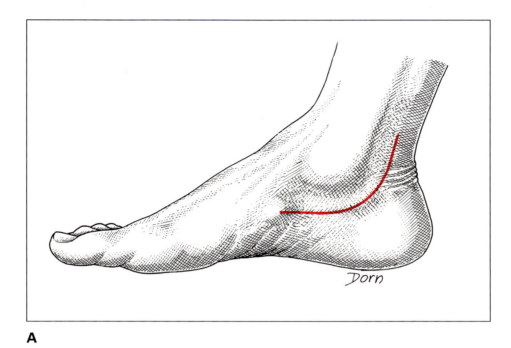

A

Posteromedial approach to the ankle

Indications

- Surgery of club foot.
- Inspection of the deltoid ligament.
- Exposure of the medial surface of the calcaneum.
- Resection of a talocalcaneal bar from the subtalar joint.

Position of the patient

The patient lies supine.

Incision

A The skin incision passes down the line of the limb from a point 5 cm above the medial malleolus in the interval between the Achilles tendon and the medial border of the tibia. At the level of the medial malleolus, there is a forward curve towards the navicular tuberosity.

Exposure

B The deep fascia and the flexor retinaculum are split longitudinally. It is essential to identify the neurovascular bundle, comprising the posterior tibial artery and tibial nerve, as early as possible and to protect it by a Silastic sling passed around it so that it can be safely retracted when necessary.

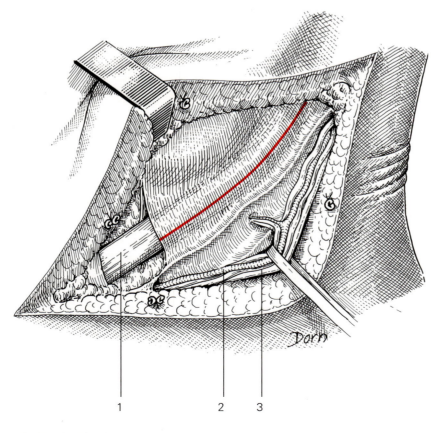

1   2   3

B

1 tibialis posterior tendon
2 posterior tibial artery
3 tibial nerve

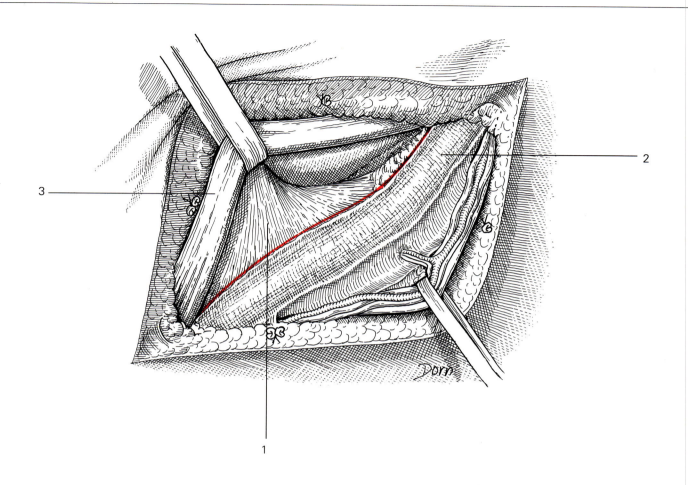

C Division of the sheath of tibialis posterior and displacement of the tendon anteriorly will expose the deltoid ligament.

c

1 deltoid ligament (tibiocalcaneal ligament)
2 tendon of flexor digitorum longus within its sheath
3 tibialis posterior tendon, retracted

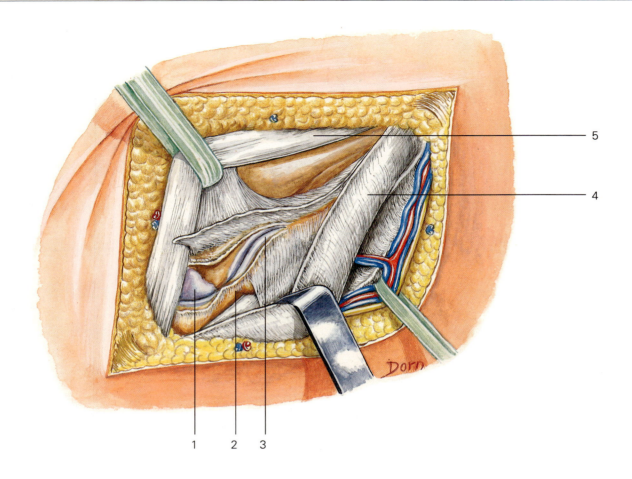

D The posterior capsule of the ankle and subtalar joint can be reached quite easily especially if the Achilles tendon has been divided, as is the case with club foot surgery.

To expose the subtalar joint to resect a talocalcaneal bar, it is necessary to open the gap between tibialis posterior and flexor digitorum longus.

To display the medial surface of the calcaneum, flexor digitorum longus, the neurovascular bundle and flexor hallucis longus are retracted anteriorly whilst abductor hallucis is mobilized by division of the fascia along the superior border of the muscle and the belly is displaced towards the plantar surface.

D

1 head of talus
2 sustentaculum tali
3 subtalar joint
4 flexor digitorum longus tendon, retracted
5 tibialis posterior tendon, retracted

Posterolateral approach to the ankle

Indications

This provides an excellent view of the posterior aspect of the ankle and subtalar joint, and is invaluable for the release of the lateral tethering structures for a club foot. It also provides access to the posterior surface of the distal tibia and fibula which is useful for internal fixation of ankle fractures.

Position of the patient

The patient should be prone with the foot hanging downwards over the edge of the operating table.

Incision

A The skin incision is placed parallel to the lateral border of the Achilles tendon posterior to the sural nerve and short saphenous vein, and extends distally below the lateral malleolus to the level of the calcaneocuboid joint (dotted line).

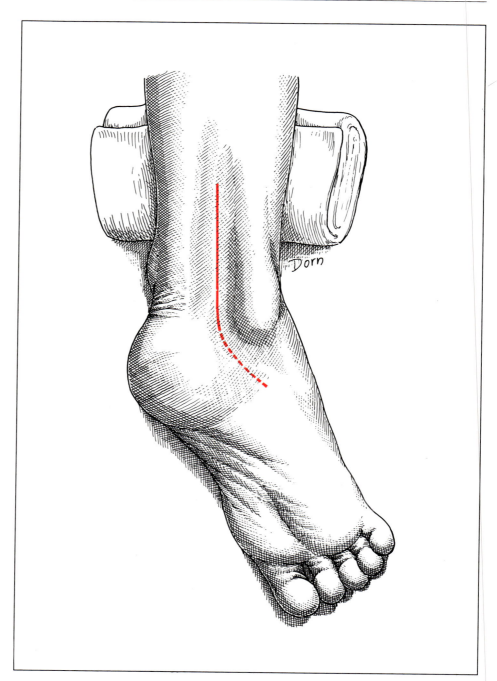

A

Exposure

B Care must be taken to avoid damage to the sural nerve which lies adjacent to the short saphenous vein. These structures are retracted laterally and the dissection continued deep to the Achilles tendon. The gap between flexor hallucis longus medially and the peroneal tendons laterally can be opened to expose the distal surface of the tibia and the posterior aspect of the ankle and subtalar joints.

B

1 sural nerve
2 short saphenous vein

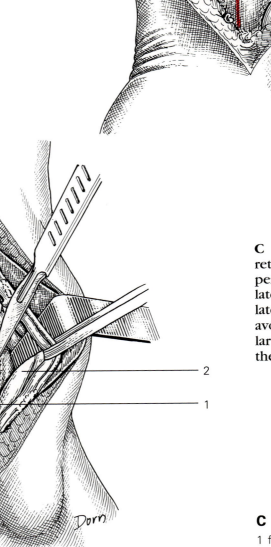

C Flexor hallucis longus is retracted medially and the peroneal tendons are retracted laterally. It is essential to remain lateral to flexor hallucis longus to avoid damage to the neurovascular bundle which runs posterior to the medial malleolus.

C

1 flexor hallucis longus
2 peroneus brevis tendon

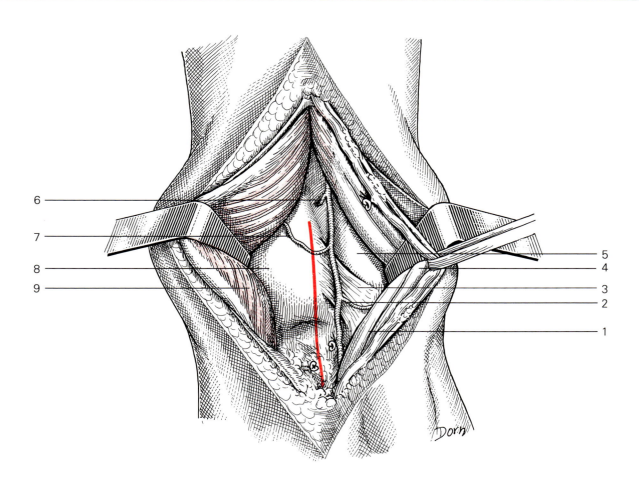

D To see the distal fibula, it is necessary to incise the peroneal tendon sheath; the tendons are retracted anteriorly. The ankle joint can be exposed via a longitudinal posterior incision.

D

1 peroneus brevis tendon
2 posterior lateral malleolar branch of peroneal artery
3 posterior tibiofibular ligament
4 peroneus longus tendon
5 fibula
6 perforating branch of peroneal artery
7 communicating branch of peroneal artery
8 tibia
9 flexor hallucis longus, retracted

E More distal dissection will allow exposure of the lateral aspect of the subtalar and calcaneocuboid joints.

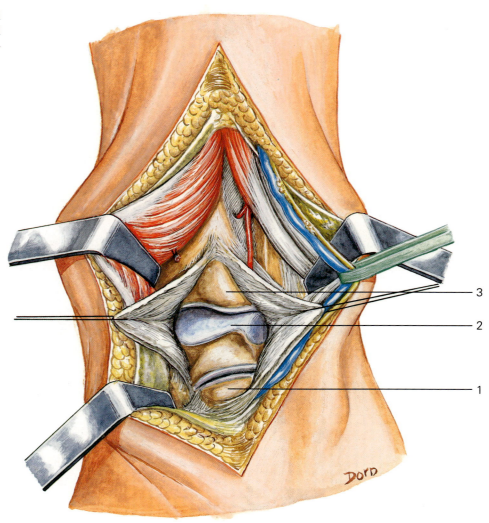

E

1 calcaneum
2 talus
3 tibia

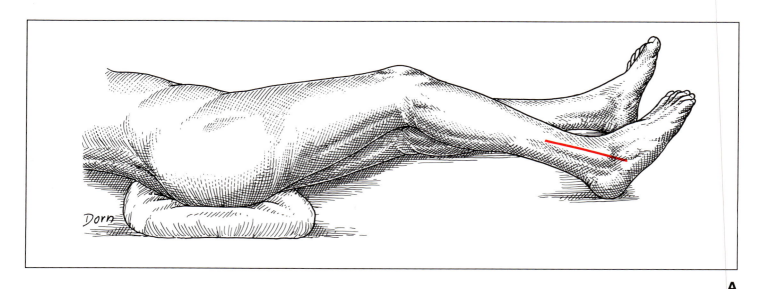

A

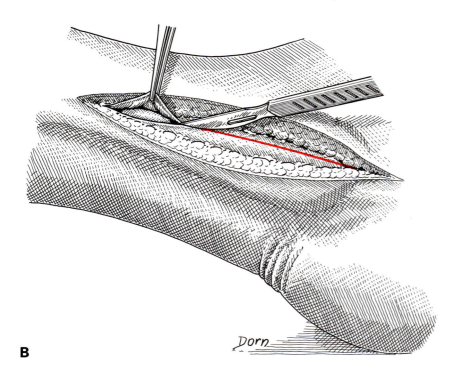

B

Position of the patient

The patient lies supine.

Incision

A The incision passes from the level of the lower third of the fibula down the lateral ridge of the malleolus into the foot to the fleshy bulk of extensor digitorum brevis.

Exposure

B The deep fascia is incised longitudinally. The fibula is to be exposed and osteotomized 5 cm proximal to the ankle joint and the distal fragment retracted distally and posteriorly. However, if there is a fracture of the lower third of the fibula, the distal fragment can be dissected free and turned distally towards the heel based on its attachments to the calcaneum and talus by the three components of the lateral ligament: the anterior talofibular, the calcaneofibular and the posterior talofibular bands.

Transfibular approach to the ankle

Indication

This is a useful approach for an ankle arthrodesis and for internal fixation of a posterior malleolar fracture. It provides a clear view of the lateral aspect of the joint and the whole anterior surface of the tibia can be seen except for the medial malleolus. If exposure of the medial malleolus is required, a separate medial incision should be made.

237

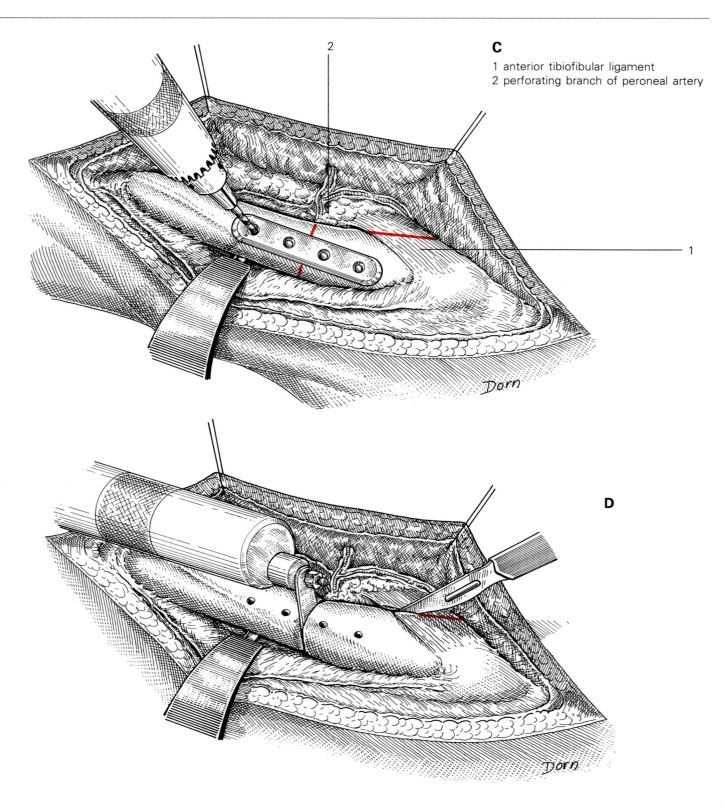

1 anterior tibiofibular ligament
2 perforating branch of peroneal artery

1

C   The plate to be used for internal fixation should be placed in position and the screw holes drilled prior to mobilization of the distal fibula. Once internal fixation of the posterior malleolus has been achieved, the fibula can be repositioned into normal alignment and fixed with a plate using the prepared screw holes.

D   The anterior tibiofibular ligament is incised to allow the rotation of the distal part of the fibula. The posterior tibiofibular ligament is left intact, as are the posterior muscular attachments of the distal fibula.

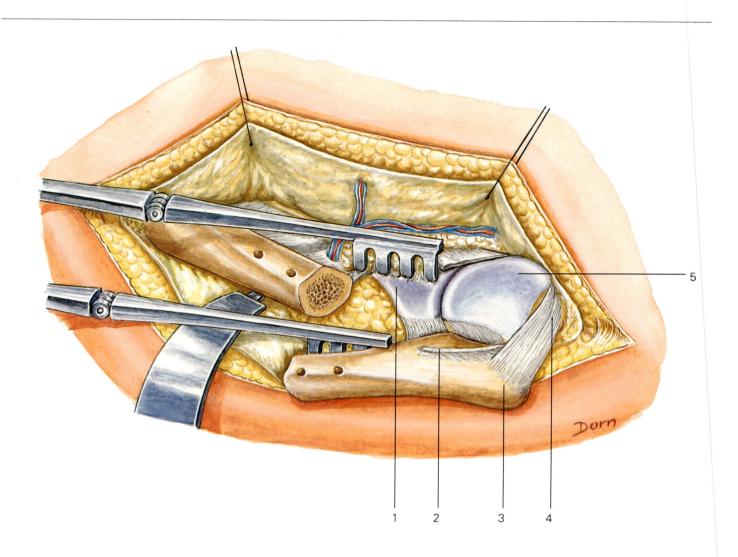

E   The lateral aspect of the ankle
joint is exposed. If the ankle joint
is to be arthrodesed, the articular
surfaces of the joint can be readily
denuded of cartilage. It is not
necessary to replace the fibula
because it is doubtful if it adds any
stability to the ankle arthrodesis.

E

1 tibia
2 anterior tibiofibular ligament, cut
3 lateral malleolus
4 anterior talofibular ligament
5 talus

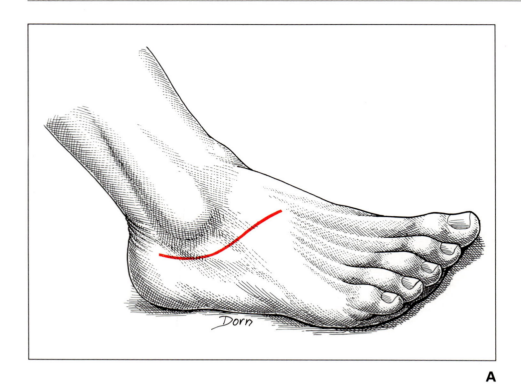

A

Lateral approach to the subtalar joint and midtarsal joints

Indications

This incision is required for a subtalar fusion which may be required after a calcaneal fracture, for a triple arthrodesis, for a Grice extra-articular arthrodesis of the subtalar joint or for resection of a calcaneonavicular bar.

Position of the patient

A sandbag placed beneath the buttock of the operated limb is used to counteract the natural tendency for the limb to rotate externally at the hip.

Incision

A The incision commences about 3–4 cm distal to the tip of the lateral malleolus; it then curves below the lateral malleolus and ends on the dorsomedial aspect of the foot over the talonavicular joint, about 1 cm proximal to the base of the first metatarsal.

Exposure

B The peroneus tertius and extensor digitorum longus tendons are exposed medially. The peroneal tendons lie parallel to the posterior flap of the incision.

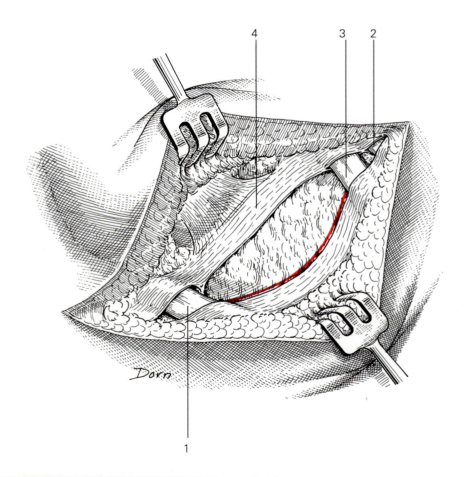

B

1 peroneus brevis and longus tendons
2 extensor digitorum longus tendon
3 peroneus tertius tendon
4 inferior extensor retinaculum

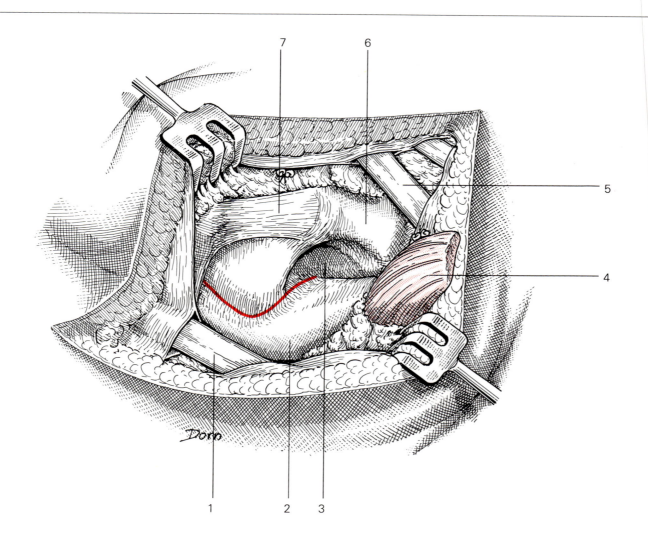

C   The extensor digitorum brevis muscle belly is clearly seen and is detached proximally from its attachment to the calcaneum. It is lifted forward towards the toes to expose the subtalar joint.

C

1 peroneus brevis and longus tendons
2 calcaneum
3 sinus tarsi
4 extensor digitorum brevis, retracted
5 peroneus tertius tendon
6 talus (head)
7 anterior talofibular ligament

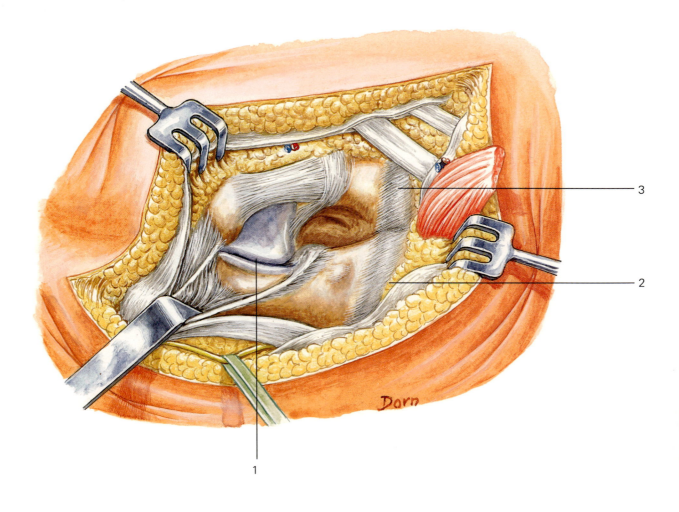

D   Further distal dissection will allow definition of the talonavicular and calcaneocuboid joints if this is required.

D

1 subtalar joint, opened
2 calcaneocuboid joint
3 talonavicular joint

Lateral approach to the calcaneum

Indications

This approach is used for calcaneal osteotomies or to expose the lateral surface of a fractured calcaneum. If used for the latter purpose, the proximal portion of the wound should be extended to allow for better exposure.

Position

The patient lies supine with a sandbag under the buttock of the operated limb.

Incision

A This is curved and passes from a point about 2–3 cm proximal to the tip of the lateral malleolus, parallel to the peroneal tendons; it ends near the base of the fifth metatarsal.

Exposure

B It is essential to avoid damage to the sural nerve which runs with the short saphenous vein in the anterior portion of the wound. The subcutaneous fat on the lateral surface of the calcaneum is divided in the line of the incision and reflected to expose the underlying bone.

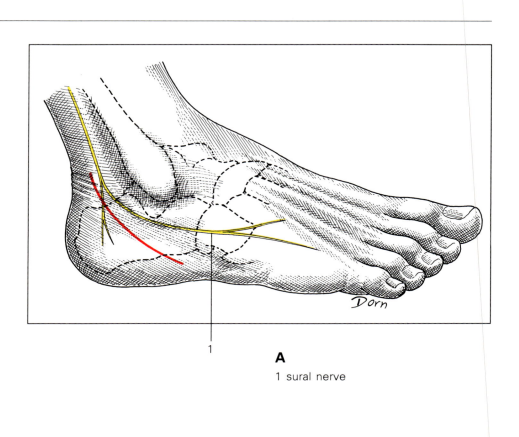

A

1 sural nerve

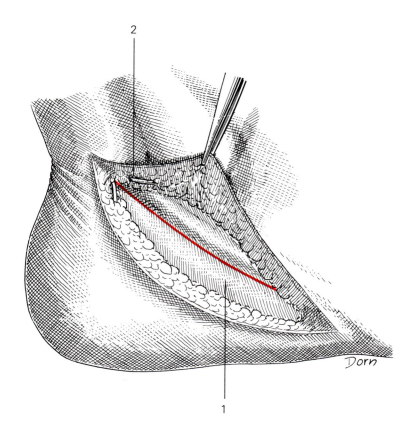

B

1 peroneal tendons
2 sural nerve

C   For a calcaneal osteotomy it is necessary to protect the insertion of the Achilles tendon by placing a bone lever superiorly between the tendon and the posterior aspect of the talus. The curved end of the lever is hooked over the medial surface of the calcaneum and marks the point where the osteotomy should start. A second lever should be inserted beneath the periosteum on the plantar surface to indicate the plantar end of the osteotomy, and the line of the osteotomy should be parallel to the peroneal tendons.

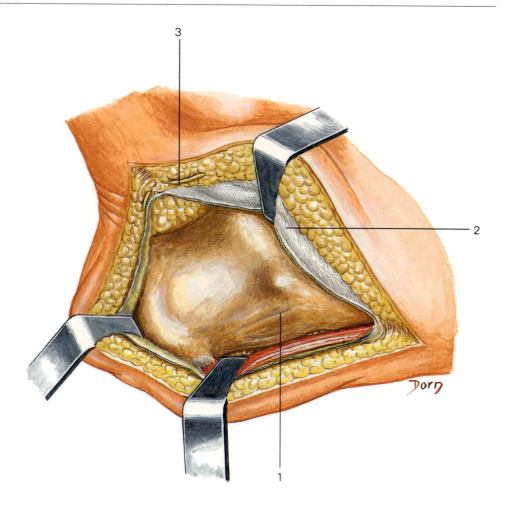

C

1 calcaneum
2 sheath of peroneus longus tendon
3 sural nerve

Dorsolateral approach to the foot

Indication

- Exposure of the calcaneocuboid joint in club foot surgery or following trauma to the base of the fifth metatarsal.

Position of the patient

The patient lies supine with a sandbag under the buttock of the operated limb.

Incision

A The incision passes from the tip of the lateral malleolus to the base of the fifth metatarsal.

Exposure

B On elevation of the skin flaps, care is taken to avoid the sural nerve which usually lies adjacent to the short saphenous vein. The insertion of peroneus brevis into the base of the fifth metatarsal is clearly seen with its articulation with the cuboid.

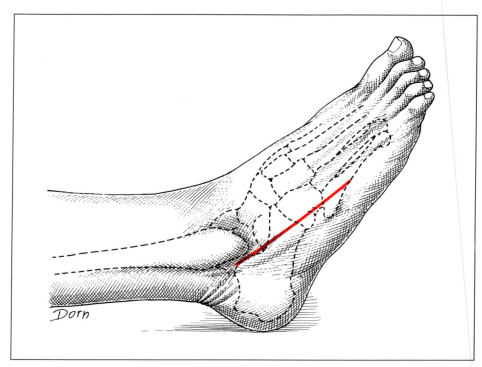

A

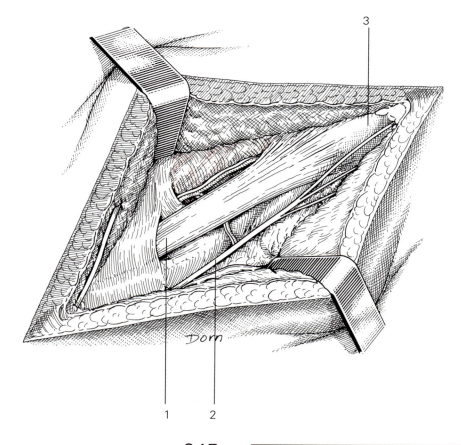

B

1 peroneus brevis tendon
2 sural nerve
3 tuberosity of fifth metatarsal

C Extensor digitorum brevis is released and retracted.

D The calcaneocuboid joint and the joint between the cuboid and the base of the fifth metatarsal are exposed.

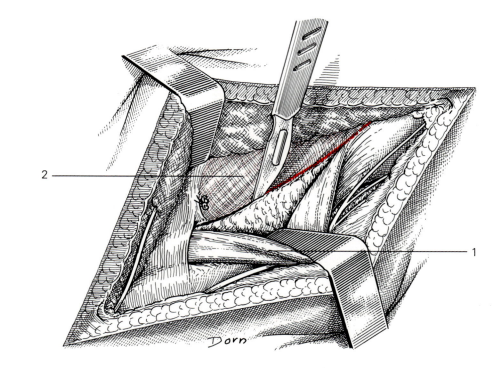

C

1 peroneus brevis tendon, retracted
2 extensor digitorum brevis

D

1 peroneus brevis tendon
2 calcaneum
3 peroneus longus tendon
4 base of fifth metatarsal
5 cuboid
6 extensor digitorum brevis, retracted

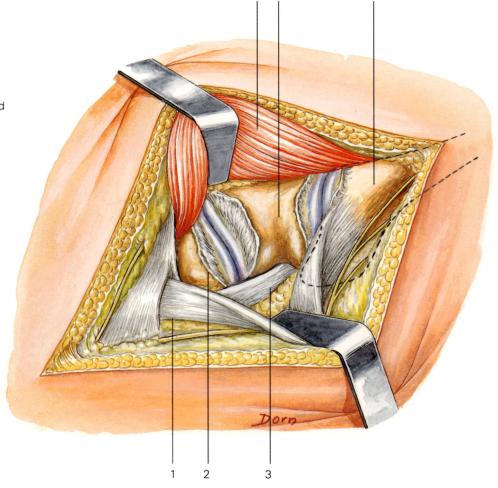

Dorsomedial approach to the foot

Indications

This incision can be used for exposure of the joints on the inner side of the foot, for bony procedures for flat foot, or soft tissue surgery to the cavus foot. In its posterior third, the incision can be used for exposure of the medial surface of the calcaneum for fracture fixation.

Position of the patient

The patient lies supine.

Incision

A The incision runs from the ball of the great toe to the heel. The most anterior part of the incision passes over the navicular tuberosity. Posteriorly the incision may be directed proximally or towards the plantar surface of the heel according to the exposure required.

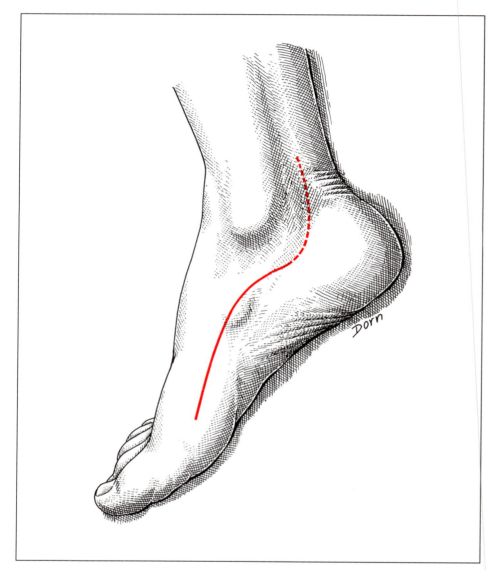

A

Ankle and foot

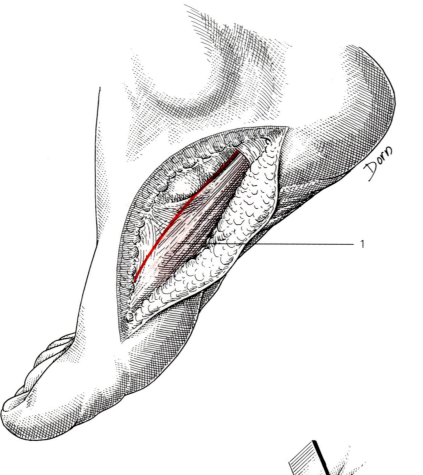

Exposure

B The skin flap is reflected towards the plantar surface and the tendon of abductor hallucis is identified on the medial side of the first metatarsal.

C The structures on the inner side of the foot can be exposed by turning abductor hallucis downwards based on its plantar attachments.

B

1 abductor hallucis

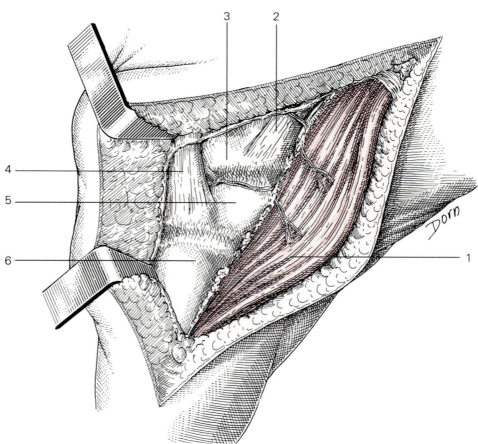

C

1 abductor hallucis, retracted
2 tibialis posterior tendon
3 navicular
4 tibialis anterior tendon
5 medial cuneiform
6 first metatarsal

D   The incision may be extended posteriorly and can be used for exposure of the medial surface of the calcaneum for open reduction of a fracture. To do this safely the neurovascular bundle must be retracted anteriorly after division of the flexor retinaculum. Blunt dissection can then be used to clear the medial surface of the calcaneum.

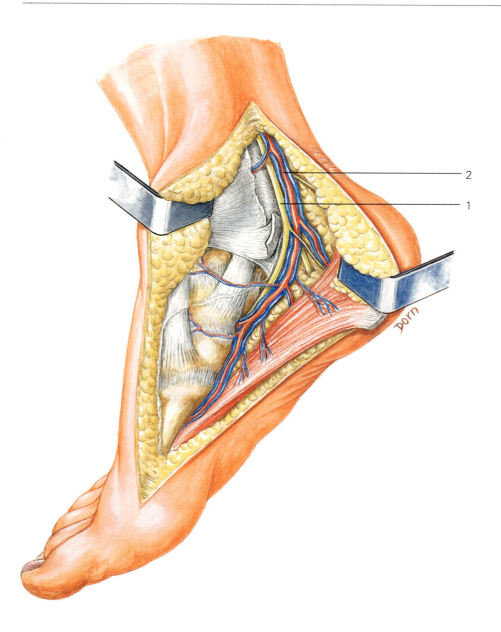

D

1 tibial nerve
2 posterior tibial artery

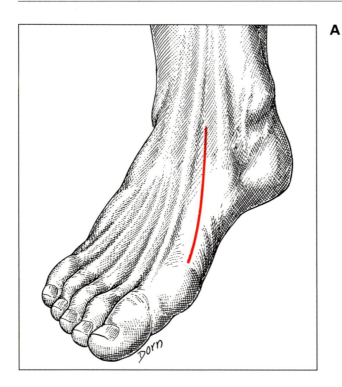

A

First tarsal column: dorsal approach

Indications

- Basal osteotomy of the first metatarsal shaft.
- Removal of an exostosis at the cuneiform metatarsal joint.

Position of the patient

The patient lies supine.

Incision

A The incision is parallel and medial to the extensor hallucis longus tendon commencing proximal to the navicular tuberosity and ending over the midshaft of the hallux metatarsal.

Exposure

B The skin is reflected. The tendon of tibialis anterior is identified at its insertion into the medial cuneiform and the base of the first metatarsal. Extensor hallucis longus lies under the lateral skin flap.

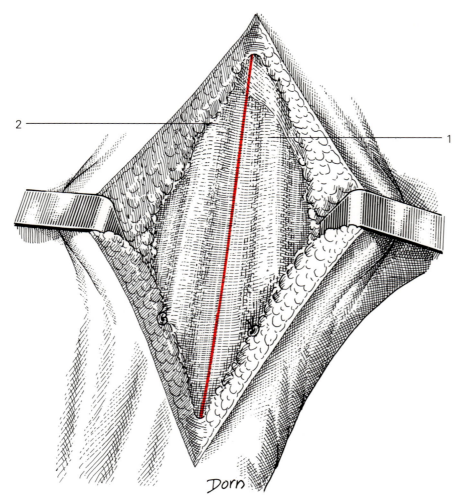

B

1 tibialis anterior tendon
2 extensor hallucis longus tendon

C It is safe to work between the two tendons which are retracted to expose the navicular, the medial cuneiform and the base of the first metatarsal.

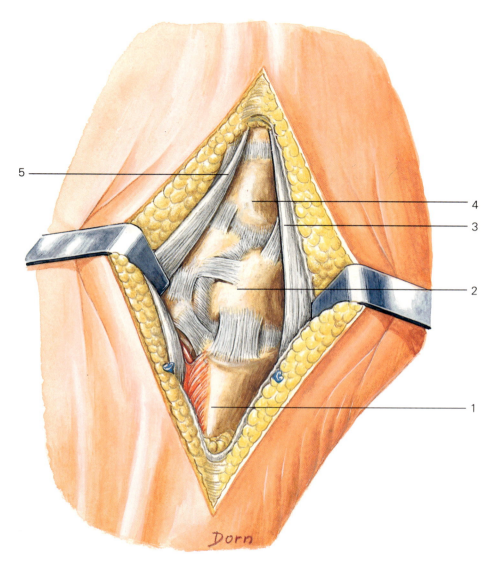

Dorn

C

1 first metatarsal
2 medial cuneiform
3 tibialis anterior tendon
4 navicular
5 extensor hallucis longus tendon

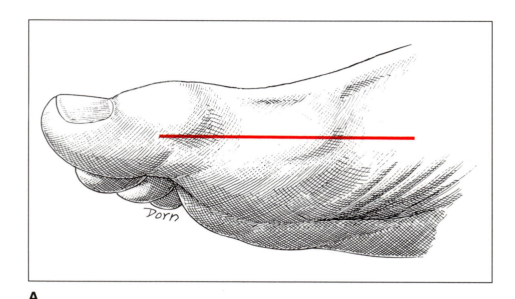

A

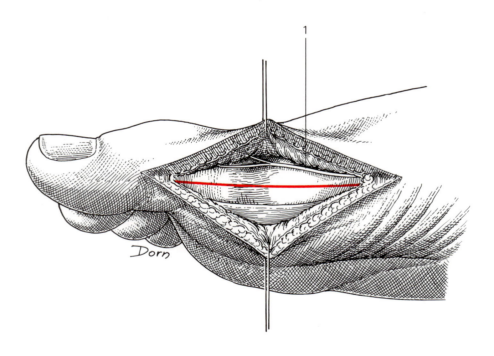

B

1 dorsal digital nerve

Exposure of the metatarsophalangeal joint of the great toe

Indications

- Distal metatarsal osteotomy.
- Arthrodesis of the joint.

Position

The patient lies supine.

Incision

A A medial longitudinal incision about 7.5 cm long is made centred over the metatarsophalangeal joint.

Exposure

B When the skin flaps are reflected care is taken to avoid damage to the dorsomedial cutaneous branch supplying the great toe.

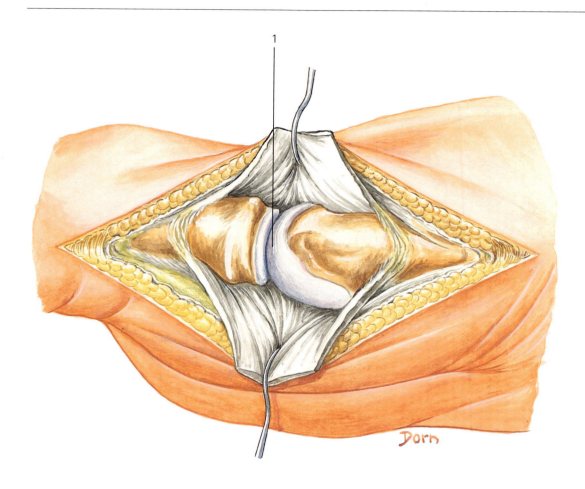

C   The metatarsophalangeal joint is readily exposed and opened in the line of the skin incision. The extensor hallucis longus tendon lies under the lateral skin flap and can easily be exposed if necessary, as, for example, for lengthening.

C

1 metatarsophalangeal joint

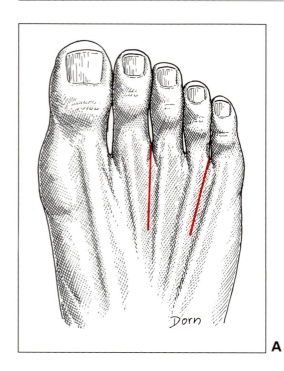

A

Exposure of the metatarsal heads for resection

Introduction

Forefoot arthroplasty in patients with rheumatoid arthritis is commonly performed to relieve metatarsalgia. Dorsal incisions are safer than those on the plantar surface because there is less likelihood of damage to the digital vessels and nerves. There is no need for a plantar approach because even marked callosities will regress spontaneously once the pressure distribution beneath the forefoot is returned to a more functional pattern.

Indication

• Relief of metatarsalgia.

Incision

A   The dorsal approach requires three incisions, one being medial to the great toe, as already described (see pages 252–3). The other two incisions are placed between the second and third metatarsal heads and the fourth and fifth metatarsal heads respectively.

Exposure

B   The incision passes in the cleft between the metatarsal heads. The extensor tendons are carefully protected. Bone levers are placed on either side of the metatarsal heads to provide exposure of the bone. The soft tissues on the dorsal aspect of the metatarsal head are cleared. The head may be difficult to see because it has prolapsed into the sole and is overlapped by the base of the proximal phalanx of the adjacent toe.

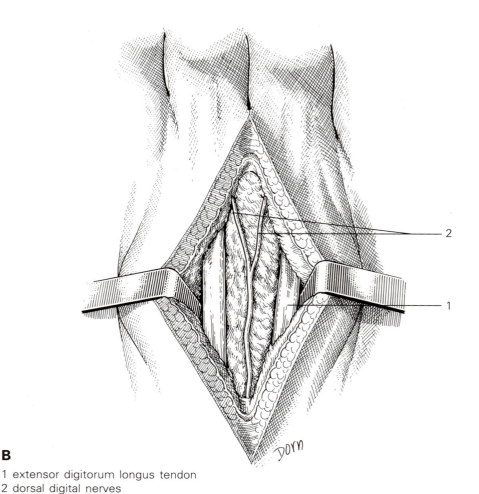

B

1 extensor digitorum longus tendon
2 dorsal digital nerves

C The neck of the metatarsal is divided with a power saw and the metatarsal head can then be extracted.

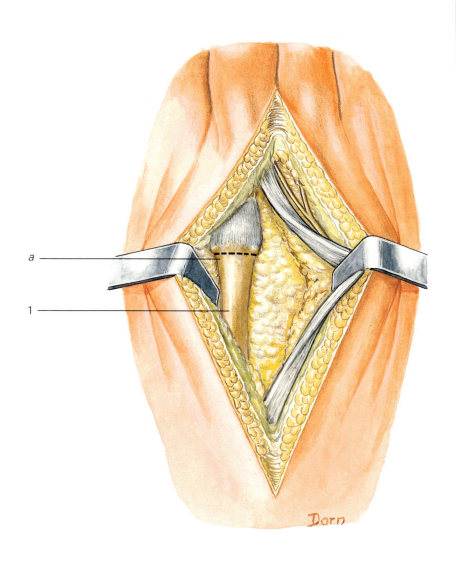

C

1 metatarsal
a level of division for head resection

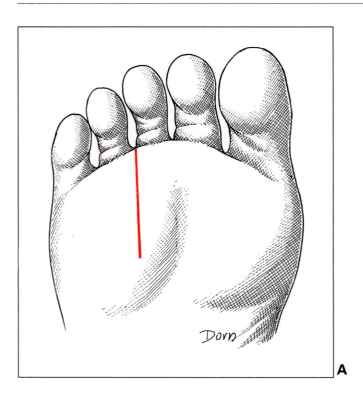

A

Approaches for the removal of digital neuromas

Introduction

There are two methods for removal of digital neuromas: plantar and dorsal. The advantage of the plantar approach is that the full length of the affected inter-metatarsal nerve can be exposed. The alleged disadvantage is that occasionally painful hypertrophic scars result. The dorsal approach provides a more limited exposure, heals rapidly and allows a rapid return to full activity.

Plantar approach

Incision

A A longitudinal incision 7.5 cm long is made on the line of the affected interspace.

Exposure

B The overlying fat must be cleared to show the space between the adjacent flexor tendon sheaths. The inter-metatarsal nerve to the affected cleft can be seen throughout its length ending in a Y-shaped bifurcation.

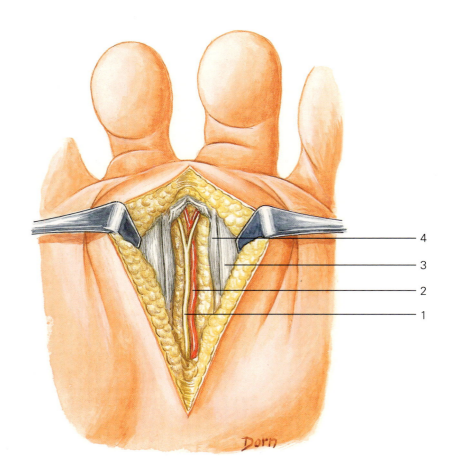

B

1 common plantar digital nerve
2 common plantar digital artery
3 flexor digitorum longus tendon
4 flexor digitorum brevis tendon

C

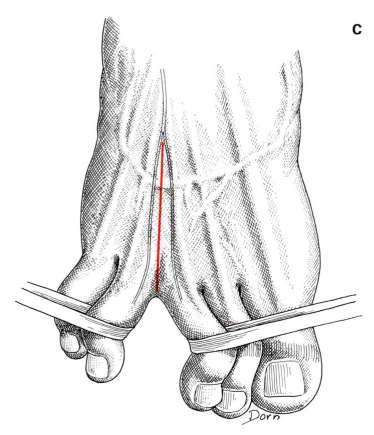

Dorsal approach

Incision

C An incision is made on the dorsal aspect of the affected interspace.

Exposure

D The deep fascia is incised in line with the skin incision.

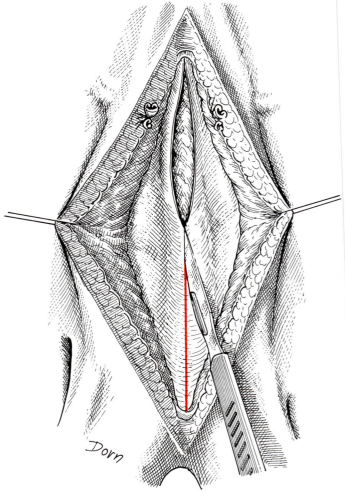

D

E

1 intermetatarsal ligament

E   The transverse intermetatarsal ligament is exposed in depth and must be divided.

F   After division of the transverse intermetatarsal ligament and separation of the metatarsal heads with a self-retaining retractor, the intermetatarsal nerve and its bifurcation can be pushed into view by pressure on the sole of the foot.

F

1 common plantar digital nerve and its bifurcation
2 intermetatarsal ligament, cut

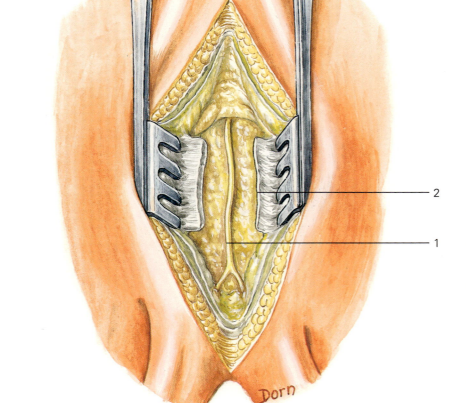

Posteromedial approach to the Achilles tendon

Introduction

Precise positioning of this incision is important because if it is placed on the lateral side of the tendon the sural nerve may be damaged. In addition, wound healing in this region is poor.

Indication

• Lengthening or repair of the Achilles tendon after a rupture.

Position of the patient

The patient should be prone with both feet hanging downwards over the edge of the operating table.

Incision

A The incision passes down the long axis of the limb slightly medial to the midline. It should end at the level of the transverse skin creases of the heel.

B Skin flaps are reflected. The Achilles tendon is readily found because it is subcutaneous in the distal third. The sheath is incised longitudinally.

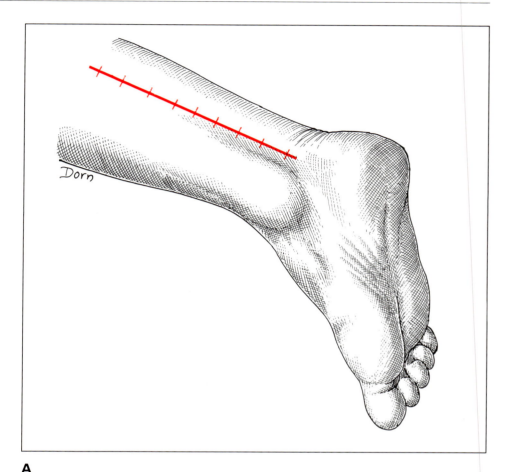

A

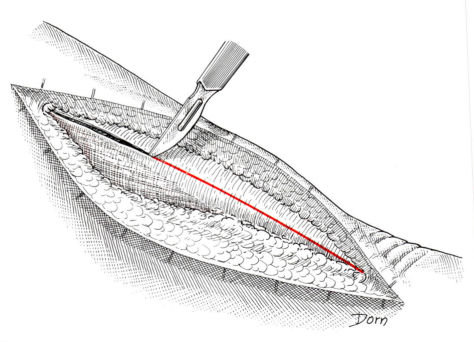

B

Ankle and foot

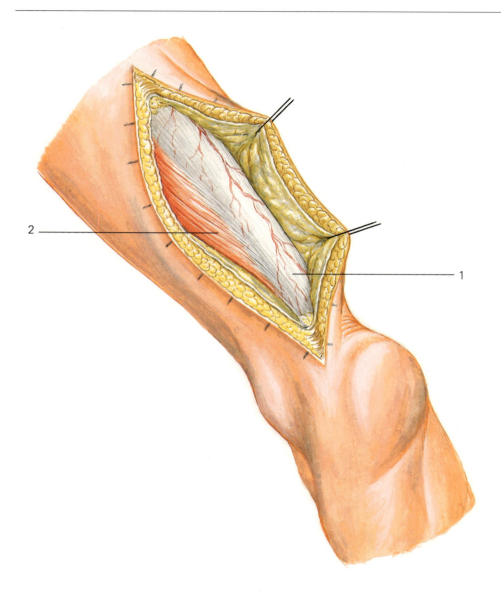

C Dissection of the lateral border should be performed with care to avoid damage to the sural nerve which runs with the short saphenous vein.

C
1 Achilles tendon
2 soleus

7

Arteries and veins

Introduction

Vascular surgery is much more frequently indicated in the lower limb than in the upper limb. Surgery for varicose veins is frequently performed. Additional procedures for the veins include thrombectomy and ligation. The long saphenous vein is often used as a graft in arterial reconstructive surgery. Arterial surgery is also commonly performed for peripheral vascular disease, traumatic lesions of the arteries and for the reconstruction of aneurysms.

Damage to the arteries of the lower limb is a relatively common occurrence. The popliteal artery may be injured by fractures or dislocations of the knee joint, whilst femoral shaft fractures may damage the femoral artery. The iatrogenic arterial lesions following hip surgery are well described. The anterior and posterior tibial arteries are often involved in severe fractures of the tibia and fibula, and compartment syndromes should also be considered in this regard.

Pathology of the venous system is largely dependent on the relationship between the deep and superficial veins. An imbalance between the two results in the development of varicosities. In the standing position, venous return depends in large part on contraction of the calf muscles. When the calf muscles contract, blood is pumped into the deep veins. The flow of blood to the superficial veins is normally prevented by valves in the perforating veins which connect the deep and superficial systems. At rest, blood can pass from the superficial to the deep veins. If the valves in the perforating veins become incompetent, the high venous pressure in the deep veins is transmitted to the superficial veins resulting in dilatation and stagnation of blood producing varicosities and ulceration of the skin. For this reason, in the operative treatment of varicose veins, the perforating veins should be ligated.

Anatomy of the arteries

The femoral artery is the continuation of the external iliac artery and commences beneath the midpoint of the inguinal ligament. It runs in the extensor compartment of the thigh to pass through the adductor hiatus and becomes the popliteal artery which traverses the popliteal fossa. In the distal fossa, it divides into the anterior and posterior tibial arteries which supply the leg and foot.

Femoral artery

A The proximal portion of the femoral artery runs in the femoral triangle (Scarpa's triangle), and the distal portion in the adductor canal (Hunter's canal). The first 3–4 cm of the artery are enclosed with the femoral vein in the femoral sheath. The surface marking of the femoral artery is from the midpoint of the inguinal ligament to a point two-thirds along a line drawn towards the adductor tubercle with the hip semi-flexed, abducted and externally rotated.

Branches

The majority of the arterial branches arise from the proximal portion of the femoral artery within Scarpa's triangle.

- The **superficial epigastric artery** runs in the superficial abdominal fascia and supplies the superficial inguinal lymph nodes and the superficial fascia and skin.
- The **superficial circumflex iliac artery** turns laterally towards the anterior superior iliac spine. It supplies a large area of skin; this artery is the pedicle for the groin flap.
- The **superficial external pudendal artery** arises medially and supplies the lower abdominal, penile, scrotal and labial skin.
- The **deep external pudendal artery** supplies the skin of the perineum.

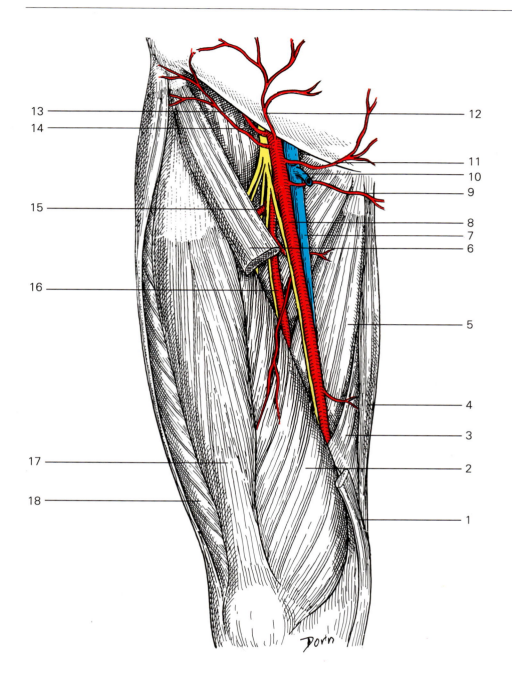

A

1 sartorius
2 vastus medialis
3 adductor magnus
4 gracilis
5 adductor longus
6 sartorius
7 femoral vein
8 femoral artery
9 deep external pudendal artery
10 long saphenous vein
11 superficial external pudendal artery
12 superficial epigastric artery
13 superficial circumflex iliac artery
14 deep circumflex iliac artery
15 lateral femoral circumflex artery
16 profunda femoris
17 rectus femoris
18 vastus lateralis

Arteries and veins

Profunda femoris

B The profunda femoris, a large branch, arises from the lateral side of the femoral artery 3–4 cm distal to the inguinal ligament. It passes between pectineus and adductor longus and then between adductor brevis and longus, and finally descends between adductor longus and adductor magnus. It pierces adductor magnus and becomes the fourth perforating artery. Its branches are as follows:

- The **lateral circumflex artery** runs posterior to sartorius and rectus femoris, and divides into ascending, transverse and descending branches. The ascending branch supplies the greater trochanter and participates in the blood supply to the femoral neck and head. The descending branch, which sometimes arises directly from the profunda femoris, descends posterior to rectus femoris along the medial border of vastus lateralis. The transverse branch pierces vastus lateralis to wind round the femur and anastomose with the medial circumflex artery.
- The **medial circumflex artery** curls medially round the femur and divides into transverse and ascending branches which anastomose with adjacent arteries.
- The **perforating arteries** pass through the insertion of adductor magnus to reach the posterior compartment of the thigh. The perforating arteries form a double chain of anastomoses in the muscle, adjacent to the linea aspera. The nutrient artery to the femur usually arises from the second perforating artery. The profunda femoris is the main arterial supply to the muscles of the thigh.

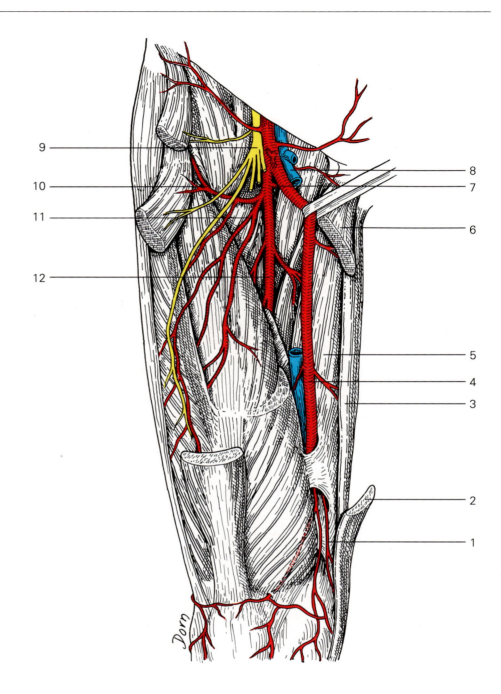

B

1 saphenous artery
2 sartorius
3 gracilis
4 femoral artery
5 adductor magnus
6 adductor longus
7 medial circumflex femoral artery

8 femoral vein
9 femoral nerve
10 ascending branch of the lateral circumflex femoral artery
11 descending branch of the lateral circumflex femoral artery
12 profunda femoris

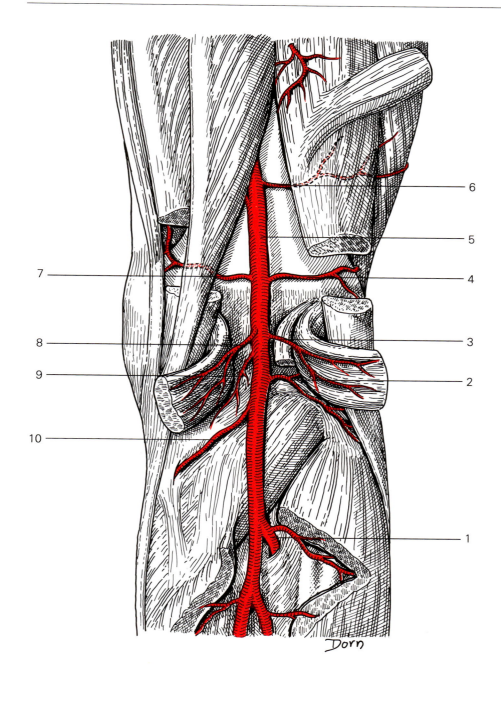

Dorn

- The **descending genicular artery** arises from the distal portion of the femoral artery, just proximal to the adductor hiatus. It supplies muscular branches, particularly to vastus medialis, articular branches and the saphenous branch which accompanies the saphenous nerve.

The popliteal artery

C The popliteal artery is a continuation of the femoral artery and crosses the popliteal fossa. The branches are muscular, articular and cutaneous.

The first branch arises from the lateral side and supplies vastus lateralis, biceps femoris and the skin of the lateral aspect of the distal third of the thigh. It anastomoses with the fourth perforating artery and constitutes an important chain of anastomoses between the profunda and popliteal arteries.

- The **sural arteries** (two in number) supply the calf muscles.
- The **superior genicular arteries** curve around both femoral condyles.
- The **middle genicular artery** pierces the oblique popliteal ligament to supply the cruciate ligament.
- The **inferior genicular arteries** arise distal to the joint and curve round the tibial condyles.
- The **popliteal artery** leaves the popliteal fossa by passing beneath the fibrous arch in soleus and immediately divides into anterior and posterior tibial arteries.

C

1 anterior tibial artery
2 lateral inferior genicular artery
3 lateral sural artery
4 lateral superior genicular artery
5 popliteal artery
6 proximal artery (Bourgery's artery)
7 medial superior genicular artery
8 medial sural artery
9 middle genicular artery
10 medial inferior genicular artery

Arteries and veins

D An extended medial dissection allows the exposure of the distal portion of the femoral artery, the popliteal artery and its division.

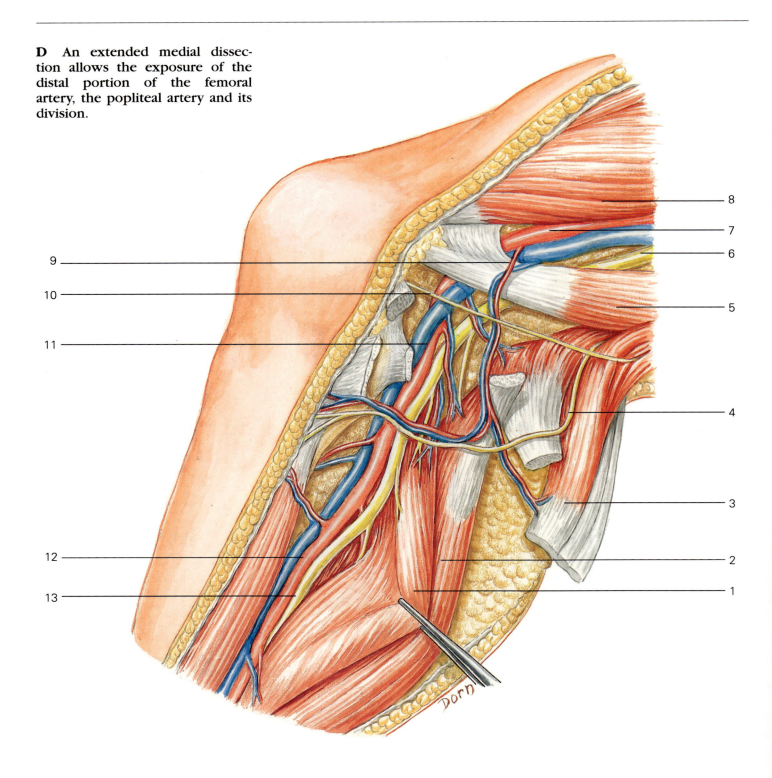

D

1 soleus
2 gastrocnemius (medial head)
3 sartorius
4 saphenous nerve
5 adductor magnus
6 sciatic nerve
7 femoral artery

8 vastus medialis
9 descending genicular artery
10 infrapatellar branch of saphenous nerve
11 popliteal vessels
12 posterior tibial vessels
13 tibial nerve

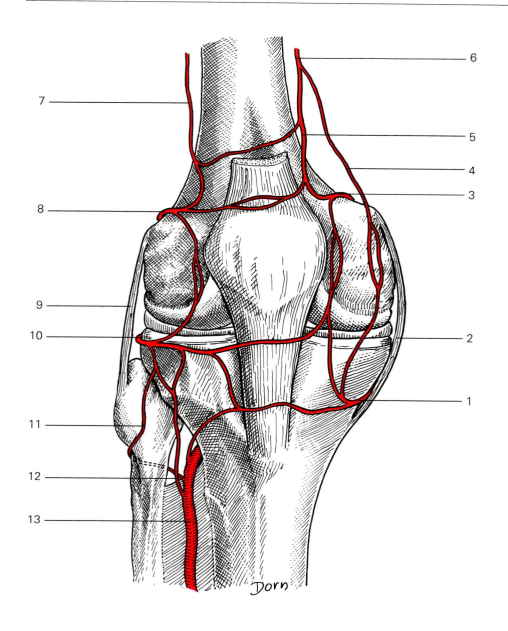

E All the structures of the knee are well vascularized by an intricate anastomosis which involves the medial and lateral genicular, the descending genicular, the descending branch of the lateral femoral circumflex, the circumflex fibular, and the anterior and posterior tibial recurrent arteries.

E

1 medial inferior genicular artery
2 tibial collateral ligament of knee joint
3 medial superior genicular artery
4 saphenous branch of descending genicular artery
5 articular branch of descending genicular artery
6 descending genicular artery
7 descending branch of lateral circumflex artery
8 lateral superior genicular artery
9 fibular collateral ligament of knee joint
10 lateral inferior genicular artery
11 circumflex fibular artery
12 anterior tibial recurrent artery
13 anterior tibial artery

Arteries and veins

The anterior tibial artery

F The anterior tibial artery is one of the terminal branches of the popliteal artery. Its origin is in the posterior compartment of the leg, but it gains access to the anterior compartment by passing forward above the proximal border of the interosseous membrane medial to the fibular neck. It descends on the anterior surface of the interosseous membrane and continues to the dorsum of the foot as the dorsalis pedis artery. Proximally, the artery lies between tibialis anterior and extensor digitorum longus, and further distally it lies between tibialis anterior and extensor hallucis longus. The surface marking commences 2.5 cm distal to the medial side of the fibular head and ends midway between the medial and lateral malleoli.

Branches

- The **posterior tibial recurrent artery** is not constant. It belongs to the posterior compartment and supplies the superior tibiofibular joint.
- The **anterior tibial recurrent artery** ascends through tibialis anterior and anastomoses with the genicular branches of the popliteal artery on the lateral side of the knee.
- The **anterior medial malleolar artery** arises just proximal to the ankle and joins with branches from the posterior tibial artery.
- The **anterior lateral malleolar artery** arises from the lateral side at a variable level. It anastomoses with the perforating branch of the peroneal artery and descends anterior to the tibiofibular ligament.

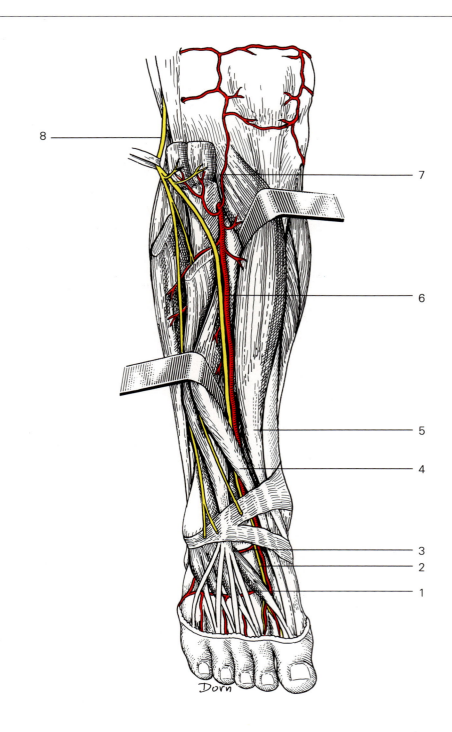

F

1 arcuate artery
2 dorsalis pedis
3 tarsal branch
4 extensor hallucis longus

5 tibialis anterior
6 anterior tibial artery
7 anterior tibial recurrent artery
8 common peroneal nerve

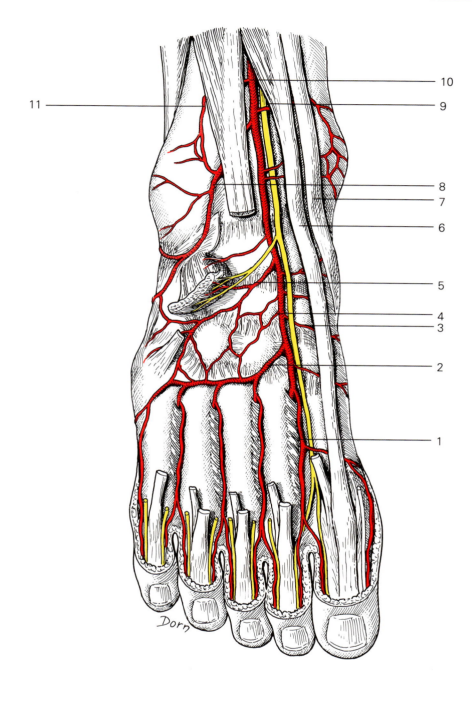

The dorsalis pedis artery

G The dorsalis pedis artery runs between the tendon of extensor hallucis longus and the medial tendon of extensor digitorum longus. It turns into the sole to complete the plantar arch. The surface marking commences midway between the malleoli and ends at the proximal end of the first intermetatarsal space. The lateral tarsal artery supplies extensor digitorum brevis and anastomoses with the perforating branch of the peroneal artery. A further branch, the arcuate artery, arises on the lateral side at the level of the metatarsal base. It provides the second, third and fourth dorsal metatarsal arteries.

G

1 first dorsal metatarsal artery
2 arcuate artery
3 medial tarsal artery
4 dorsalis pedis
5 lateral tarsal artery
6 extensor hallucis longus

7 tibialis anterior
8 anterior lateral malleolar artery
9 anterior medial malleolar artery
10 anterior tibial artery
11 perforating branch of peroneal artery

Arteries and veins

The posterior tibial artery

H The posterior tibial artery commences at the distal border of popliteus descending in the deep posterior compartment and terminates by dividing into the medial and lateral plantar arteries. It is accompanied by two veins and the tibial nerve.

Branches

- The **circumflex fibular artery** curves laterally round the neck of the fibula.
- The **peroneal artery** arises 3 cm distal to popliteus and descends along the medial crest of the fibula between tibialis posterior and flexor hallucis longus. At the level of the inferior tibiofibular syndesmosis, it divides into the calcaneal branches. It supplies a nutrient artery to the fibula, a perforating branch, which traverses the interosseous membrane and may replace the dorsalis pedis artery, and a communicating branch to the posterior tibial artery.
- A **nutrient artery** to the tibia and muscular branches to soleus.

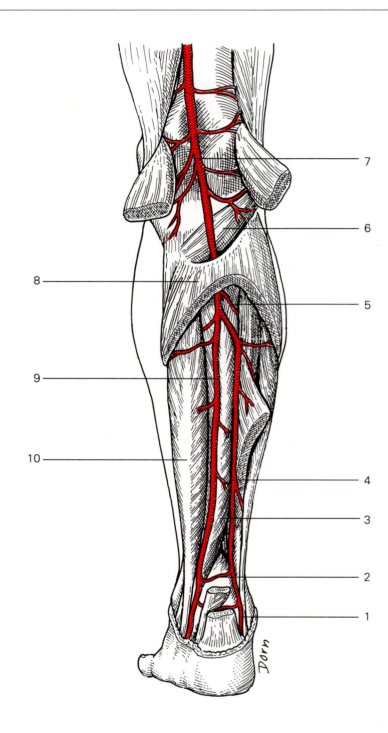

H

1 calcaneal branch	6 popliteus
2 communicating branch	7 popliteal artery
3 flexor hallucis longus	8 soleus
4 peroneal artery	9 posterior tibial artery
5 anterior tibial artery	10 flexor digitorum longus

The medial and lateral plantar arteries

I The medial plantar artery runs along the medial border of the foot, initially deep to abductor hallucis and then between this muscle and flexor digitorum brevis. It is accompanied by the medial plantar nerve. It bifurcates into a branch which reaches the medial border of the hallux and a branch which supplies three superficial digital branches.

The lateral plantar artery, which is a larger branch, curves distally and medially and, between the first and second metatarsals, unites with the dorsalis pedis artery to form the plantar arch. The plantar arch supplies three perforating branches, anastomosing with the dorsal metatarsal arteries and four plantar metatarsal arteries which each divide into two plantar digital arteries.

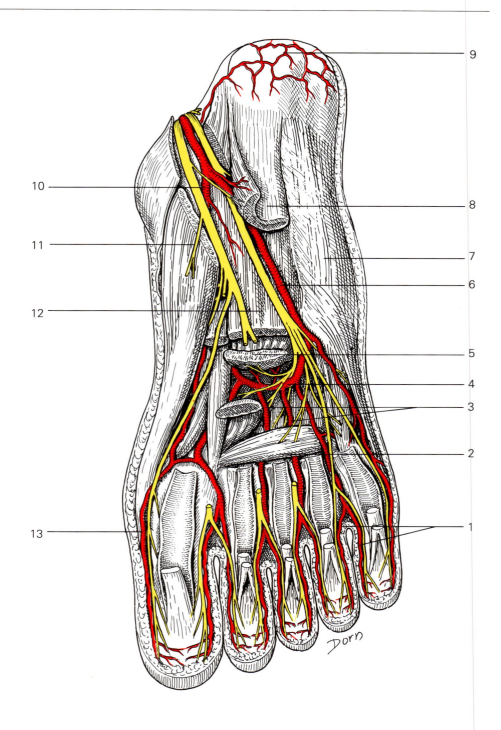

I

1 plantar digital arteries
2 adductor hallucis, transverse head
3 plantar metatarsal arteries
4 plantar arch
5 adductor hallucis, oblique head
6 lateral plantar artery
7 abductor digiti minimi

8 flexor digitorum brevis
9 calcaneal branches
10 medial plantar artery
11 cutaneous branch
12 flexor accessorius
13 digital branch of first plantar
    metatarsal artery

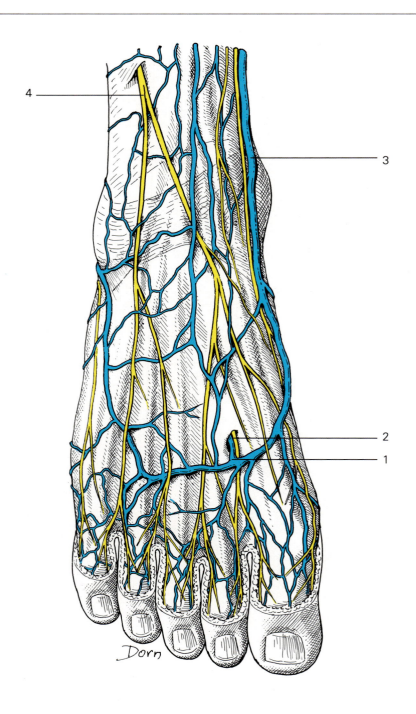

Dorn

J The main superficial veins are the long and short saphenous veins. In the foot, the dorsal digital veins join to form the dorsal metatarsal veins which unite to form the dorsal venous arch. On each side of the foot, the dorsal venous arch drains into the lateral and medial marginal veins. The plantar cutaneous arch also drains into these marginal veins.

The long saphenous vein

K,L The long saphenous vein is a continuation of the medial marginal vein and runs anterior to the medial malleolus before crossing the distal third of the tibia. It ascends just posterior to the medial border of the knee, over the medial aspect of the thigh, to enter the femoral vein proximal to the inguinal ligament. There are considerable variations in the size and position of the saphenous vein. It is accompanied in the thigh by the medial femoral cutaneous nerve, at the knee by the saphenous branch of the descending genicular artery, and in the leg and foot by the saphenous nerve. It has many connections with the deep veins, especially in the leg. Perforating veins drain into the posterior tibial venae comitantes, whilst other perforating veins are present in the upper calf and lower thigh. Three large tributaries exist just distal to the knee and arise from the anterior aspect of the leg, from the tibial malleolar region and from the calf. In the thigh, two large tributaries—the posteromedial and anterolateral veins of the thigh—drain large areas of skin and subcutaneous tissue. In the upper part of the thigh, just before entering the fascia, the long saphenous vein is joined by the superficial epigastric, the superficial circumflex iliac and the superficial pudendal veins.

J

1 dorsal arch
2 deep peroneal nerve, sensory branch
3 long saphenous vein
4 superficial peroneal nerve

Anatomy of the veins

The veins of the lower limb can be divided into superficial and deep groups, the deep veins accompanying the main arteries of the limb.

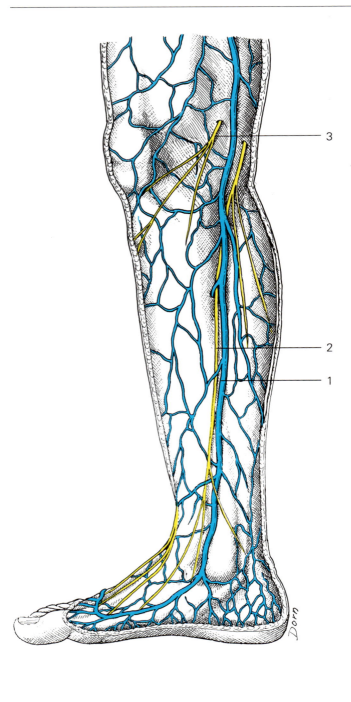

3

2

1

L

1 long saphenous vein
2 medial cutaneous nerve of thigh
   L2, 3
3 superficial external pudendal vein
4 superficial epigastric vein
5 superficial circumflex vein
6 lateral cutaneous nerve of thigh
   L2, 3
7 femoral branch of genitofemoral
   nerve L1, 2
8 infrapatellar branch of saphenous
   nerve

5

6

7

4

3

2

1

8

K

1 long saphenous vein
2 saphenous nerve
3 infrapatellar branch of saphenous
   nerve

Arteries and veins

The short saphenous vein

M The lateral marginal veins of the foot continue proximally as the short saphenous vein. In the lower third of the leg, it ascends lateral to the Achilles tendon, lying on the deep fascia, accompanied by the sural nerve. It runs through a tunnel in the deep fascia to lie on gastrocnemius. In the popliteal fossa it joins the popliteal vein. The short saphenous vein receives many tributaries in the leg.

Deep veins

The deep veins accompany the arteries and have numerous valves. The plantar digital veins join to form four plantar metatarsal veins; these then form the deep venous plantar arch, from which arise lateral and medial plantar veins that form the posterior tibial veins.

- The **posterior tibial veins** accompany the posterior tibial artery and receive veins from soleus.
- The **anterior tibial veins** follow the anterior tibial artery and join the posterior tibial veins to form the popliteal vein at the distal border of popliteus.
- The **popliteal vein** ascends through the popliteal fossa and becomes the femoral vein proximal to the adductor hiatus. It lies medial to the artery distally, superficial between the two heads of gastrocnemius and posterolateral in the upper part of the popliteal fossa.
- The **femoral vein** is posterolateral to the artery in the adductor canal and posterior to it as it enters Scarpa's triangle. It becomes medial to lie with the artery in the femoral sheath before passing under the

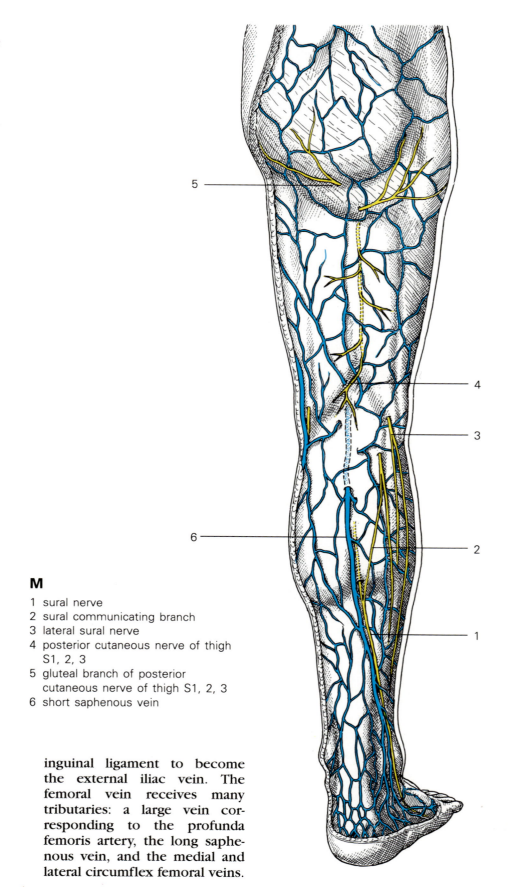

M
1 sural nerve
2 sural communicating branch
3 lateral sural nerve
4 posterior cutaneous nerve of thigh S1, 2, 3
5 gluteal branch of posterior cutaneous nerve of thigh S1, 2, 3
6 short saphenous vein

inguinal ligament to become the external iliac vein. The femoral vein receives many tributaries: a large vein corresponding to the profunda femoris artery, the long saphenous vein, and the medial and lateral circumflex femoral veins.

274

Femoral artery: Scarpa's triangle

Anatomy

Scarpa's triangle is bounded proximally by the inguinal ligament, medially by pectineus and the adductors, and laterally by the medial border of sartorius. The femoral artery enters the thigh from the pelvis at a point midway between the anterior superior iliac spine and the symphysis pubis. It is enclosed in the femoral sheath which is a distal prolongation of the extraperitoneal fascia and persists for about 2.5 cm distal to the inguinal ligament. The sheath is divided by two septa into arterial, venous and lymphatic compartments.

Indications

- Control of the femoral artery.
- Embolectomy.
- Treatment of traumatic arterial lesions.

Position of the patient

The patient is supine, with the thigh in abduction and slight external rotation.

Incision

A The incision is placed over the site of arterial pulsation. If there is no pulse, the incision is made from the midpoint of the inguinal ligament running towards the adductor tubercle. The incision is curved medially as it crosses the inguinal ligament and runs along the medial border of sartorius.

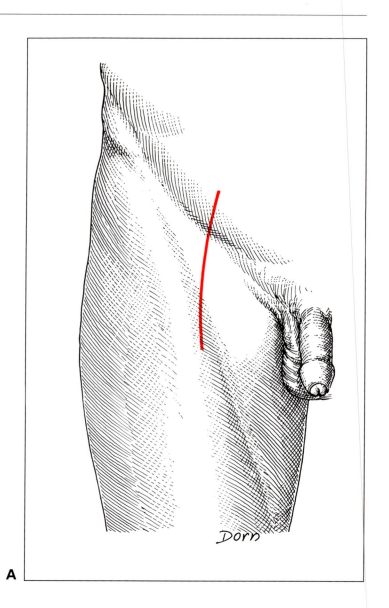

A

275

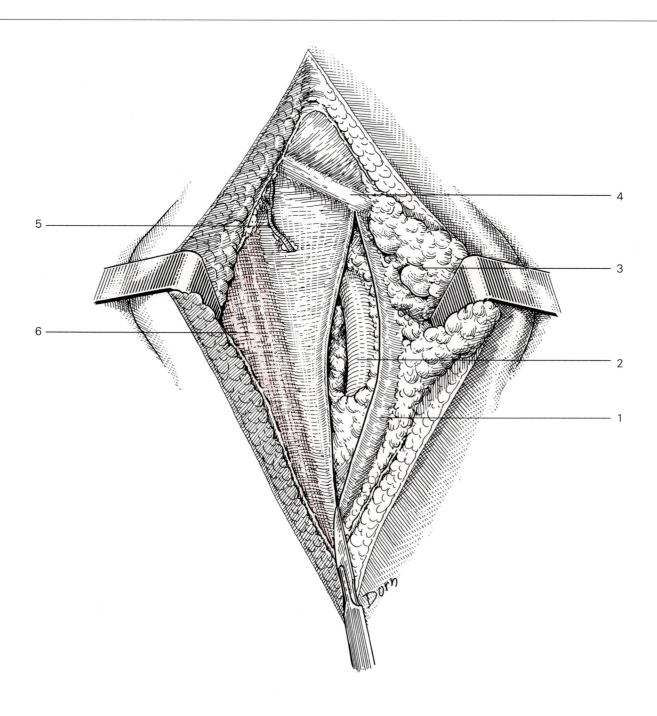

Exposure

B The edges of the skin are gently retracted. When incising the subcutaneous tissue, care should be taken to avoid damage to the inguinal nodes which are gently retracted medially. Before incising the fascia, it is usually necessary to divide the lateral venous branches, particularly the superficial circumflex iliac vein. The deep fascia is incised on the medial border of sartorius. The femoral sheath is just beneath the fascia. It is opened along its entire length to mobilize the artery. Proximally, care should be taken to avoid injuring the epigastric and superficial circumflex iliac arteries.

B

1 deep fascia
2 femoral artery
3 lymphatic nodes
4 inguinal ligament
5 superficial circumflex iliac artery
6 sartorius

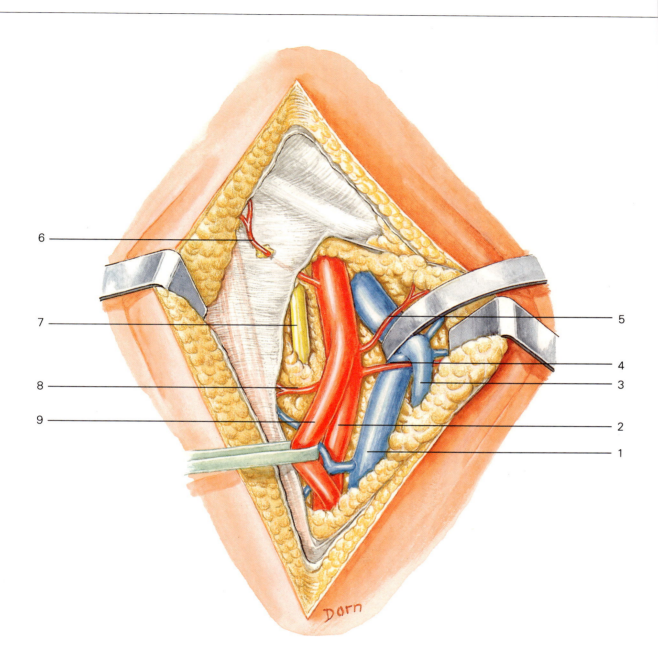

C A tape is placed around the proximal artery and the artery is then mobilized distal to the origin of the profunda femoris. A further tape is placed around the artery distally. Gentle traction on the two tapes will allow the identification of the origin of the profunda femoris which is posterior. A fibrous band anterior to the origin must be divided. Some branches of the profunda femoris vein may have to be ligated. Other branches of the femoral artery have to be controlled before any surgical procedure is undertaken. By retraction of the lymphatic tissue medially, the saphenous vein can be dissected.

c
1 femoral vein
2 profunda femoris
3 long saphenous vein
4 deep external pudendal artery
5 superficial external pudendal artery
6 superficial circumflex iliac artery
7 femoral nerve
8 lateral femoral circumflex artery
9 femoral artery

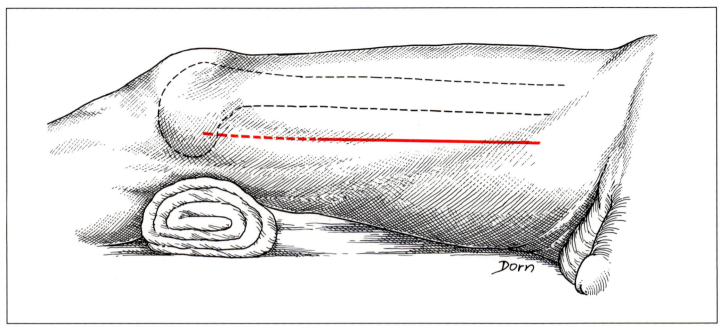

A

Femoral artery: Hunter's canal

Anatomy

Hunter's canal extends from the apex of Scarpa's triangle to the adductor hiatus. It is bounded laterally by vastus medialis, posteriorly by adductor longus proximally and adductor magnus distally. The roof is a layer of deep fascia over which lies sartorius. Hunter's canal contains the femoral artery and vein, and the saphenous nerve which is anterior to the vessels.

Indications

- Arterial reconstructive surgery.
- Traumatic lesions of the artery.

Position of the patient

The patient is supine, with the knee flexed and the limb in external rotation.

Incision

A The incision is made in the middle third of the thigh along a line running from the midpoint of the inguinal ligament to the adductor tubercle.

B

1 long saphenous vein
2 sartorius

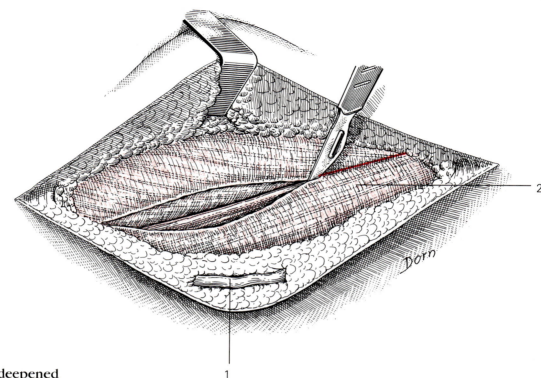

Exposure

B The incision is deepened through the subcutaneous tissue and the superficial fascia overlying sartorius.

C The long saphenous vein is retracted medially, sartorius is mobilized, and retracted medially and posteriorly. The deep fascia which constitutes the roof of the canal is cautiously opened.

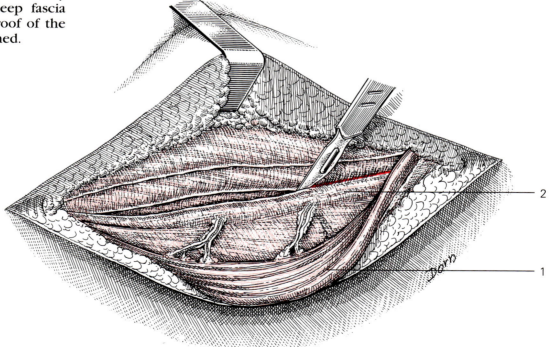

C

1 sartorius, retracted
2 femoral sheath

279

Arteries and veins

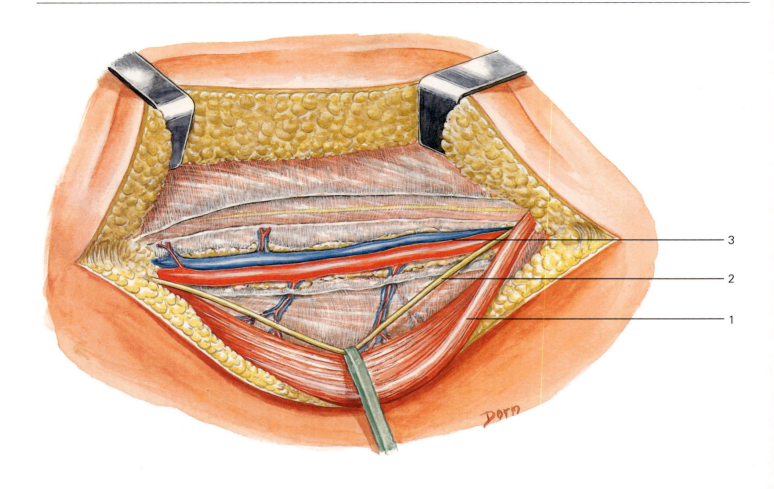

3

2

1

D The femoral vessels are exposed. The saphenous nerve is protected and retracted medially with a tape.

D
1 sartorius
2 saphenous nerve
3 femoral artery and vein

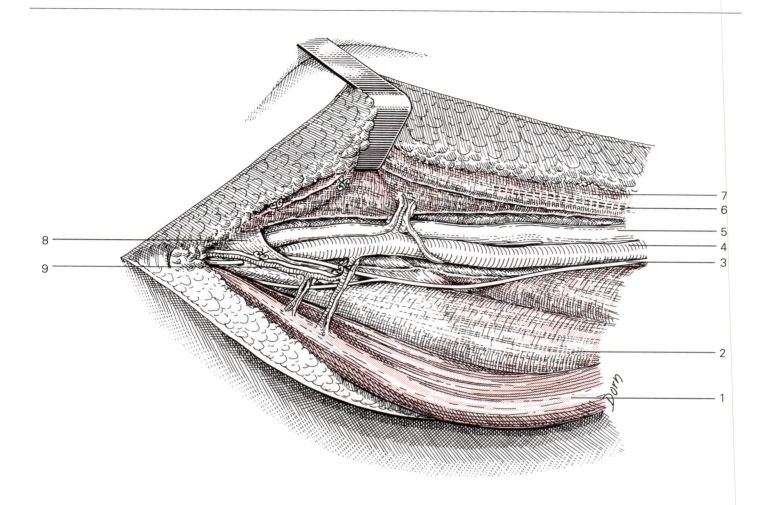

E Care should be taken to preserve the origin of the descending genicular artery at the distal end of the incision. This approach can be extended proximally and distally to allow the exposure of the entire femoral artery and the femoropopliteal junction.

E

1 sartorius
2 adductor magnus
3 saphenous nerve
4 femoral artery
5 femoral vein
6 motor nerve to vastus medialis
7 vastus medialis
8 adductor hiatus
9 descending genicular artery

281

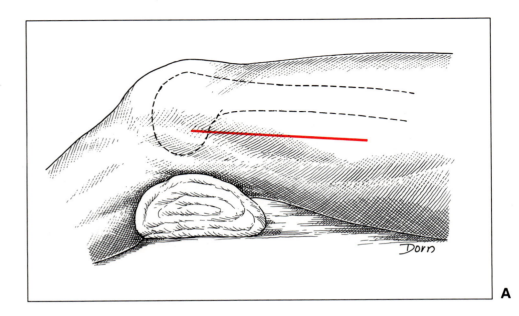

A

Popliteal artery

Anatomy

The popliteal artery is the distal continuation of the femoral artery and enters the popliteal fossa, which is a diamond-shaped space, via the adductor hiatus. The artery is deep and lies in direct contact with the posterior capsule of the knee. It descends vertically and ends at the distal border of popliteus, dividing into the anterior and posterior tibial arteries. In the popliteal fossa, the branches of the popliteal artery are five genicular arteries and branches to the muscles of the fossa, the most constant of which is a Y-shaped vessel to the two heads of gastrocnemius. The popliteal vein is adjacent to the artery, which explains the frequency of their dual injury and the formation of an arteriovenous fistula. In the popliteal fossa, the sciatic nerve divides into the tibial nerve, which follows the course of the popliteal vessels, and the common peroneal nerve, which runs laterally towards the head of the fibula. By dissecting the subcutaneous fat, the sciatic nerve and its bifurcation can be identified, being relatively superficial. Deep to the nerves is a thick layer of adipose tissue which must be dissected to expose the vessels.

The popliteal artery can be considered as consisting of two main segments: the proximal which lies on the femur and the distal which lies on the tibia. Each segment can be exposed alone or the vessel can be exposed in its entirety. There are four main exposures of the popliteal artery, depending on which segment of the artery is to be displayed. The femoropopliteal junction can be exposed by a limited medial approach. The popliteal artery lying on the posterior tibia can be exposed by a more distal limited medial approach. The entire popliteal artery can be exposed via either an extended medial approach or a posterior approach, although the latter does not allow a view of the femoropopliteal junction, and hence the femoral artery cannot be controlled. Both the extended approaches afford exposure of the popliteal bifurcation.

Femoropopliteal junction: limited medial approach

Indication

- Reconstructive vascular surgery of strictly localized lesions.

Position of the patient

The patient is supine, with the limb externally rotated and the knee supported in 30° flexion by a rolled towel.

Incision

A The incision represents the distal third of a line running from the midpoint of the inguinal ligament to the adductor tubercle. It runs slightly anterior to the anterior border of sartorius.

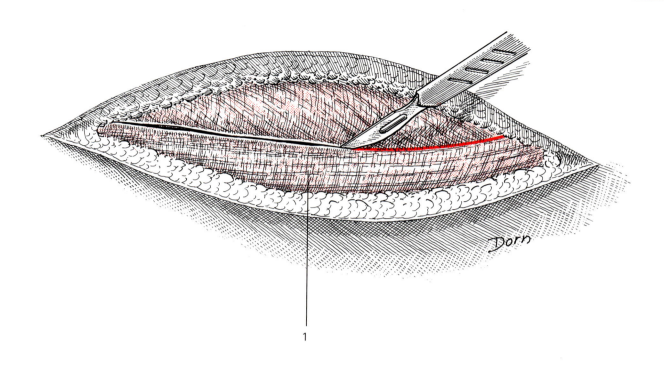

1

Exposure

B The subcutaneous tissue is incised and the posterior skin flap is reflected taking care to protect the long saphenous vein. The deep fascia is opened, which allows sartorius to be reflected posteriorly. Care should be taken to preserve the saphenous nerve which runs deep to sartorius and the saphenous artery.

B
1 sartorius

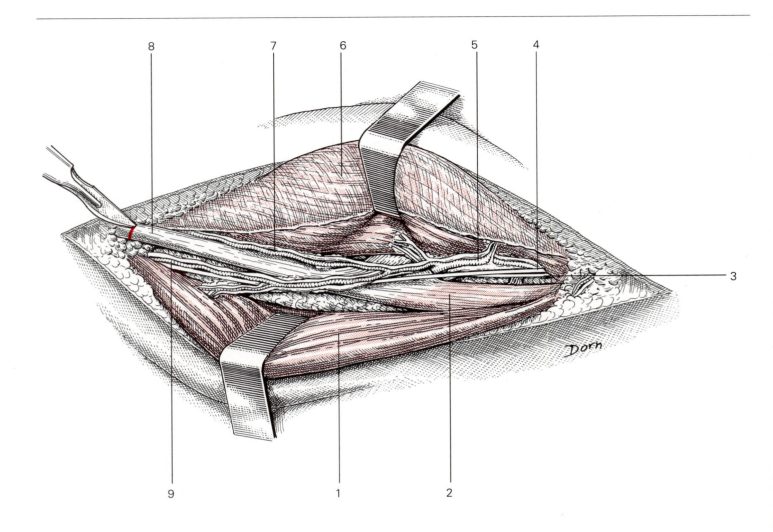

C   The posterior border of vastus medialis and the tendon of adductor magnus are identified. The aponeurosis of the muscle is incised close to the tendon. Vastus medialis is released from the floor of the tendon and retracted anteriorly and medially. The lower end of the femoral artery, the adductor hiatus and the insertion of the tendon into the medial femoral condyle are successively exposed. The descending genicular artery arises from the femoral artery just proximal to the hiatus.

C
1 sartorius
2 adductor magnus
3 motor nerve to vastus medialis
4 saphenous nerve
5 femoral artery
6 vastus medialis
7 articular branch of descending genicular artery
8 distal tendon of adductor magnus
9 saphenous branch of descending genicular artery

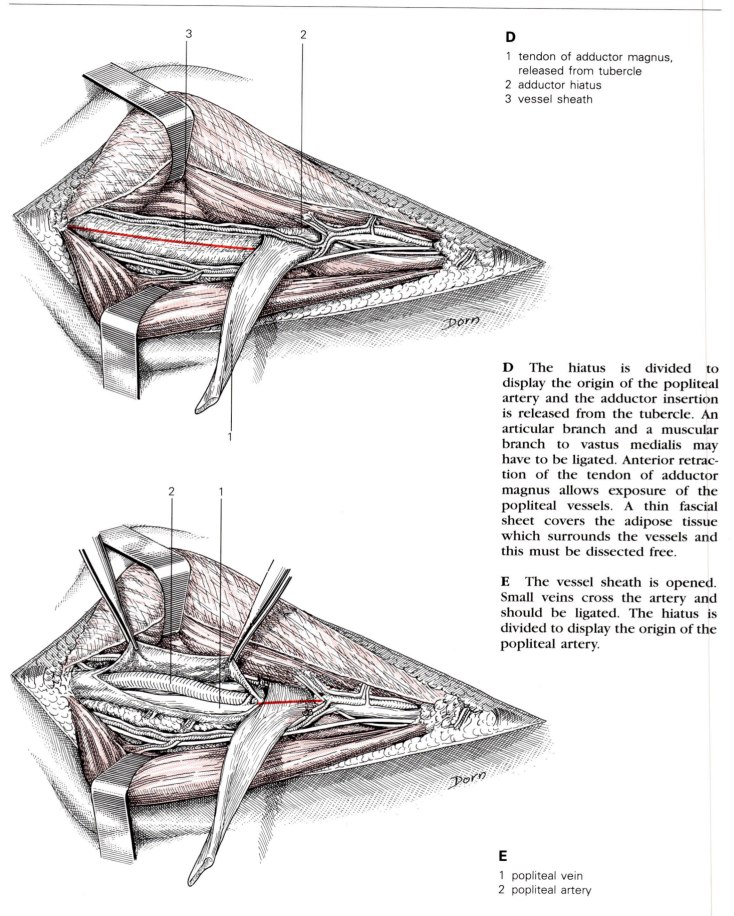

D
1 tendon of adductor magnus, released from tubercle
2 adductor hiatus
3 vessel sheath

D The hiatus is divided to display the origin of the popliteal artery and the adductor insertion is released from the tubercle. An articular branch and a muscular branch to vastus medialis may have to be ligated. Anterior retraction of the tendon of adductor magnus allows exposure of the popliteal vessels. A thin fascial sheet covers the adipose tissue which surrounds the vessels and this must be dissected free.

E The vessel sheath is opened. Small veins cross the artery and should be ligated. The hiatus is divided to display the origin of the popliteal artery.

E
1 popliteal vein
2 popliteal artery

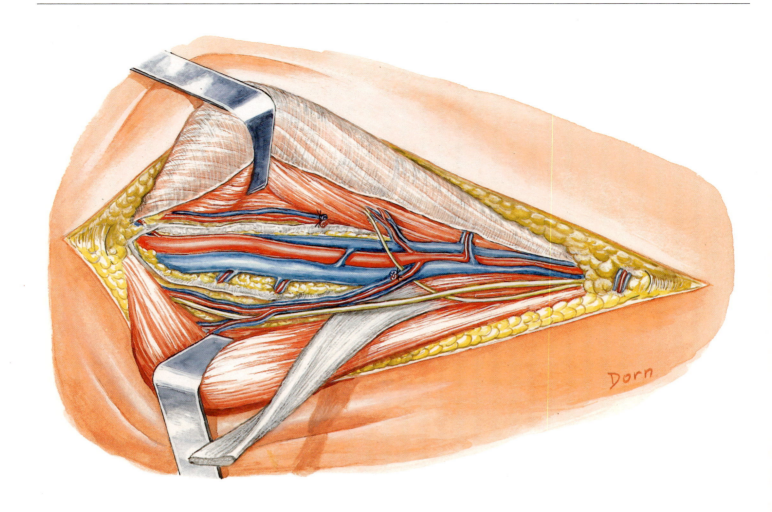

F Dense tissue intimately attached to the artery and vein can make separation of the two vessels difficult. The advantage of the medial exposure is the ease of access to the femoral artery and saphenous vein.

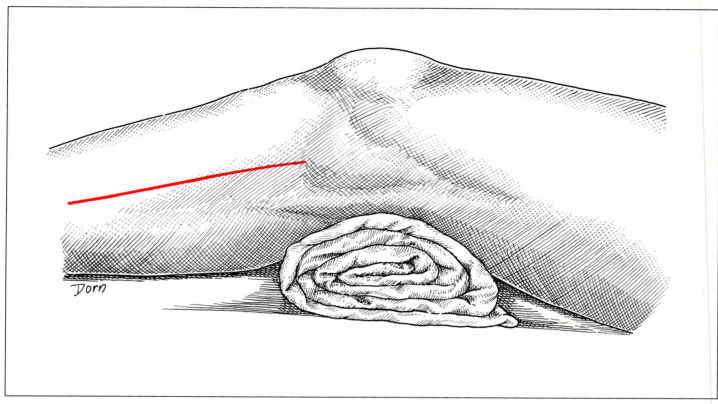

A

Distal popliteal artery: limited medial approach

Indication

- Reconstructive vascular surgery for strictly localized lesions.

Position of the patient

The patient is supine, with the limb slightly externally rotated and the knee flexed at 30° and supported by a rolled towel.

Incision

A The straight incision commences distal to the medial joint line and follows the posteromedial border of the upper third of the tibia for 8–10 cm. The incision can be extended proximally for the exposure of the entire popliteal vessels.

B

1 long saphenous vein
2 saphenous nerve

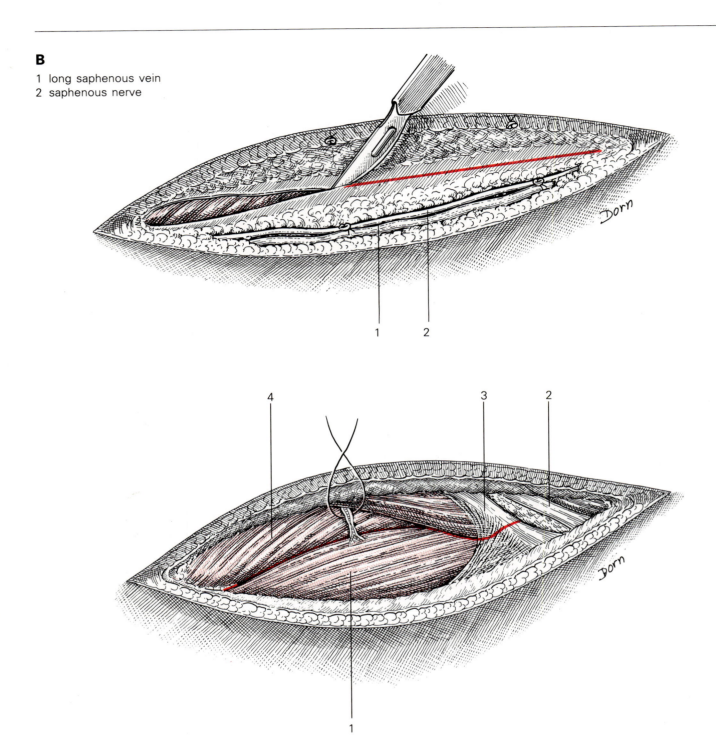

Exposure

B The subcutaneous tissue is incised, taking care to protect the long saphenous vein which is reflected posteriorly with the posterior skin flap. Several small veins should be ligated. The deep fascia is incised in line with the incision, distal to the tendons of gracilis and semitendinosus.

C The plane between soleus and gastrocnemius is developed. The tendon of semitendinosus can be cut without impairment or divided in a Z fashion.

C

1 gastrocnemius (medial head)
2 gracilis tendon
3 semitendinosus tendon
4 soleus

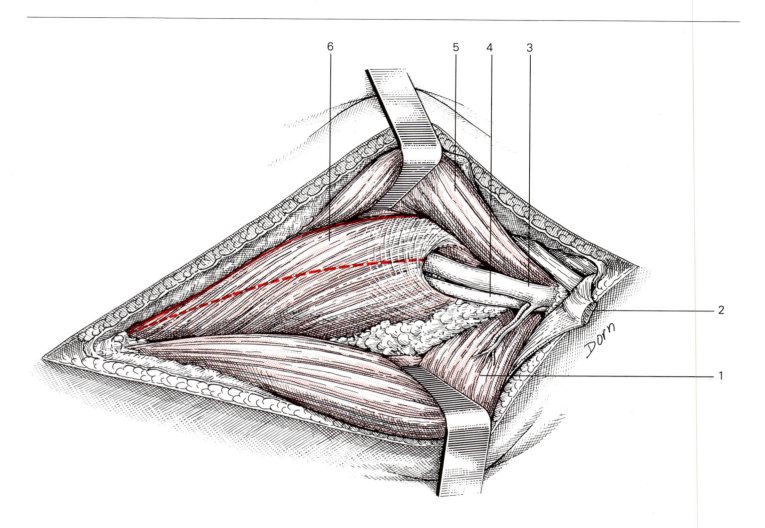

D The medial head of gastrocnemius is retracted posteriorly, exposing soleus and the vessels. The neurovascular bundle is deep and lies on the posterior surface of the tibia which is covered at this level by popliteus. Numerous veins cross the artery and should be divided and ligated. The tibial nerve runs posterior to the vessels and should be protected. The popliteal artery and vein can be mobilized distally either by dividing the soleus arcade or by releasing it from the tibia. The muscle fibres of soleus can be split.

D

1 gastrocnemius, retracted
2 semitendinosus
3 popliteal vein
4 tibial nerve
5 popliteus
6 soleus

Arteries and veins

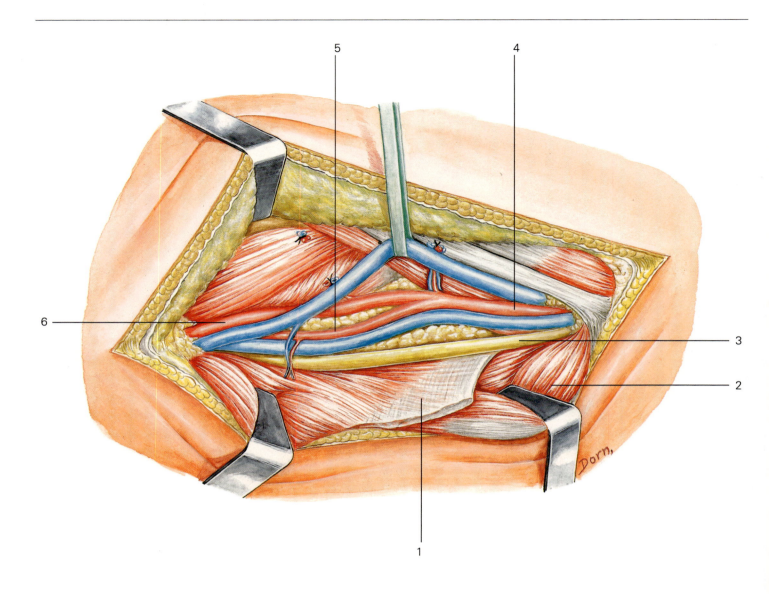

E There are usually no significant branches arising from the popliteal, posterior tibial and anterior tibial arteries.

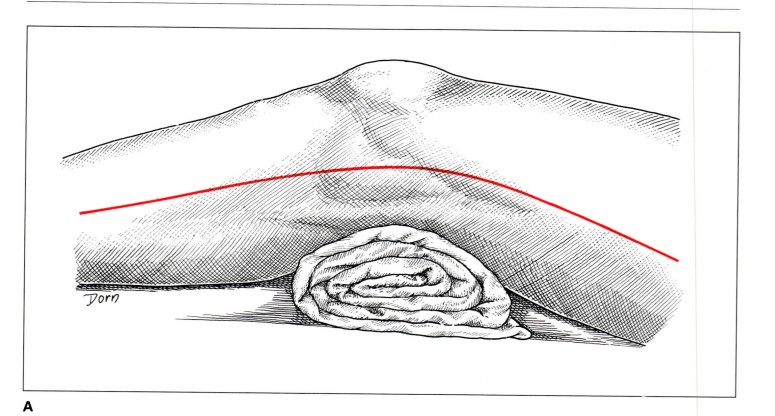

A

Popliteal artery: extended medial approach

Introduction

This approach allows exposure of the popliteal artery in its entirety and is of particular value in lesions of the artery resulting from fractures or dislocations around the knee. In these circumstances, the artery can be compressed distally by the arcade of soleus. The extended medial approach allows control of the bifurcation of the popliteal artery. Associated fractures or dislocations around the knee can probably also be treated through this approach.

Indications

- Reconstructive vascular surgery.
- Treatment of traumatic vascular lesions.

Position of the patient

The patient is supine, with the limb in external rotation and the knee flexed to 30° and supported with a rolled towel.

Incision

A The incision commences over the distal third of the thigh anterior to sartorius, reaches the posteromedial border of the knee and continues along the posteromedial border of the tibia.

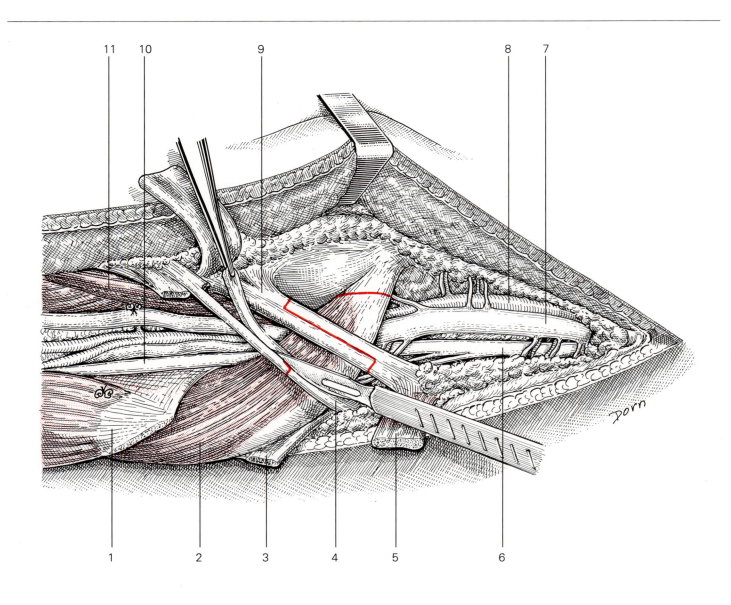

Exposure

B The incision is deepened through the subcutaneous tissue, taking care to protect the long saphenous vein which is retracted posteriorly. The deep fascia is incised anterior to sartorius and the popliteal space is entered below the tendon which may be released from its distal insertion to be retracted anteriorly with vastus medialis. The insertion of the pes anserinus and semimembranosus are divided from the tibia to expose the medial head of gastrocnemius which is also released from the distal femur. Retraction of this muscle allows an exposure of the popliteal vessels. The saphenous nerve and artery, which run deep to sartorius, but superficial to the other tendons, are protected. Distally, the popliteal artery and vein pass beneath the arcade of soleus, which should be released to expose the popliteal bifurcation into the anterior and posterior tibial arteries.

B

1 soleus, split
2 gastrocnemius
3 semitendinosus
4 gracilis
5 sartorius
6 tibial nerve
7 popliteal vein
8 popliteal artery
9 semimembranosus
10 tibial nerve
11 popliteus

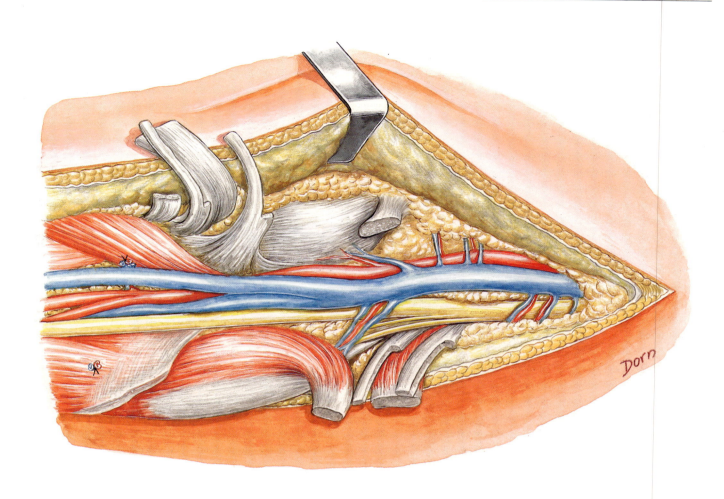

C To expose the artery, it should be dissected from the adipose tissue and the venous plexus which surrounds it. The posterior tibial nerve which is superficial to the artery should be protected. At the end of the surgical procedure, the continuity of the tendons must be restored and gastrocnemius repaired using nonabsorbable sutures.

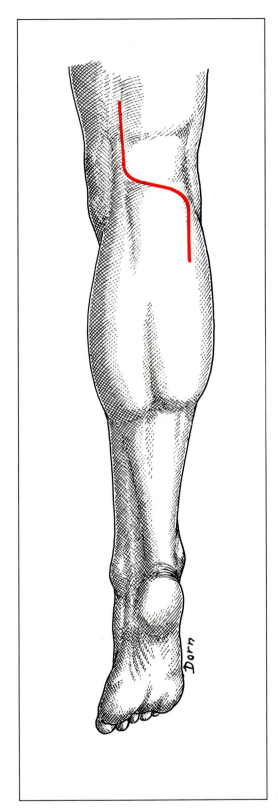

A

Popliteal artery: posterior approach

Introduction

The posterior approach to the popliteal artery offers obvious advantages. No muscles or tendons need be divided and the neurovascular structures are relatively superficial. However, the approach does not facilitate the control of the femoral artery and access to the long saphenous vein is difficult. The popliteal bifurcation can be exposed by splitting soleus and its arcade. Associated orthopaedic injuries cannot be treated by this approach.

Indication

• Reconstructive vascular surgery.

Position of the patient

The patient is prone.

Incision

A A curved incision is made, commencing over the posterior thigh adjacent to the tendons of semimembranosus and semitendinosus. It is angled as it crosses the popliteal skin crease, and runs distally and laterally towards the lateral head of gastrocnemius. The incision can then be extended further distally and reach the midline of the calf if the artery is to be exposed deep to soleus.

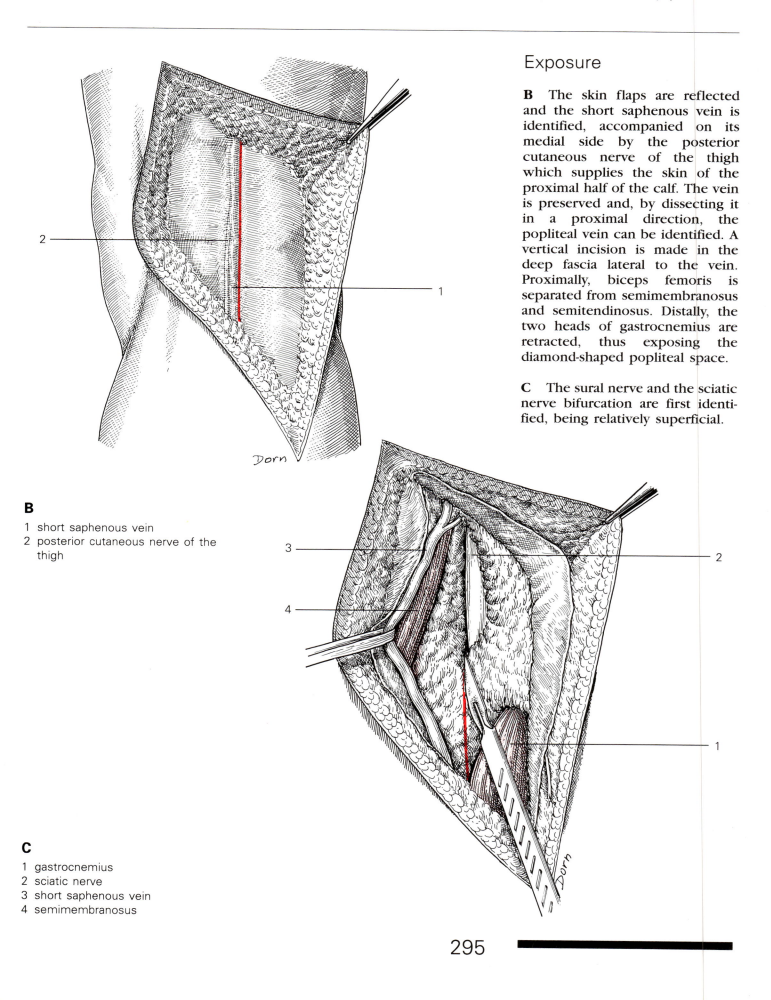

Exposure

B The skin flaps are reflected and the short saphenous vein is identified, accompanied on its medial side by the posterior cutaneous nerve of the thigh which supplies the skin of the proximal half of the calf. The vein is preserved and, by dissecting it in a proximal direction, the popliteal vein can be identified. A vertical incision is made in the deep fascia lateral to the vein. Proximally, biceps femoris is separated from semimembranosus and semitendinosus. Distally, the two heads of gastrocnemius are retracted, thus exposing the diamond-shaped popliteal space.

C The sural nerve and the sciatic nerve bifurcation are first identified, being relatively superficial.

B

1 short saphenous vein
2 posterior cutaneous nerve of the thigh

C

1 gastrocnemius
2 sciatic nerve
3 short saphenous vein
4 semimembranosus

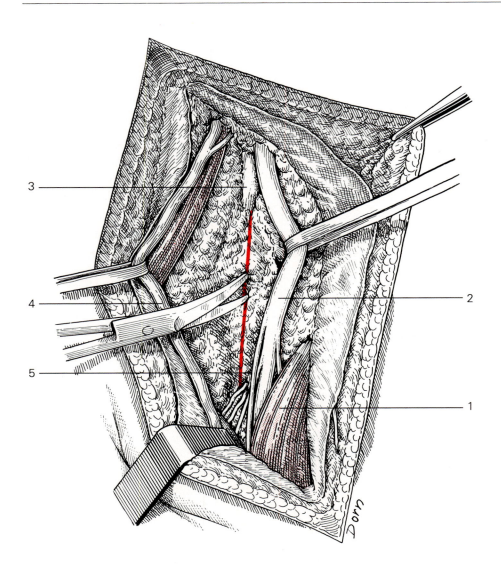

D The nerves are retracted and, by careful dissection of the fat, the popliteal vein is progressively exposed. The short saphenous vein can be traced as it enters the popliteal vein.

D

1 gastrocnemius
2 tibial nerve
3 popliteal vein
4 short saphenous vein
5 sural nerve

E   The sheath is opened and the popliteal artery identified deep to the vein and on its medial side. The popliteal artery can be traced distally by dividing the arcade of soleus and splitting the muscle fibres after retracting the two heads of gastrocnemius. The sural nerve should be identified and protected.

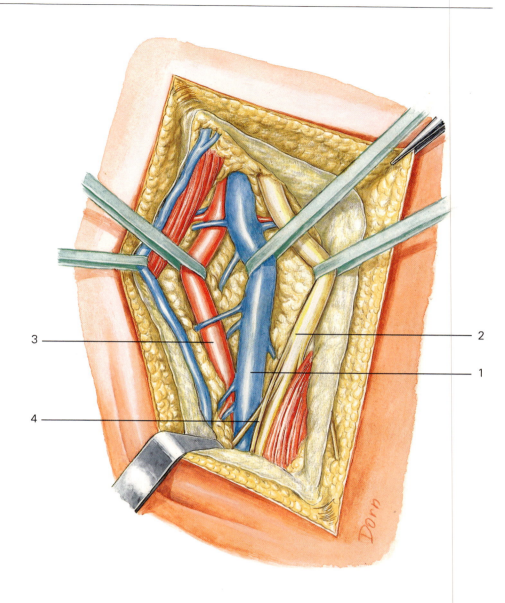

E

1   popliteal vein
2   tibial nerve
3   popliteal artery
4   sural nerve

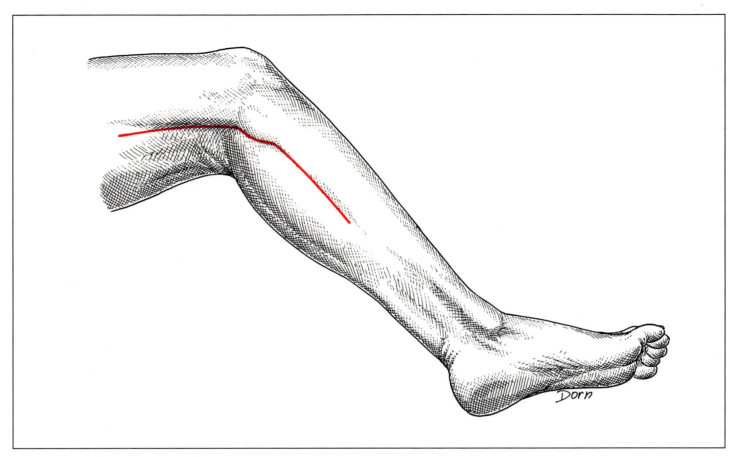

A

Popliteal artery and bifurcation: lateral approach

Introduction

The lateral approach is rarely used. However, it provides access to the arch of the anterior tibial artery. An endarterectomy of the distal popliteal artery and its three branches can be carried out under direct vision.

Indications

- Direct control of the bifurcation of the popliteal artery.
- Reconstructive vascular surgery of strictly localized lesions.

Position of the patient

The patient is supine, with a sandbag under the ipsilateral buttock. The limb is internally rotated and adducted, the knee being flexed to 30°.

Incision

A The biceps tendon and the head of the fibula are easily palpated. The incision commences 6 cm proximal to the head of the fibula, over the lower part of the biceps tendon, and descends over the shaft of the fibula for 12–15 cm.

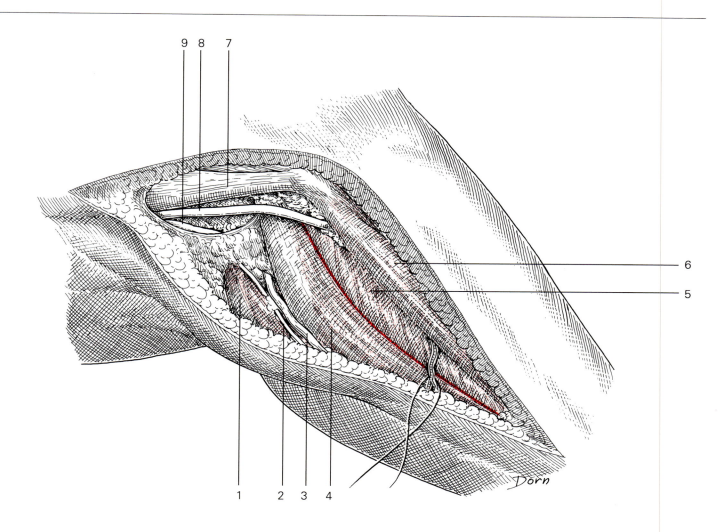

Exposure

B The subcutaneous tissue is incised in line with the incision. The deep fascia is cautiously opened along the posterior border of biceps femoris. The common peroneal nerve is identified as far distally as the neck of the fibula. The lateral head of gastrocnemius, the lateral border of soleus and peroneus longus are identified.

B

1 gastrocnemius (medial head)
2 sural nerve
3 short saphenous vein
4 gastrocnemius (lateral head)
5 soleus
6 peroneus longus
7 biceps femoris
8 common peroneal nerve
9 tibial nerve

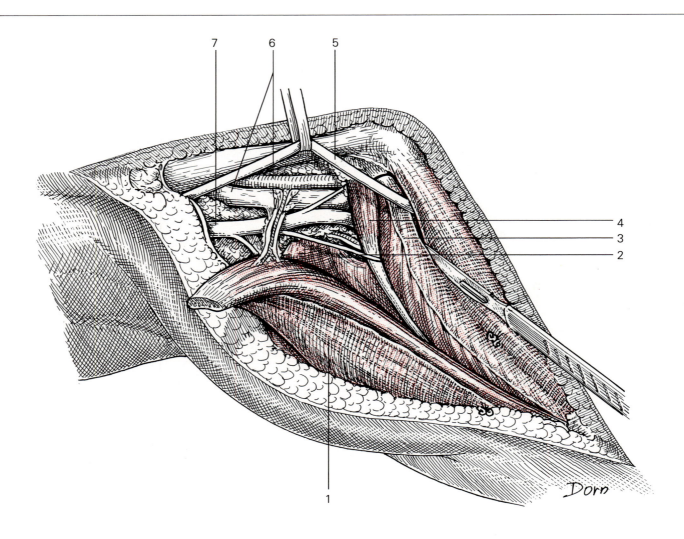

C The plane between gastrocnemius and soleus is developed
and the lateral head of gastrocnemius is released from its
origin.

C

1 gastrocnemius, retracted
2 motor nerve to soleus
3 soleus
4 plantaris
5 common peroneal nerve
6 popliteal vein and artery
7 tibial nerve

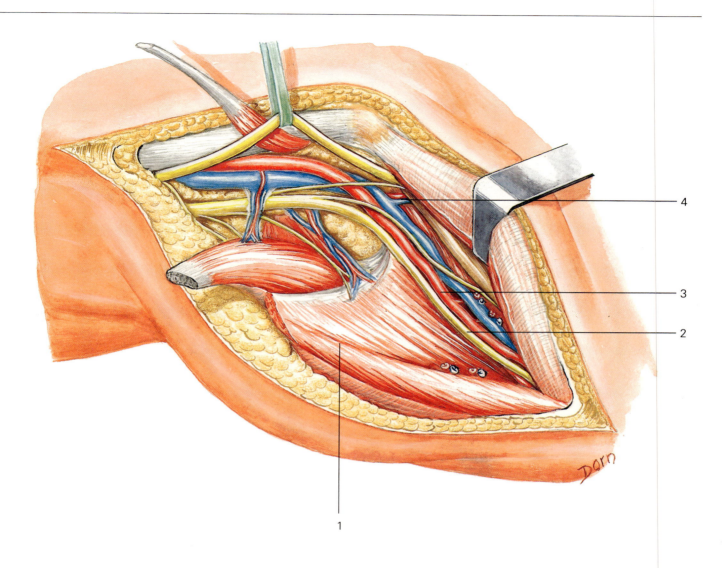

D The lateral head of gastro-cnemius is released from the femoral condyle, exposing the proximal portion of the popliteal vessels. The plane between soleus and peroneus longus is developed and soleus is detached from its insertion on the fibula. Retraction of soleus allows the exposure of the posterior tibial vessels and the tibial nerve. If necessary, the excision of the fibula—the proximal cut being immediately distal to the head—allows the exposure of the distal popliteal artery and its three main branches.

D

1 soleus, released from the fibula and retracted
2 tibial nerve
3 peroneal artery
4 anterior tibial artery

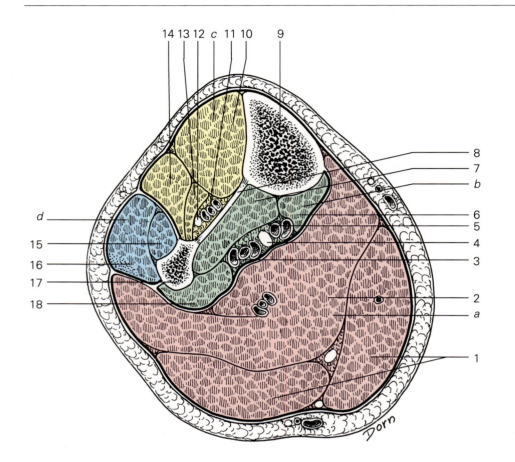

14 13 12 *c* 11 10   9

A

1 medial and lateral heads of gastrocnemius
2 soleus
3 peroneal artery and veins
4 tibial nerve
5 posterior tibial artery and veins
6 flexor digitorum longus
7 tibialis posterior
8 interosseous membrane
9 tibia
10 tibialis anterior
11 anterior tibial artery and veins
12 deep peroneal nerve
13 extensor hallucis longus
14 extensor digitorum longus
15 peroneus brevis
16 peroneus longus
17 fibula
18 flexor hallucis longus
a superficial } posterior compartment
b deep
c anterior compartment
d lateral compartment

The arteries of the leg

Introduction

A The neurovascular bundles of the leg run in the compartments of the leg which are formed by the deep fascia and its septae. A cross-section through the middle third of the leg shows the four compartments.

• The **anterior or extensor compartment** is bounded anteriorly by the fascia, posteriorly by the interosseous membrane and the anterior aspect of the tibia,

medially by the lateral aspect of the tibia, and laterally by the anterior intermuscular septum. It contains tibialis anterior, extensor digitorum longus, extensor hallucis longus and peroneus tertius, the anterior tibial vessels and the deep peroneal nerve.

• The **lateral compartment** (evertors) is situated between two intermuscular septae which insert into the fibula. It contains peroneus longus and brevis and the superficial peroneal nerve.

• The **posterior compartment** is bounded medially by the medial border of the posterior aspect of the tibia, laterally by the inter-

muscular septum and the fibula, anteriorly by the interosseous membrane, and posteriorly by the deep fascia. The posterior compartment is divided into superficial and deep sections by a fascial septum which extends between the fibula and the medial border of the tibia. The superficial compartment contains soleus, gastrocnemius, plantaris and the sural nerve.

• The **deep posterior compartment** contains tibialis posterior, flexor hallucis longus, flexor digitorum longus, the posterior tibial and peroneal arteries with their venae comitantes and the tibial nerve.

Posterior tibial artery: introduction

The posterior tibial artery is the most important artery of the leg. It may often be damaged in dislocations of the knee and fractures of the tibia. The origin of the peroneal artery is a vulnerable area and its deep location makes its repair difficult. For that reason there are two different approaches to the proximal segment of the main trunk according to the pathology. The medial approach is the same as the extended medial approach to the distal popliteal artery; the posterior approach is achieved by splitting the soleus muscle. The distal portion of the posterior tibial artery behind the medial malleolus is also vulnerable by virtue of its superficial position and can be lacerated by sharp wounds. At that level, the medial approach is easy.

Posterior tibial artery: medial approach to the proximal segment

This approach is the same as the extended medial approach to the distal portion of the popliteal artery (see pages 291-3). The control of the distal popliteal artery is always necessary.

Indications

- Ligation of the artery.
- Repair of the artery.

Position of the patient

The patient is supine, the limb externally rotated.

Incision

The incision is designed over the upper third of the leg being posterior to the posteromedial border of the tibia.

Exposure

The long saphenous vein is identified, preserved and retracted either anteriorly or posteriorly. Care should also be taken of the saphenous nerve. The deep fascia is opened and the plane between soleus and gastrocnemius is developed. The medial head of gastrocnemius is retracted, exposing the distal portion of the popliteal artery, allowing its control. Soleus is then detached from the medial border of the tibia or split in line with popliteal vessels to expose the posterior tibial vessels. The vein is immediately deep to the artery and the tibial nerve is lateral to the vein.

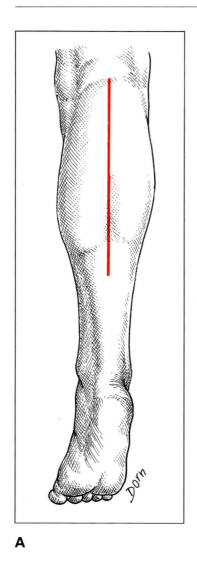

A

B
1 short saphenous vein
2 sural nerve
3 gastrocnemius

Posterior tibial and peroneal arteries: posterior approach splitting soleus

Indication

• Repair of the division of the posterior tibial and peroneal arteries.

Position of the patient

The patient is prone.

Incision

A The incision is longitudinal. It starts at the popliteal skin crease and runs along the midline of the calf to reach the common aponeurosis between the medial and lateral heads of gastrocnemius. The incision can be extended proximally to control the entire popliteal artery.

Exposure

B The fascia is incised and care should be taken to identify and to isolate the short saphenous vein and the sural nerve, which are retracted by a tape. The two heads of gastrocnemius are exposed.

C In the upper part of the incision, the popliteal fossa is opened and the neurovascular axis is identified. The tibial nerve is lying superficial on the lateral side of the popliteal vein. The popliteal artery is deeper. Thus the midline fascia of gastrocnemius is incised to separate the two heads of the muscle, which are retracted, exposing the extensive surface of soleus.

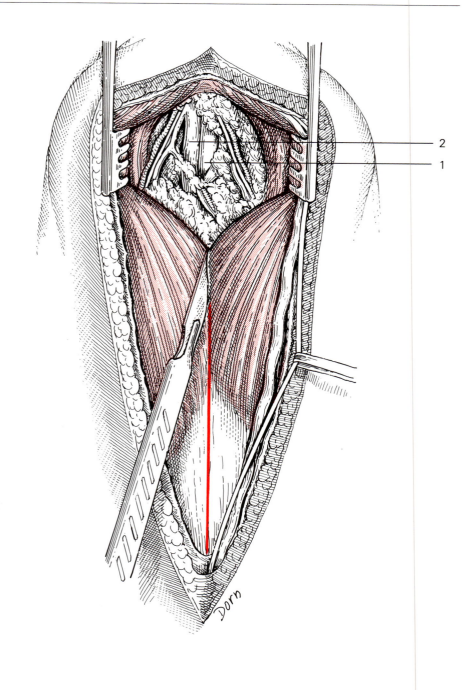

c

1 tibial nerve
2 popliteal vein

D   Soleus is divided by a midline longitudinal incision, taking care to protect the underlying neurovascular structures. The muscle is split progressively and cautiously and numerous transverse anastomoses must be ligated and divided.

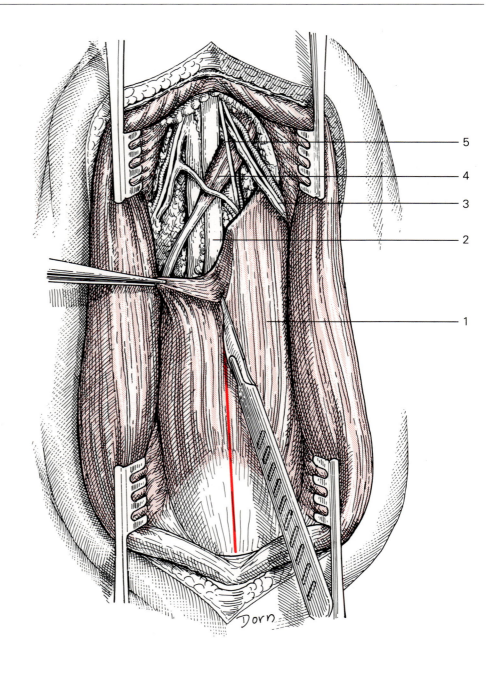

D

1 soleus
2 tibial nerve
3 neurovascular bundle to the lateral head of gastrocnemius
4 plantaris
5 motor nerve to soleus

E This approach allows the entire exposure of the distal portion of the popliteal artery, the origin of the anterior tibial artery, the posterior tibial artery and its branch, the peroneal artery. Care should also be taken to spare the neurovascular pedicles of gastrocnemius, soleus, flexor hallucis longus, tibialis posterior and flexor digitorum communis.

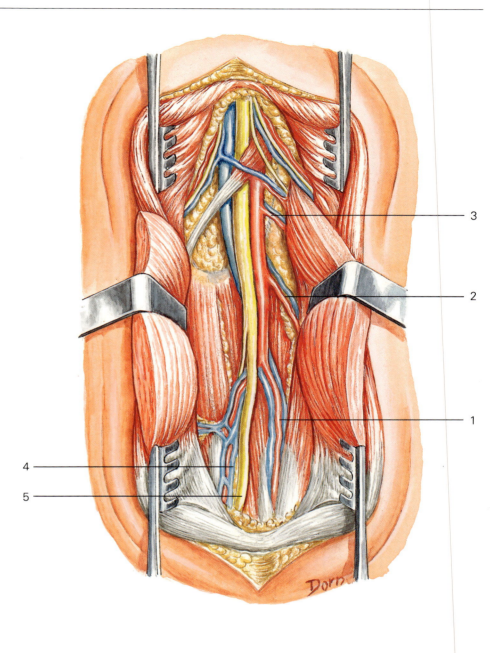

E

1 peroneal vessels
2 anterior tibial vessels
3 vascular pedicle to soleus
4 posterior tibial vessels
5 tibial nerve

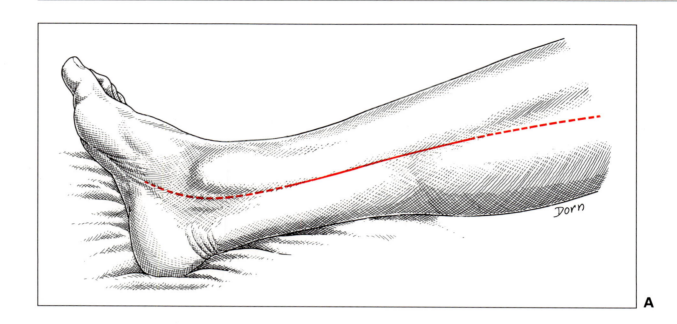

A

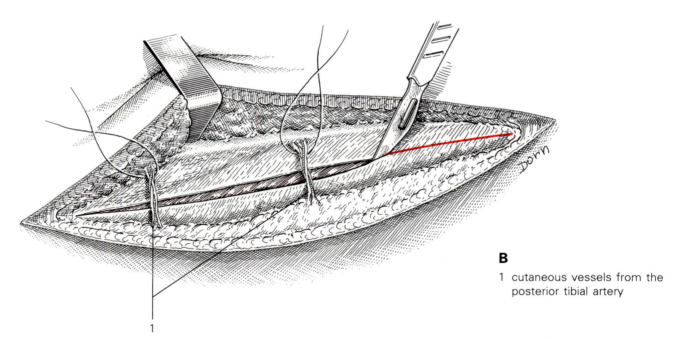

B

1 cutaneous vessels from the posterior tibial artery

Posterior tibial artery: medial approach to the distal segment

Indications

• Ligation of the artery.
• Repair of the artery.

Position of the patient

The patient is supine, with the limb in external rotation.

Incision

A The longitudinal incision is made over the distal two-thirds of the leg, just behind the postero-medial border of the tibia. It can be extended proximally and distally.

Exposure

B The deep fascia is incised after ligation of small cutaneous vessels which cross the incision.

C

1 soleus
2 deep aponeurosis

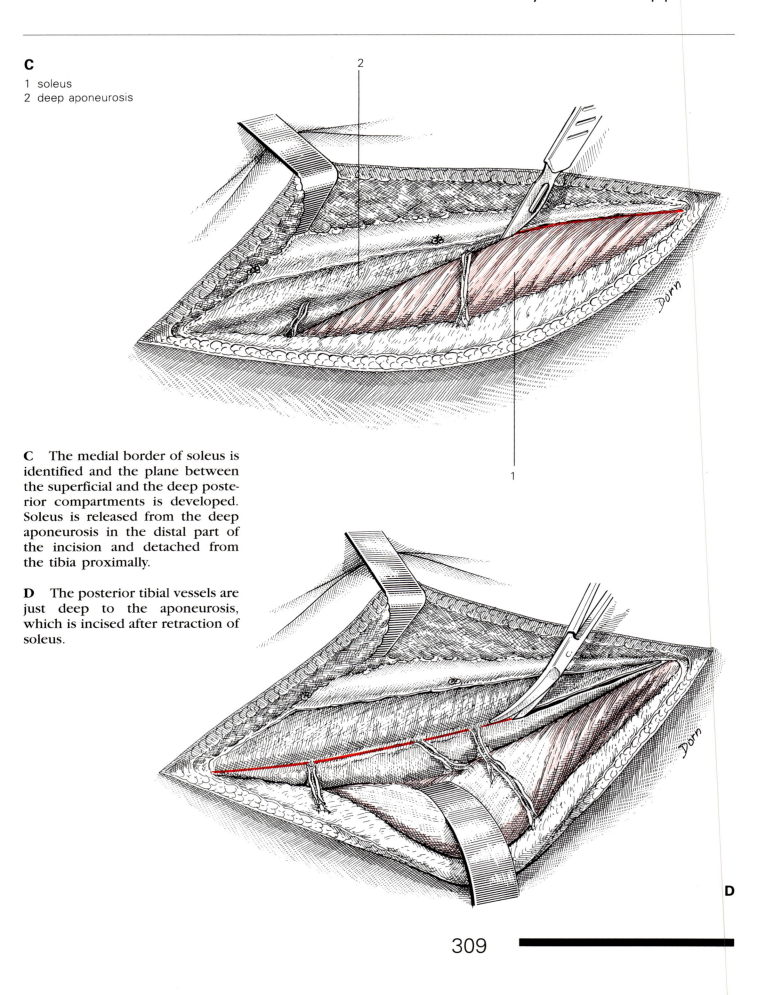

C The medial border of soleus is identified and the plane between the superficial and the deep posterior compartments is developed. Soleus is released from the deep aponeurosis in the distal part of the incision and detached from the tibia proximally.

D The posterior tibial vessels are just deep to the aponeurosis, which is incised after retraction of soleus.

D

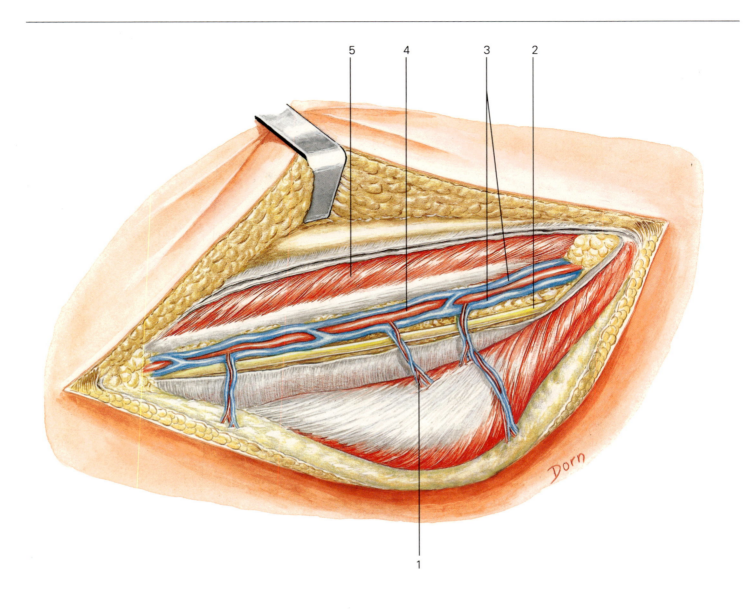

E The neurovascular axis is exposed lying on the muscles of the deep compartment of the leg.

E

1 vascular pedicle to the distal third of soleus
2 tibial nerve
3 posterior tibial veins
4 posterior tibial artery
5 flexor digitorum longus

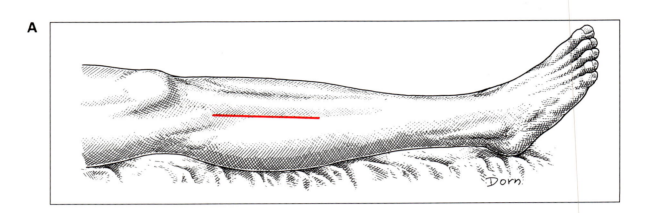

A

Anterior tibial artery: proximal segment

Introduction

The anterior tibial artery can be considered to consist of two segments: the upper which comprises its origin and the arch, and the lower comprising the distal two-thirds of the artery. The best access to the origin and arch is via the lateral transfibular approach. The anterior approach here described does not give such a good exposure of the bifurcation and is limited to the upper third.

Indications

- Ligation of the artery.
- Repair of the artery.

Position of the patient

The patient is supine, with a sandbag under the ipsilateral buttock to maintain the limb in slight internal rotation.

Incision

A The incision is made on the line drawn from the medial aspect of the fibular head to the lateral border of the tendon of tibialis anterior at the ankle.

Exposure

B The deep fascia is incised in the groove between tibialis anterior and extensor digitorum longus.

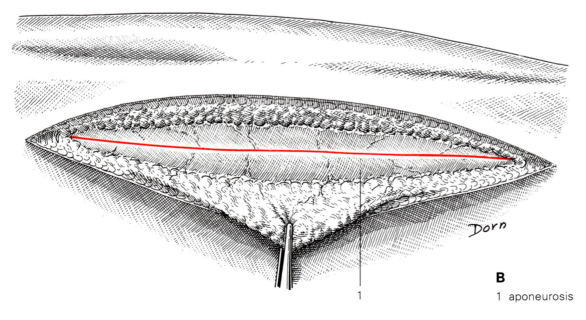

1

B

1 aponeurosis

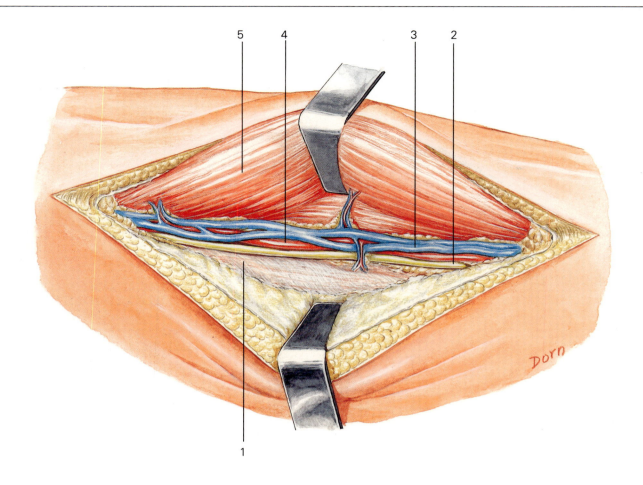

C The two muscles are gently separated, exposing the neurovascular bundle lying on the floor of the anterior compartment. The artery is freed from its venous plexus and the deep peroneal nerve should be identified and preserved.

c
1 extensor digitorum longus
2 deep peroneal nerve
3 anterior tibial veins
4 anterior tibial artery
5 tibialis anterior

Anterior tibial artery: distal segment

Indications

The indications for surgery and positioning of the patient are the same as for the proximal segment.

Incision

A The incision is made along the same line as for the proximal segment, but placed more distally.

Exposure

B The deep fascia is opened and care should be taken in the lower part of the incision to protect the medial branch of the superficial peroneal nerve. The muscles are identified.

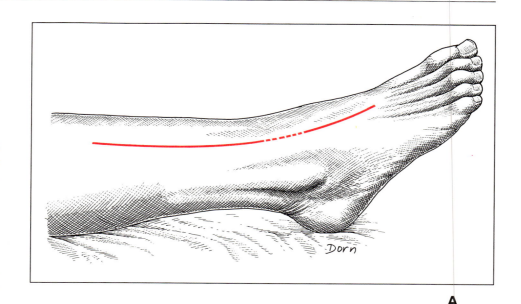

A

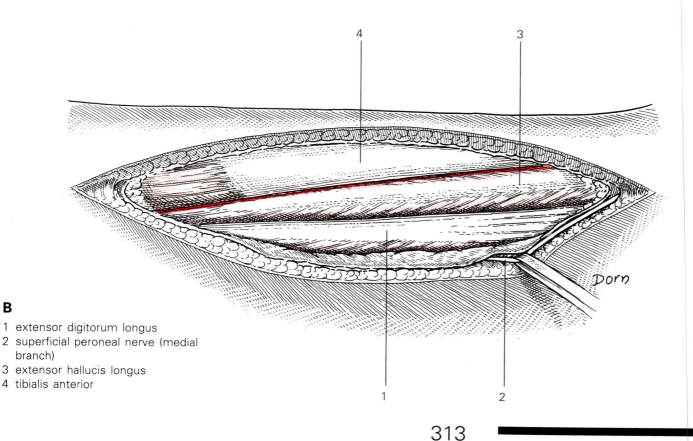

B

1 extensor digitorum longus
2 superficial peroneal nerve (medial branch)
3 extensor hallucis longus
4 tibialis anterior

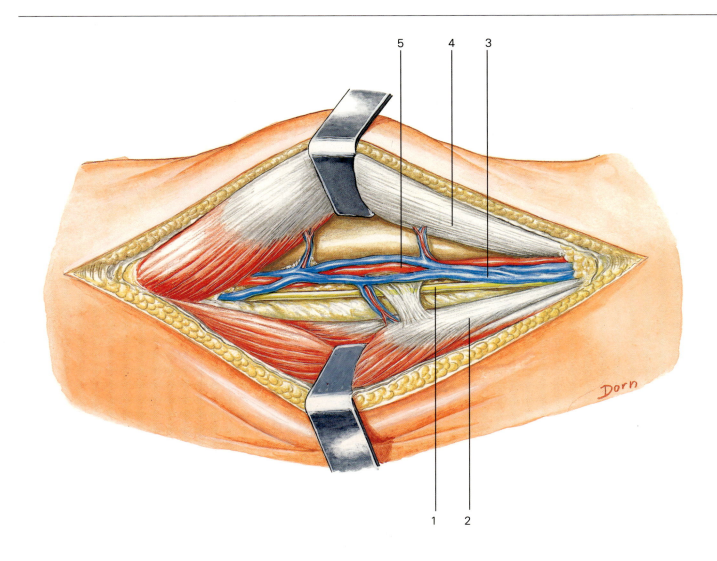

C The tendon of tibialis anterior is retracted medially and extensor hallucis longus laterally, thus exposing the neurovascular bundle. To expose the artery more distally, it is necessary to divide the superior extensor retinaculum. The branches of the deep peroneal nerve should be preserved. At that level, the artery is very deep and is found beneath the tendon of extensor hallucis longus which crosses the course of the artery.

C
1 deep peroneal nerve
2 extensor hallucis longus
3 anterior tibial veins
4 tibialis anterior
5 anterior tibial artery

Dorsalis pedis artery

Anatomy

The dorsalis pedis artery is the continuation of the anterior tibial artery. It lies on the capsule of the ankle joint, the talus, the navicular and the intermediate cuneiform. It runs between the tendon of extensor hallucis longus medially and the tendon of extensor digitorum longus laterally. It ends at the base of the first web space, plunging between the metatarsals to join the lateral plantar artery and completing the plantar arch. Near its termination, it is crossed by the tendon of extensor digitorum brevis. This artery is now of great importance when considering the microvascular transfer of tissue from the foot.

Indications

- Ligation or repair.
- Composite tissue transfer.

Incision

A The course of the artery can be marked preoperatively by palpation or Doppler examination. If it is not palpable, the incision is placed medial to extensor hallucis longus and commences distal to the superior extensor retinaculum.

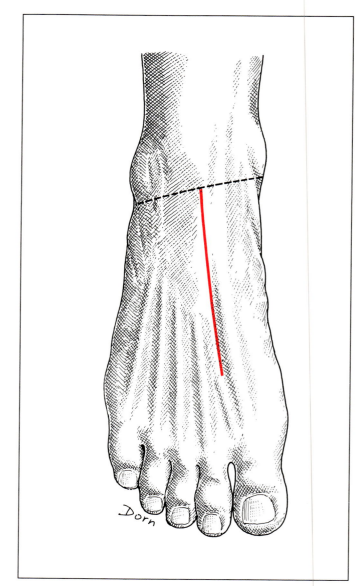

A

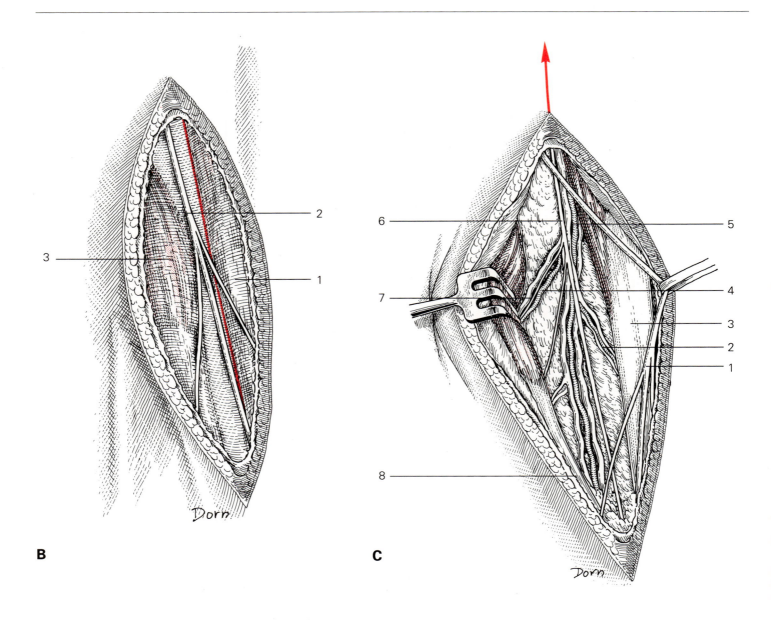

B

C

Exposure

B Care should be taken for the superficial peroneal nerve. The inferior extensor retinaculum is incised between the tendons of extensor hallucis longus (medially) and extensor digitorum longus and extensor digitorum brevis (laterally). The latter are retracted laterally and the former medially, thus exposing the vessels.

C The artery is accompanied by two veins and the deep peroneal nerve which should be isolated and preserved. The exposure of the distal end of the artery requires the division of the first tendon of extensor digitorum brevis.

B

1 extensor hallucis longus
2 superficial peroneal nerve
3 extensor digitorum brevis

C

1 superficial peroneal nerve
2 medial tarsal vessels
3 extensor hallucis longus
4 lateral tarsal artery
5 dorsalis pedis artery
6 deep peroneal nerve
7 motor branch to extensor digitorum brevis
8 first tendon of extensor digitorum brevis

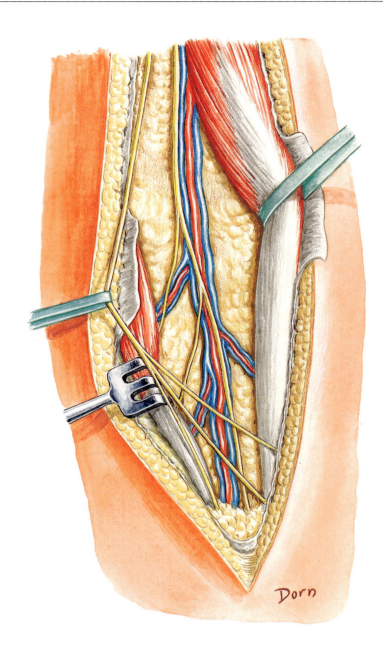

D The approach can be extended proximally by dividing the superior extensor retinaculum. The distal portion of the tibialis anterior artery is thus exposed.

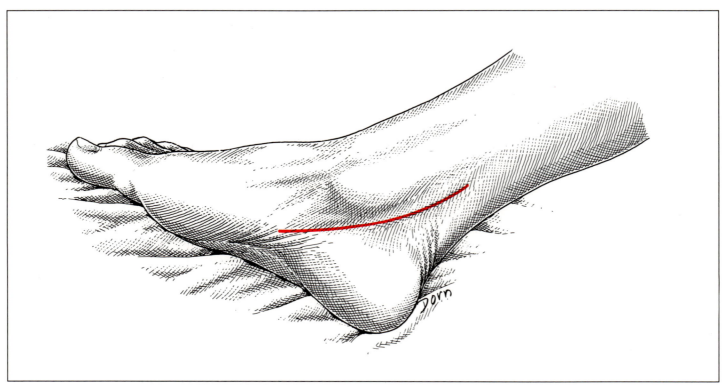

A

Posterior tibial and plantar arteries

Indications

- Ligation or repair of the arteries.
- Reconstructive vascular surgery.
- The elevation of skin flaps.

Position of the patient

The patient is supine, with the limb in external rotation. Rotation can be increased by a sandbag under the contralateral buttock.

Incision

A The longitudinal incision is made over the distal quarter of the leg, midway between the posterior border of the tibia and the Achilles tendon. It runs posterior to the medial malleolus towards the arch of the sole of the foot.

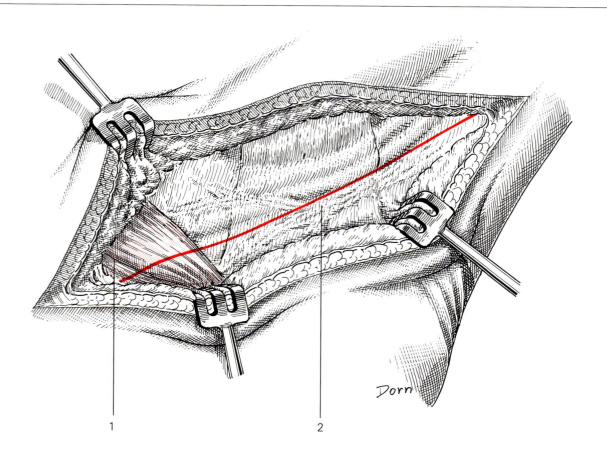

Exposure

B The superficial veins are diathermied and the skin edges reflected to expose the flexor retinaculum in the proximal part of the incision. Distally, the deep fascia is incised to expose, in part, abductor hallucis. The flexor retinaculum is cautiously incised to demonstrate the neurovascular bundle. The isolation of the artery requires excision of the surrounding venous plexus. The tibial nerve is posterior and deep to the artery.

B
1 abductor hallucis
2 flexor retinaculum

319

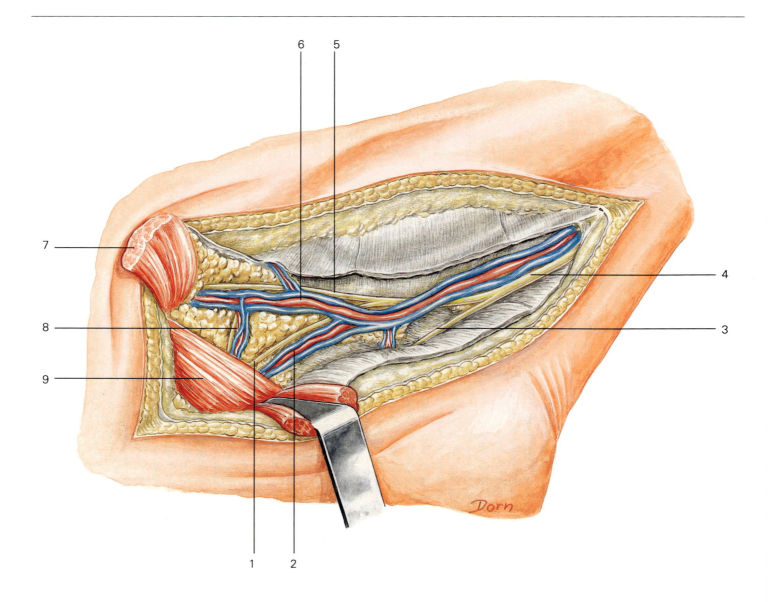

C The bifurcation of the posterior tibial artery into the medial
and lateral plantar arteries is just
proximal to the proximal border
of abductor hallucis. The fibres of
the muscle and the deep aponeurosis are separated to expose the
proximal portion of the medial
and lateral plantar arteries.

The incision can be extended
proximally. The deep aponeurosis
of the leg is incised in continuity
with the flexor retinaculum to
expose the neurovascular axis. In
the lower part of the leg flexor
digitorum longus and flexor hallucis longus are anterior to the
vessels.

C

1 lateral plantar nerve
2 lateral plantar artery
3 calcaneal branch
4 tibial nerve
5 medial plantar nerve
6 medial plantar artery
7 abductor hallucis, split and retracted
8 neurovascular pedicle to flexor
    digitorum brevis
9 flexor digitorum brevis

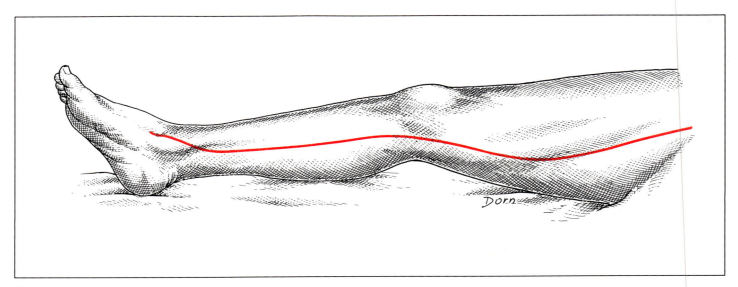

A

Exposure of the long saphenous vein

Indications

- Reconstructive vascular surgery.
- The long saphenous vein is harvested to provide vascular grafts.

Incision

A The course of the long saphenous vein can be located preoperatively by slight inflation of the tourniquet.

The incision commences just anterior to the medial malleolus, runs along the posteromedial border of the tibia, curves round the medial femoral condyle and runs upwards on the medial aspect of the thigh to reach the femoral vein a few centimetres below the inguinal ligament.

Arteries and veins

Exposure

B,C In the distal part of the incision the vein is beneath the aponeurosis and there is a small superficial vein, which should not be confused with the long saphenous vein.

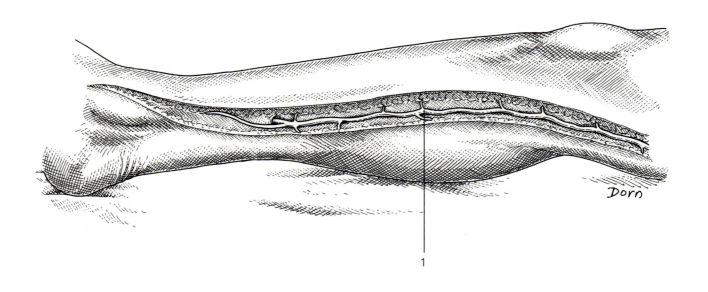

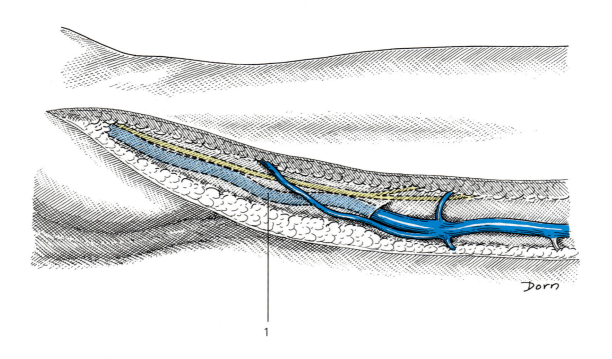

C

1 long saphenous vein beneath the aponeurosis

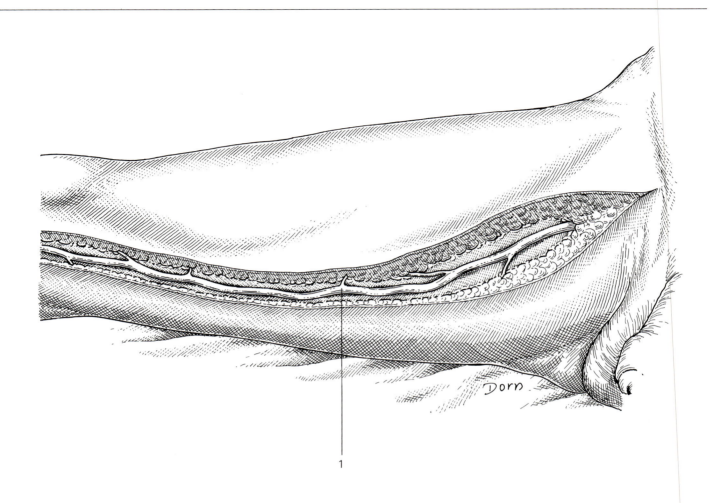

Dorn

1

D The entire course of the vein is progressively exposed to the desired length. Numerous collaterals must be ligated and divided.

D

1 long saphenous vein and tributaries

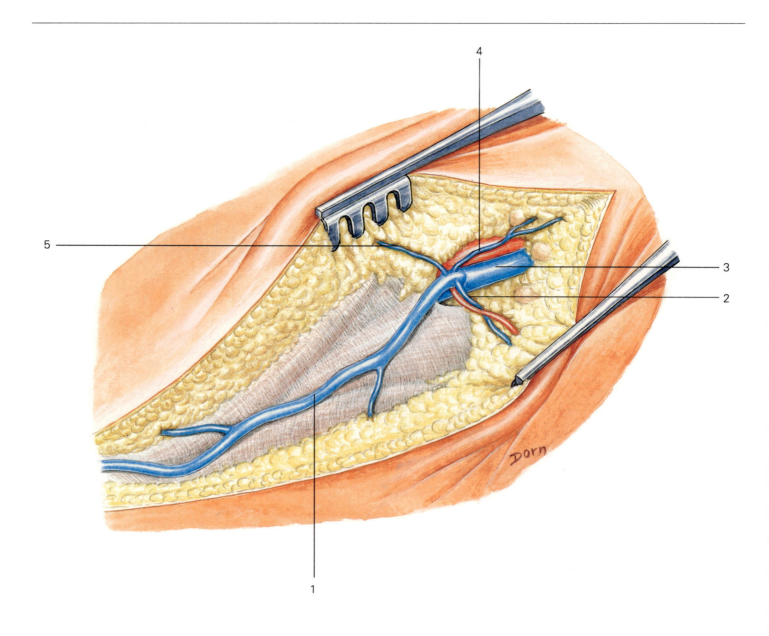

E The origin of the saphenous vein can be dissected and exposed in the groin. The long saphenous vein lies superficial to the deep aponeurosis, except in the distal quarter of the leg.

E
1 long saphenous vein and tributaries
2 superficial external pudendal vein
3 femoral vein
4 superficial epigastric vein
5 superficial circumflex iliac vein

8

Peripheral nerves

Peripheral nerves

Introduction

The indications for the surgical exposure of the nerves of the lower limb are less frequent than for the upper limb. For this reason, the approaches to the nerves are less well known. However, lesions of the peripheral nerves of the lower limb are not uncommon, resulting from gunshot or knife wounds, traction lesions following dislocation of the hip or knee, compression by haematoma, or nerve tumours. The sciatic, femoral and common peroneal nerves are most frequently involved. The sural nerve is commonly used as a donor nerve graft. Nerves of the lower limb arise from the lumbosacral and coccygeal plexuses (**A**).

A

1 sciatic nerve
2 posterior cutaneous nerve of thigh
3 perineal nerve
4 dorsal nerve of penis/clitoris
5 inferior rectal nerve
6 obturator nerve
7 pudendal nerve (S2, 3, 4)
8 perineal branch of fourth sacral nerve
9 to levator ani and coccygeus (S3, 4)
10 posterior cutaneous nerve of thigh (S1, 2, 3)
11 sciatic nerve
12 S4
13 inferior gluteal nerve (L5, S1, 2)
14 S3
15 to piriformis (S1, 2)
16 S2
17 superior gluteal nerve (L4, 5, S1)
18 S1
19 to obturator internus and superior gemellus (L5, S1, 2)
20 to quadratus femoris and inferior gemellus (L5, S1, 2)
21 lumbosacral trunk
22 L5
23 L4
24 L3
25 L2
26 L1
27 subcostal nerve
28 transversus abdominis
29 iliohypogastric nerve (T12, L1)
30 ilioinguinal nerve (L1)
31 to psoas
32 quadratus lumborum
33 femoral branch of genitofemoral nerve
34 genital branch of genitofemoral nerve
35 lateral cutaneous nerve of thigh
36 iliacus
37 psoas
38 femoral nerve (L2, 3, 4)
39 accessory obturator nerve (L3, 4)

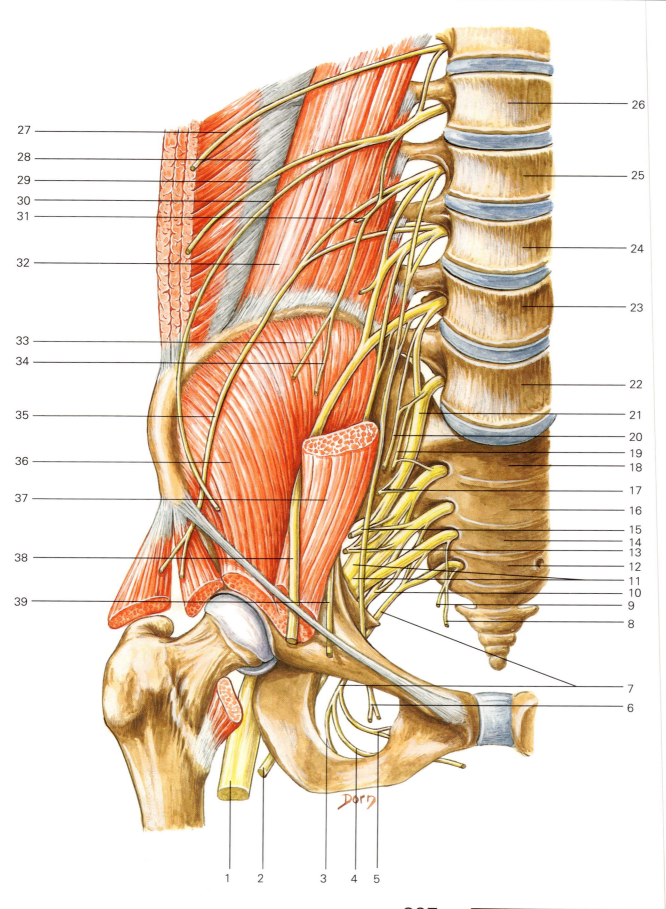

27
28
29
30
31
32
33
34
35
36
37
38
39

26
25
24
23
22
21
20
19
18
17
16
15
14
13
12
11
10
9
8

7
6

Dorn

1   2   3   4   5

Anatomical considerations

The lumbar plexus (B)

The lumbar plexus lies between the anterior and posterior parts of psoas major. It is formed by the anterior primary rami of the first three lumbar nerves and the greater part of the anterior primary ramus of the fourth lumbar nerve. The first lumbar nerve receives a branch from the twelfth thoracic nerve and bifurcates into an upper and lower branch. The upper branch divides into the iliohypogastric and ilio-inguinal nerves. The lower branch receives a branch from the second lumbar nerve to form the genitofemoral nerve.

The larger part of the second and third lumbar nerves, and most of the fourth lumbar nerve, divide into ventral and dorsal branches. All three ventral branches join together to form the obturator nerve. The dorsal branches of the second and third nerves each form a small and large division. The small divisions join together to form the lateral cutaneous nerve of the thigh. The large divisions join with the dorsal branch of the fourth lumbar nerve to form the femoral nerve.

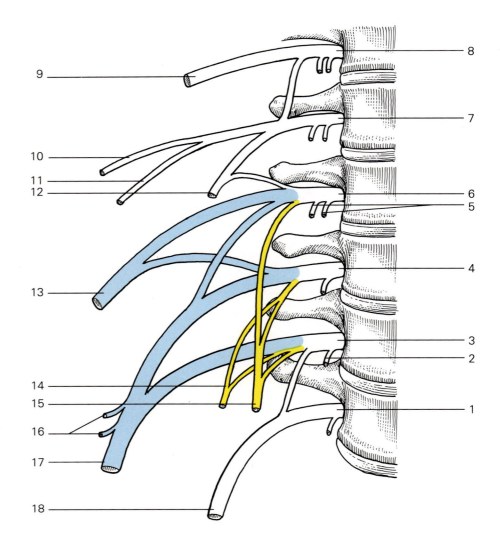

B

1 L5
2 grey rami communicantes
3 L4
4 L3
5 white and grey rami communicantes
6 L2
7 L1
8 T12
9 subcostal nerve
10 iliohypogastric nerve

11 ilioinguinal nerve
12 genitofemoral nerve
13 lateral cutaneous nerve of thigh
14 accessory obturator nerve (often absent)
15 obturator nerve
16 muscular branches to psoas and iliacus
17 femoral nerve
18 lumbosacral trunk

Branches of the lumbar plexus (C)

- **Muscular branches** supply psoas, iliacus and quadratus lumborum.
- The **iliohypogastric nerve (L1)** perforates transversus abdominis supplying this muscle, and divides into lateral and anterior cutaneous branches. The lateral branch supplies the posterolateral gluteal skin, whilst the anterior branch is distributed to the suprapubic skin.
- The **ilioinguinal nerve (L1)** supplies the internal oblique muscle, traverses the inguinal canal and is distributed to the proximal medial skin of the thigh, the penile root and the upper part of the scrotum (mons pubis and labium major).
- The **genitofemoral nerve (L1, L2)** divides close to its origin into two branches. The genital branch enters the inguinal canal and supplies the cremaster and the scrotal skin (mons pubis and labium major). The femoral branch passes beneath the inguinal ligament, enters the femoral sheath which it pierces with the fascia lata and supplies the anterior skin over the upper part of Scarpa's triangle.
- The **lateral cutaneous nerve of the thigh (L2, L3)** crosses iliacus and runs towards the anterior superior iliac spine. It passes behind or through the inguinal ligament, medial to the anterior iliac spine, and divides into anterior and posterior branches. The anterior branch becomes superficial about 10 cm distal to the spine and is distributed to the skin of the anterior and lateral thigh as far distally as the knee. It joins with the infrapatellar branch of the saphenous nerve forming the parapatellar plexus. The posterior branch pierces the fascia lata and supplies the skin on the lateral aspect of the greater trochanter.

The obturator nerve (L2, L3, L4)

This nerve passes lateral to the internal iliac vessels and descends on obturator internus entering the upper part of the thigh. It divides into anterior and posterior branches, which are separated by obturator externus and adductor brevis. The anterior branch descends deep to pectineus and adductor longus. It supplies the skin of the medial thigh and innervates adductor longus, pectineus, gracilis and adductor brevis. It occasionally supplies a communicating branch to the medial cutaneous nerve of the thigh and the saphenous nerve. The posterior branch pierces obturator externus, which it supplies and passes deep to adductor brevis.

The femoral nerve (L2, L3, L4)

This nerve is the most important branch of the lumbar plexus. It descends through psoas major and passes between psoas and iliacus. It enters the thigh beneath the inguinal ligament, just lateral to its midpoint and lateral to the femoral artery, and divides into anterior and posterior branches.

The anterior branch innervates sartorius and supplies the intermediate and medial cutaneous nerves of the thigh. The intermediate cutaneous nerve pierces the fascia lata about 10 cm distal to the inguinal ligament, and supplies the anterior aspect of the thigh as far distally as the knee. The medial cutaneous nerve accompanies the femoral artery until the apex of Scarpa's triangle, and then divides into anterior and posterior branches. The anterior branch pierces the fascia lata in the midthigh and supplies the medial side of the thigh and knee. The posterior branch descends to the knee and links with the saphenous nerve. The saphenous nerve and muscular branches of the quadriceps arise from the posterior branch.

The saphenous nerve descends with the femoral artery in the adductor canal of Hunter. It then leaves the vessels, piercing the aponeurotic sheath with the saphenous branch of the descending genicular artery. It descends deep to sartorius and emerges in the leg anterior or posterior to this muscle. It becomes subcutaneous and descends along the medial side of the tibia with the long saphenous vein. It divides distally into a branch passing anterior to the ankle and another continuing along the posterior border of the tibia. It supplies an infrapatellar branch at the level of the adductor canal.

Muscular branches innervate the quadriceps. Each head of the quadriceps is supplied by a well-defined branch, the largest being to vastus lateralis which forms a neurovascular bundle with the descending branch of the lateral circumflex artery.

Peripheral nerves

c

1 deep peroneal nerve
2 tibialis anterior
3 recurrent branch of deep peroneal
   nerve
4 saphenous nerve
5 infrapatellar branch of saphenous
   nerve
6 vastus medialis
7 sartorius, cut
8 gracilis
9 saphenous nerve
10 cutaneous branch of obturator
    nerve
11 adductor magnus
12 adductor longus, cut
13 adductor brevis
14 anterior division of obturator nerve
15 pectineus
16 quadratus femoris
17 posterior division of obturator nerve
18 obturator externus
19 obturator nerve
20 lateral cutaneous nerve of thigh
21 femoral nerve and its divisions
22 rectus femoris, cut
23 motor branches from the femoral
    nerve
24 vastus lateralis
25 common peroneal nerve
26 peroneus longus
27 extensor digitorum
28 superficial peroneal nerve

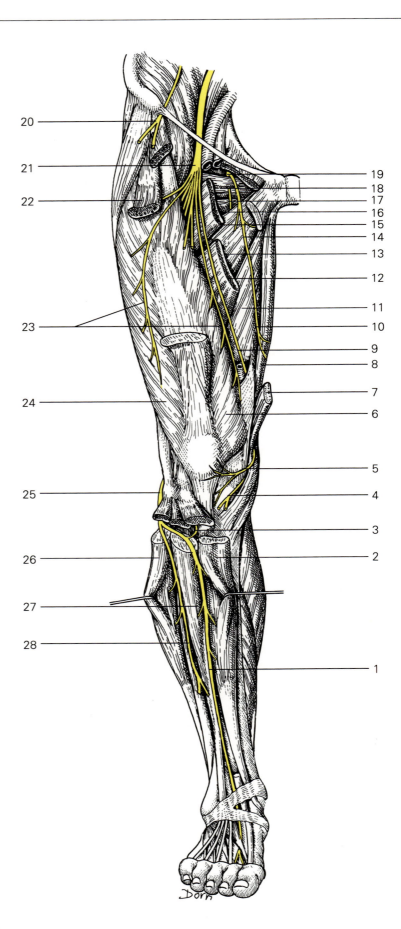

The sacral plexus (**D**)

The sacral plexus is formed from the lumbosacral trunk and the anterior primary rami of the first three sacral nerves. The lumbosacral trunk itself comprises a part of the anterior primary ramus of the fourth lumbar nerve and the whole of the anterior primary ramus of the fifth lumbar nerve. It appears at the medial border of psoas major, and crosses the pelvic brim in front of the sacroiliac joint to join the first sacral nerve. The anterior primary ramus of the fourth sacral nerve divides into two branches, the upper joining the sacral plexus and the lower descending to assist in forming the coccygeal plexus.

The sacral plexus lies on the posterior pelvic wall on piriformis, behind the internal iliac vessels, the ureters and the bowel. The nerves converge towards the greater sciatic notch as a flattened band at which point several branches arise. The continuation of this band into the posterior thigh is the sciatic nerve.

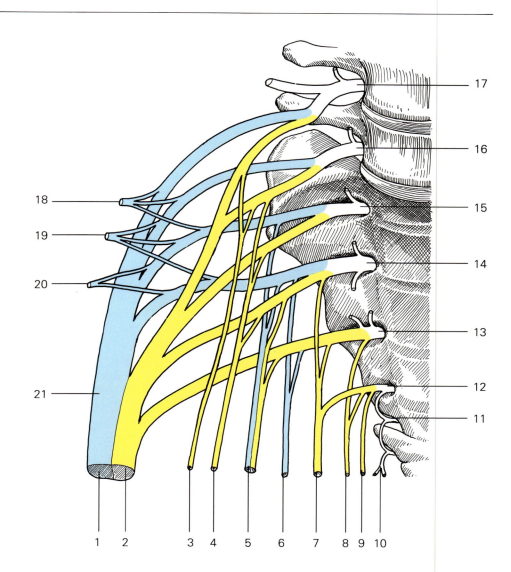

D

1 common peroneal nerve
2 tibial nerve
3 nerve to quadratus femoris and inferior gemellus
4 nerve to obturator internus and superior gemellus
5 posterior cutaneous nerve of thigh
6 perforating cutaneous nerve
7 pudendal nerve
8 nerve to levator ani and coccygeus
9 perineal branch of fourth sacral nerve

10 anococcygeal nerve
11 S5
12 S4
13 S3
14 S2
15 S1
16 L5
17 L4
18 superior gluteal nerve
19 inferior gluteal nerve
20 nerve to piriformis
21 sciatic nerve

Branches of the sacral plexus (E)

- The **superior gluteal nerve (L4, L5, S1)** leaves the pelvis via the greater sciatic foramen with the gluteal vessels and divides into superior and inferior branches. The superior branch innervates gluteus medius and the inferior branch supplies gluteus medius and minimus and tensor fasciae latae.
- The **inferior gluteal nerve (L4, S1, S2)** supplies gluteus maximus.
- The **nerve to piriformis (S1, S2)**.
- The **nerve to obturator internus and gemellus superior (L5, S1, S2)** leaves the pelvis via the greater sciatic foramen, innervates gemellus superior and re-enters the pelvis via the lesser sciatic foramen to supply obturator internus.
- The **nerve to quadratus femoris and gemellus inferior (L4, L5, S1)** also leaves the pelvis via the greater sciatic foramen.
- The **posterior cutaneous nerve of the thigh (S1, S2, S3)** leaves the pelvis via the greater sciatic foramen and descends deep to gluteus maximus with the inferior gluteal vessels. It runs in the thigh deep to the fascia, perforating it behind the knee. Then it accompanies the short saphenous vein as far as the midcalf and joins the sural nerve. Its branches supply large areas of skin: the inferolateral area of the lower border of gluteus maximus, the scrotum or labial skin, the back and the medial side of the thigh, the popliteal fossa and the proximal part of the posterior aspect of the leg.

The sciatic nerve (L4, L5, S1, S2, S3)

The sciatic nerve is the thickest nerve in the body, being 2 cm in breadth as it passes through the greater sciatic foramen, and is the main nerve arising from the sciatic plexus. It leaves the pelvis via the greater sciatic foramen below piriformis and runs between the greater trochanter and ischial tuberosity to descend along the back of the thigh, at first deep to gluteus maximus, crossing the posterior surfaces of obturator internus, the gemelli and quadratus femoris. It is accompanied by the posterior cutaneous nerve of thigh and the inferior gluteal artery. In the thigh, it lies deep to adductor magnus and is covered in the upper part by the long head of biceps femoris. The sciatic nerve supplies articular branches to the hip joint and muscular branches that innervate biceps femoris, semitendinosus, semimembranosus and the ischial portion of adductor magnus. The sciatic nerve usually divides in the distal thigh into the tibial and common peroneal nerves. Studies of the neuroanatomy demonstrate that the tibial nerve is formed from the ventral branches of the anterior primary rami of the fourth and fifth lumbar nerves and the first three sacral nerves, whilst the common peroneal nerve is formed from the dorsal branches of the anterior primary rami of the fourth and fifth lumbar nerves and the first and second sacral nerves. The consequence of this configuration is that the sciatic nerve may divide at any point between the sacral plexus and the distal third of the thigh. It is common, however, for the division into the tibial and common peroneal nerves to be distal.

The tibial nerve (L4, L5, S1, S2, S3, ventral divisions)

The tibial nerve runs deep to the hamstrings in the thigh and becomes superficial in the popliteal fossa lateral to the vessels. It is covered in the distal fossa by the gastrocnemii and passes anterior to the arch of soleus to lie on the interosseous membrane accompanied by the posterior tibial vessels. In the leg, the nerve is at first medial to the vessels, but becomes lateral distally, and supplies articular and muscular branches and the sural and medial calcaneal nerves before dividing into the medial and lateral plantar nerves.

- **Articular branches** accompany the genicular arteries to the knee and also supply the ankle.
- **Muscular branches** innervate gastrocnemius, plantaris, soleus and popliteus. The branch to popliteus also supplies tibialis posterior. More distally, flexor digitorum longus and flexor hallucis longus are supplied by the tibial nerve.
- The **sural nerve** descends between the two heads of gastrocnemius and perforates the fascia in the upper third of the leg. It is sometimes enclosed in a fascial tunnel before emerging subcutaneously. It runs from the midline of the calf towards the ankle midway between the lateral malleolus and the Achilles tendon, and is accompanied by the short saphenous vein. At the ankle, the sural nerve curves round the lateral malleolus and branches on the lateral border of the foot as far as the little toe. It supplies the posterior and lateral skin of the distal third of the leg and the lateral border of the foot and little toe. The medial calcaneal branch pierces the flexor retinaculum to supply the skin of the heel.

E

1 flexor hallucis longus
2 tibial nerve
3 sural nerve
4 nerve to lateral head of
 gastrocnemius
5 sural communicating nerve
6 common peroneal nerve
7 tibial nerve
8 common peroneal nerve
9 biceps femoris, cut
10 motor branches from sciatic nerve
11 sciatic nerve
12 quadratus femoris
13 inferior gemellus
14 obturator internus
15 superior gemellus
16 piriformis
17 gluteus minimus
18 superior gluteal nerve
19 gluteus medius, cut
20 inferior gluteal nerve
21 pudendal nerve
22 nerve to superior gemellus and
 obturator internus
23 posterior cutaneous nerve of thigh
24 perineal branches of posterior
 cutaneous nerve of thigh
25 posterior cutaneous nerve of thigh
26 gracilis
27 adductor magnus
28 semitendinosus
29 semimembranosus
30 nerve to medial head of
 gastrocnemius
31 motor branches from the tibial
 nerve
32 flexor digitorum
33 medial calcaneal nerve

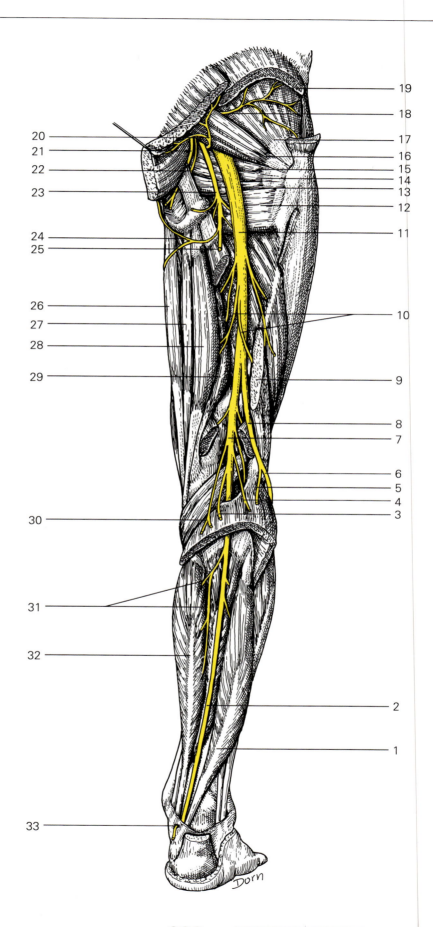

- The **medial plantar nerve (F)** passes deep to abductor hallucis, supplies the medial digital nerve to the hallux and divides near the metatarsal bases into three common plantar digital nerves. Cutaneous branches supply the sole of the foot between abductor hallucis and flexor digitorum brevis. Muscular branches innervate abductor hallucis, flexor digitorum brevis, flexor hallucis brevis and the first lumbrical. The common plantar digital nerves pass between the slips of the plantar aponeurosis and each divides into two digital branches supplying adjacent borders of the toes.
- The **lateral plantar nerve** divides into deep and superficial branches between flexor digitorum brevis and abductor digiti minimi, which is supplied by the nerve. Before division, it supplies a cutaneous branch to the lateral part of the sole. The superficial branch splits into two common plantar digital nerves, and the deep branch accompanies the lateral plantar artery, supplying the second to fourth lumbricals, adductor hallucis and the interossei. This distribution is similar to that of the ulnar nerve in the hand.

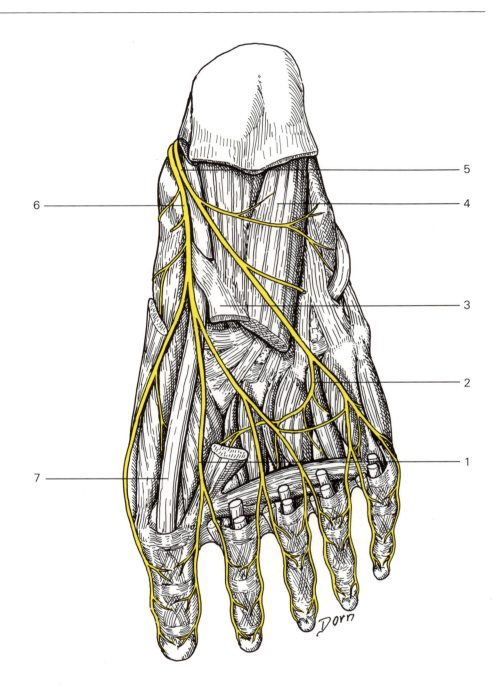

F
1 common plantar digital nerves
2 deep branch to interossei
3 flexor digitorum longus tendon
4 flexor digitorum accessorius
5 lateral plantar nerve
6 medial plantar nerve
7 flexor hallucis longus tendon

The common peroneal nerve (L4, L5, S1, S2, dorsal divisions) (see C)

The common peroneal nerve descends along the lateral side of the popliteal fossa to the fibular head lying between the tendon of biceps femoris and the lateral head of gastrocnemius. It passes deep to peroneus longus and divides to form the superficial and deep peroneal nerves, after supplying articular and cutaneous branches.

- The **lateral cutaneous nerve** of the calf supplies the skin of the anterior and posterolateral surfaces of the proximal leg.
- The **sural communicating nerve** crosses the lateral head of gastrocnemius to join the sural nerve.

- The **deep peroneal nerve** passes deep to extensor digitorum longus and reaches the anterior tibial artery in the proximal third of the leg. It accompanies the artery as far as the ankle, and divides into lateral and medial terminal branches. Before division, it innervates tibialis anterior, extensor hallucis longus, extensor digitorum longus and peroneus tertius. The lateral terminal branch curves deep to extensor digitorum brevis which it supplies. The medial terminal branch runs on the dorsum of the foot lateral to the dorsalis pedis artery and joins the medial branch of the deep peroneal nerve. It supplies the first interosseous and divides distally into two dorsal digital nerves to the first toe web.

- The **superficial peroneal nerve**, at first deep to peroneus longus, passes between the peronei and extensor digitorum longus and pierces the crural fascia in the distal third of the leg. It supplies peroneus longus, peroneus brevis and the skin of the lateral lower leg. Distally, it divides into lateral and medial branches. The medial branch passes anterior to the ankle and divides again into two branches: one to the medial side of the hallux and the other to the dorsal aspect of the second web. The lateral branch crosses the dorsum of the foot and supplies the lateral aspect of the ankle and the dorsal aspect of the third and fourth toe webs. It joins the sural nerve.

G,H Cutaneous nerves of the lower limb

G

1 dorsal digital branch of deep peroneal nerve
2 saphenous nerve
3 infrapatellar branch of saphenous nerve
4 cutaneous branch of obturator nerve
5 intermediate and medial cutaneous nerves of thigh (from femoral nerve)
6 genital branch of genitofemoral nerve
7 femoral branch of genitofemoral nerve
8 lateral cutaneous branch of subcostal nerve
9 lateral cutaneous nerve of thigh
10 lateral cutaneous nerve of thigh
11 branches of lateral cutaneous nerve of calf (from common peroneal nerve)
12 superficial peroneal nerve
13 lateral branch of superficial peroneal nerve
14 medial branch of superficial peroneal nerve
15 sural nerve, terminal branch

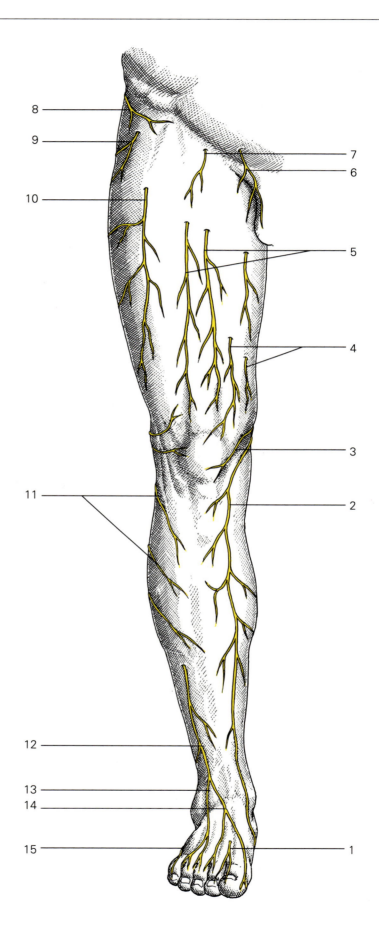

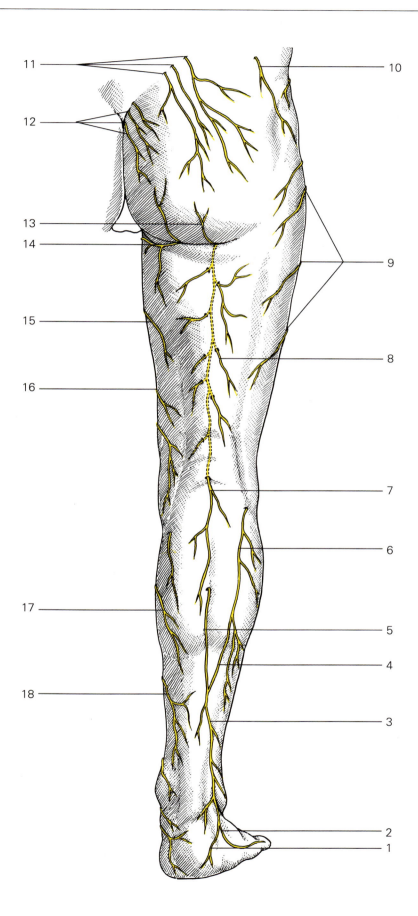

H

1 lateral calcaneal branches of sural nerve
2 sural nerve, terminal branch
3 sural nerve
4 peroneal communicating nerve
5 sural nerve (from tibial nerve)
6 lateral cutaneous nerve of calf
7 terminal branch of posterior cutaneous nerve of thigh
8 branches of posterior cutaneous nerve of thigh
9 branches of lateral cutaneous nerve of thigh
10 lateral cutaneous branch of iliohypogastric nerve
11 superior gluteal nerves (from dorsal rami of L1, 2, 3)
12 middle gluteal nerves (from dorsal rami of S1, 2, 3)
13 inferior gluteal nerves (from posterior cutaneous nerve of thigh)
14 perforating cutaneous nerve (from dorsal rami of S1, 2, 3)
15 branch of medial cutaneous nerve of thigh
16 cutaneous branch of obturator nerve
17 branch of saphenous nerve
18 branch of saphenous nerve

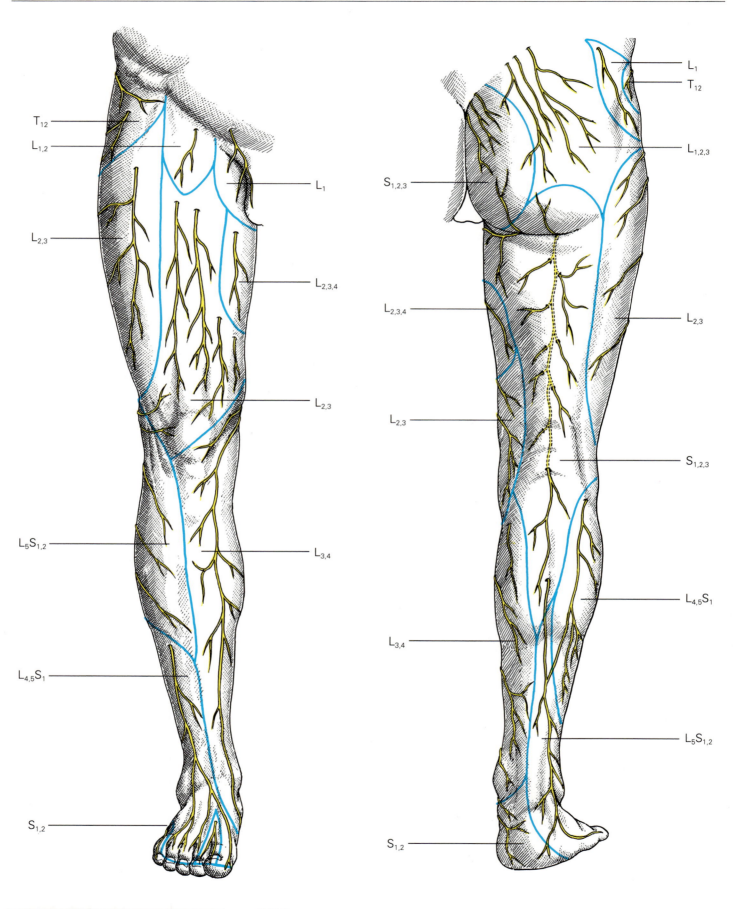

T_{12}

$L_{1,2}$

$L_{2,3}$

$L_{5}S_{1,2}$

$L_{4,5}S_{1}$

$S_{1,2}$

L_{1}

$L_{2,3,4}$

$L_{2,3}$

$L_{3,4}$

$S_{1,2,3}$

$L_{2,3,4}$

$L_{2,3}$

$L_{3,4}$

$S_{1,2}$

L_{1}

T_{12}

$L_{1,2,3}$

$L_{2,3}$

$S_{1,2,3}$

$L_{4,5}S_{1}$

$L_{5}S_{1,2}$

Lumbosacral plexus: lateral approach

Introduction

Traumatic avulsion of the lumbosacral plexus is very uncommon and the place of surgical treatment is not yet clear. However, the lumbar and sacral nerves may be compressed by fractures of the sacrum or a dislocation of the sacroiliac joint. The anterior extraperitoneal approach carries considerable risks and is difficult because of the depth of the dissection and the proximity of the vessels, particularly those of the internal iliac venous plexus. The lateral approach avoids the vessels, although its disadvantage is the osteotomy of the ilium.

Indication

• Traumatic compression of the lumbosacral plexus.

Position of the patient

The patient is in the midlateral position, with the affected side uppermost.

Incision

A A straight longitudinal incision is made beginning proximal to the iliac crest and extending for about 15 cm over the buttock posterior to the greater trochanter.

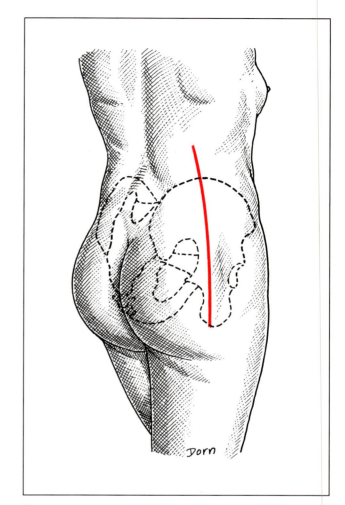

A

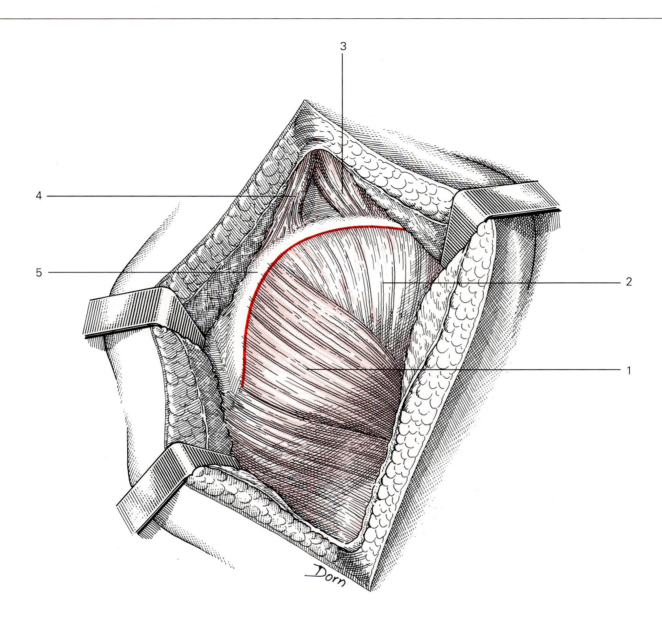

Exposure

B The subcutaneous dissection is deepened until the abdominal wall is reached with the external and internal oblique muscles proximally and gluteus maximus distally. Quadratus lumborum is left attached to the ilium posteriorly.

B

1 gluteus maximus
2 gluteus medius
3 external and internal oblique
4 quadratus lumborum
5 iliac crest

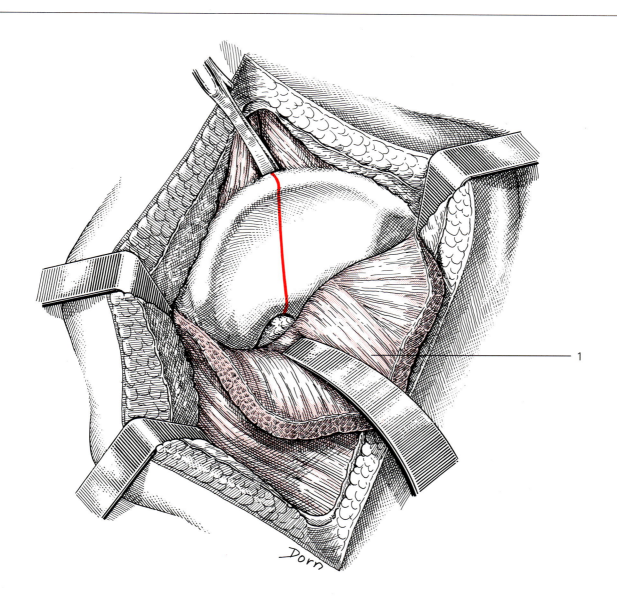

C The posterior aspect of the sacroiliac joint and the lateral ilium are freed subperiosteally from the insertions of gluteus maximus posteriorly and part of gluteus medius anteriorly. Proximally, the muscles are detached anterior to the insertion of quadratus lumborum. Distally, the greater sciatic foramen is progressively exposed. The superior gluteal vessels are protected by the subperiosteal dissection. Gluteus maximus and the vessels are gently retracted anteriorly. The thoracolumbar fascia is then incised and a plane developed between the abdominal wall muscles anteriorly and quadratus lumborum posteriorly. The inner aspect of the ilium is then released subperiosteally to expose the greater sciatic foramen.

c

1 gluteus maximus and medius, retracted

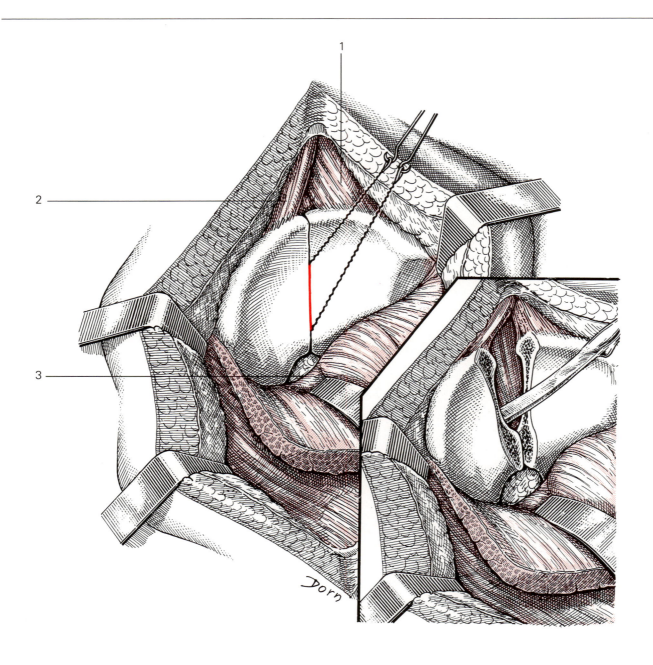

D The ilium is then osteotomized with a Gigli saw. The posterior part of the bone is retracted progressively like a door on a hinge. The posterior sacroiliac ligaments should be preserved, but the anterior ligaments should be divided to allow dislocation of the joint and to complete the opening of the bone flap posteriorly. Quadratus lumborum remains attached to the iliac crest.

D

1 external and internal oblique
2 quadratus lumborum
3 greater sciatic foramen

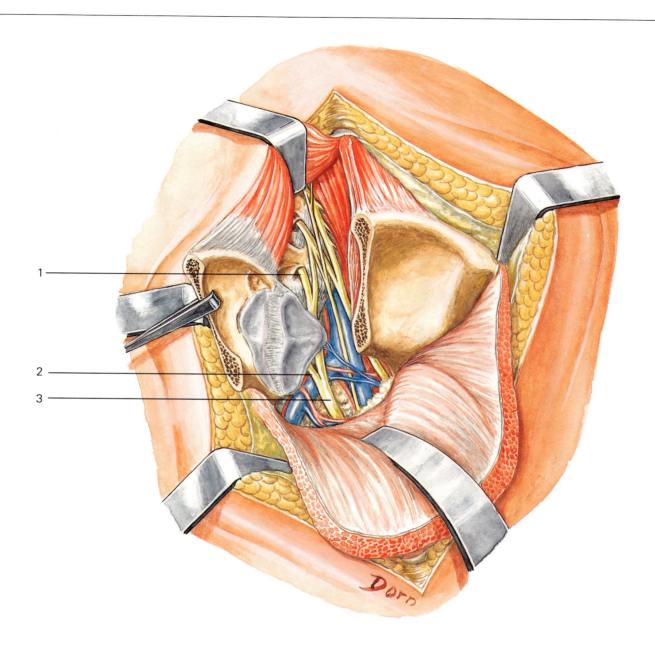

E The lateral aspect of the fifth lumbar vertebral body is thus exposed and, distally, the lumbosacral trunk and the first and second sacral nerves can be seen. The closure of the wound requires the osteosynthesis of the ilium by a combination of staples and plates.

E

1 fifth lumbar nerve
2 first sacral nerve
3 lumbosacral trunk

343

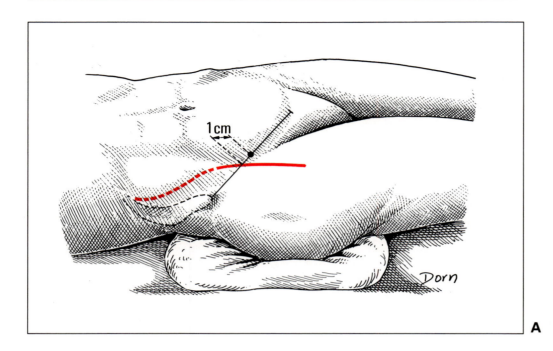

A

Femoral nerve

Introduction

Damage to the femoral nerve is relatively rare, but usually results from one of the following three causes:

1 Compression by a haematoma in the psoas sheath, usually resulting from anticoagulants.

2 During hip arthroplasty, traction on the leg may cause the injury or the nerve may be damaged directly by a retractor placed over the anterior lip of the acetabulum. To avoid damage to the femoral nerve, it is important to place such a retractor deep to the reflected head of rectus femoris.

3 Stab wounds are not uncommon.

Anatomy

The femoral nerve emerges from the pelvis on the lateral border of psoas major and descends between psoas and iliacus deep to the iliac fascia. Posterior to the inguinal ligament, it is separated by a portion of psoas. It is lateral to the femoral artery which separates it from the femoral vein. For a neurolysis to be effective, the nerve needs to be exposed in the pelvis and the thigh.

Indications

• Neurolysis.
• Repair of lacerations.

Position of the patient

The patient is supine.

Incision

A The incision runs proximally and distally from a point about 3 cm medial to the anterior superior iliac spine on the inguinal ligament. Proximally, it extends along the ligament and angles to run medial to the iliac crest. Distally, it descends along the medial border of sartorius for about 10 cm.

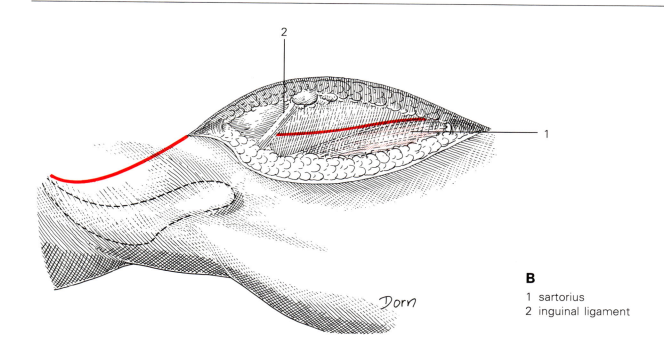

Dorn

B
1 sartorius
2 inguinal ligament

Exposure in the thigh

B The nerve is first exposed in the thigh. The fascia is incised in line with the skin incision, thus exposing sartorius. Just medial to this, psoas is seen within its own fascia.

C Sartorius is retracted laterally, exposing the femoral nerve, which is separated from the femoral artery by the distal part of iliopsoas. The branches of the nerve can be seen in the base of the wound, and a tape is placed around the nerve.

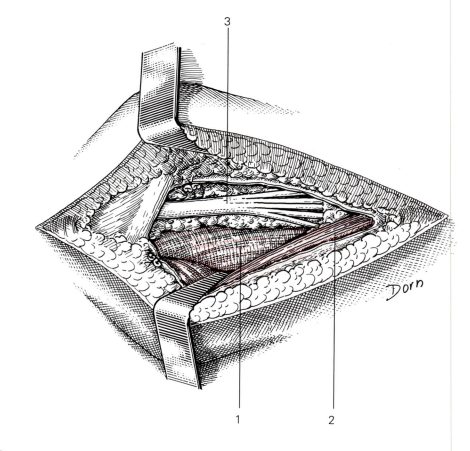

Dorn

C
1 iliopsoas
2 sartorius
3 femoral nerve

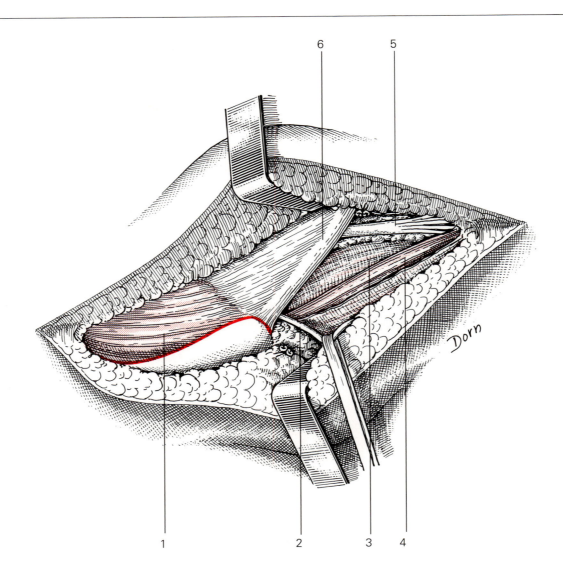

Dorn

Intrapelvic exposure

D The subcutaneous tissue is dissected to expose the free edge of the inguinal ligament and the aponeurosis of the external oblique. Medial to the anterior superior iliac spine, care should be taken to preserve the lateral cutaneous nerve of thigh. It must be identified before detaching the inguinal ligament from the pelvis. Then the three muscles of the abdominal wall (the external and internal oblique, and transversus abdominus) are divided, leaving a fringe of muscle on the iliac crest for their later reinsertion.

D
1 external oblique
2 lateral cutaneous nerve of thigh
3 iliopsoas
4 sartorius
5 femoral nerve
6 inguinal ligament

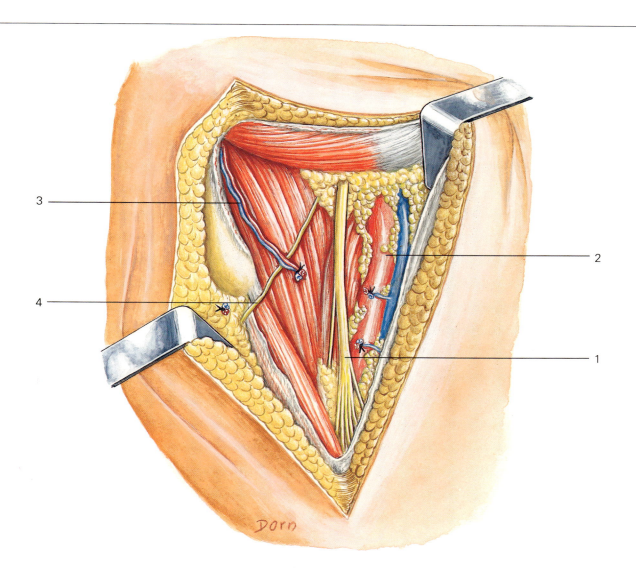

E The muscles are retracted medially, exposing the preperitoneal adipose tissue. The peritoneum is separated from psoas, care being taken to avoid injury to the deep circumflex iliac vessels which cross the retroperitoneal space. However, these vessels can be ligated without prejudice. The femoral nerve lies beneath the deep iliac fascia which should be incised to expose the nerve. The closure of the wound necessitates meticulous reattachment of the muscles and the inguinal ligament to the iliac crest and anterior superior iliac spine.

E
1 femoral nerve
2 femoral sheath, retracted
3 deep circumflex iliac vessels
4 lateral cutaneous nerve of thigh

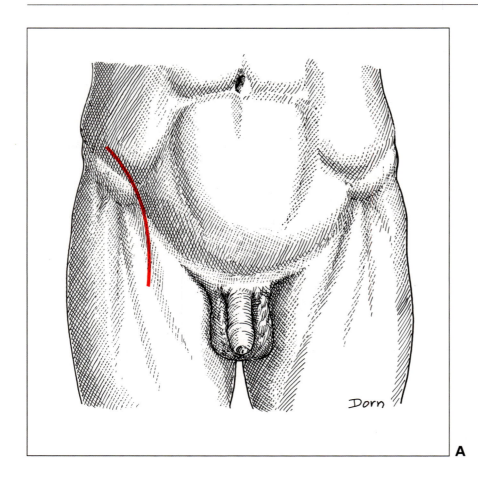

A

Lateral cutaneous nerve of thigh

Introduction

The lateral cutaneous nerve may be compressed in the inguinal ligament, to produce the syndrome of meralgia paraesthetica.

Anatomy

The lateral cutaneous nerve of the thigh runs a varied course adjacent to the anterior superior iliac spine. It passes either behind or through the inguinal ligament at a variable distance from the spine, but usually 1 cm medial to it. It runs anterior and frequently medial to sartorius before becoming superficial. The identification of the nerve is necessary in all the anterior approaches to the hip. Division of the nerve can cause burning discomfort in its cutaneous distribution. As its position is not absolute, a careful exploration is often required.

Indication

• Neurolysis.

Position of the patient

The patient is supine.

Incision

A The incision starts 1 cm medial to the anterior superior iliac spine and runs distally along the proximal thigh for about 4 cm. It may be extended proximally, the incision running parallel to the medial border of the iliac crest. Alternatively, a transverse skin crease incision can be made, centred over a point 1 cm medial to the anterior superior iliac spine.

348

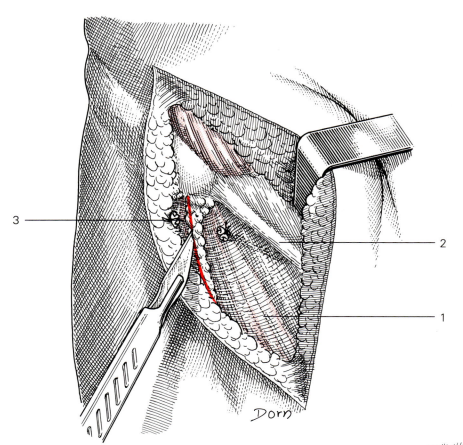

B

1 sartorius
2 inguinal ligament
3 tensor fasciae latae

C

1 external oblique
2 lateral cutaneous nerve of thigh

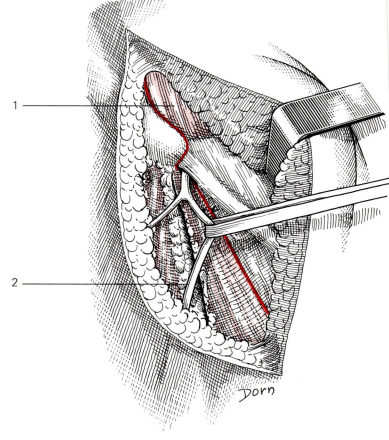

Exposure

B The fascia is incised cautiously because the nerve may lie just beneath it. The nerve is first looked for medial to tensor fasciae latae and lateral to sartorius. It runs in a fascial tunnel. If it is not found in this space, it should be looked for more medially. Sometimes it turns around a fibrous band at the level of the femoral nerve, superficial to it.

C The intrapelvic exposure requires the detachment of the inguinal ligament from the anterior superior iliac spine and the release of the external oblique from the iliac crest.

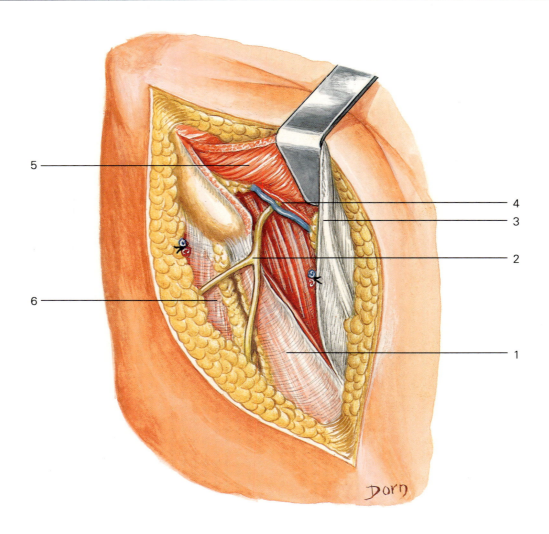

D In the pelvis, care should be taken to protect the deep circumflex iliac vessels which cross superficial to the nerve.

D
1 sartorius
2 lateral cutaneous nerve of thigh
3 inguinal ligament, retracted
4 deep circumflex iliac vessels
5 external oblique
6 tensor fasciae latae

Obturator nerve

Anatomy

The anterior branch of the obturator nerve runs anterior to adductor brevis, deep to pectineus and adductor longus. Its exposure requires the development of a plane between pectineus and adductor longus. The posterior branch lies deep to adductor brevis on the anterior surface of adductor magnus which is supplied by the nerve.

Indication

This exposure is indicated for division of the anterior branch to relieve adductor spasm in spastic paralysis. In the operation of adductor release, adductor brevis may be divided and the nerve retracted. Care should be taken, when dividing adductor brevis, not to divide the posterior branch of the obturator nerve which lies deep to it.

Position of the patient

The patient is supine, with the operated limb in external rotation and the hip flexed and abducted.

Incision

A A longitudinal 5 cm incision is made over the proximal medial thigh.

Exposure

B The fascia is incised in line with the skin incision, and the plane between pectineus and adductor longus is developed.

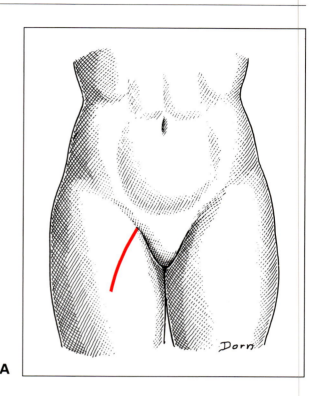

A

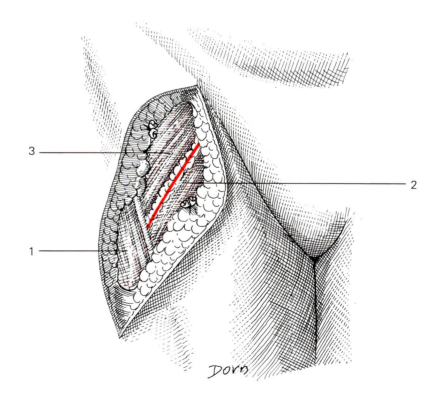

B

1 sartorius
2 adductor longus
3 pectineus

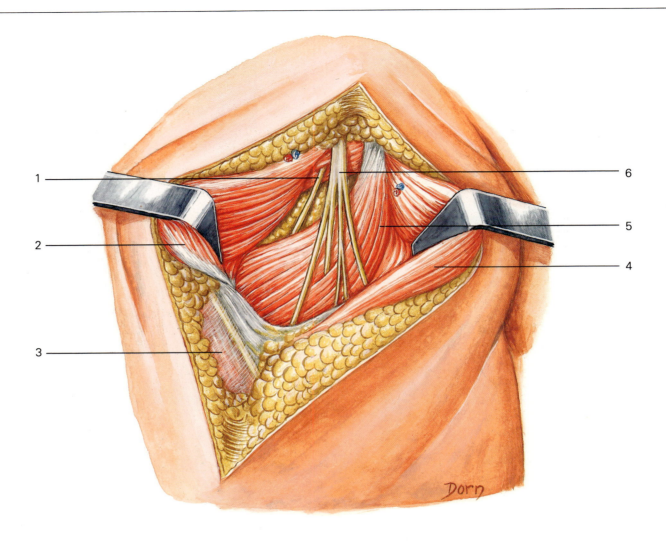

C   Pectineus is retracted laterally
and adductor longus medially,
exposing the anterior branch of
the obturator nerve which lies on
adductor brevis.

C

1 posterior division of obturator nerve
2 pectineus
3 sartorius
4 adductor longus
5 adductor brevis
6 anterior division of obturator nerve

Sciatic nerve: introduction

The sciatic nerve may be damaged in many ways.

- Gunshot or stab wounds.
- Dislocations of the hip and fractures of the acetabulum.
- Traction lesions of the nerve or compression by a retractor may occur during surgical reconstruction of the hip.
- Compression by haematoma, either anticoagulant-induced or postoperative.
- Injection.

The repair of the lacerated nerve may require cable grafts.

Anatomy

The anatomy of the sciatic nerve should be considered in two sections: the buttock and the thigh.

In the buttock the sciatic nerve emerges from the deep aspect of piriformis, accompanied by the posterior cutaneous nerve of thigh. It descends between the greater trochanter and ischial tuberosity lying sequentially on obturator internus, the gemelli and quadratus femoris. In the buttock it lies deep to gluteus maximus and is surrounded by vascular adipose tissue.

In the thigh, the course of the nerve runs from a line drawn from the midpoint between the ischial tuberosity and greater trochanter to the apex of the popliteal fossa. Distal to quadratus femoris, it lies beneath adductor magnus and is crossed superficially by the long head of biceps femoris. Muscular branches to semitendinosus, semimembranosus and the ischial part of adductor magnus arise from the medial aspect of the nerve. Only one branch, that of biceps femoris, arises from the lateral aspect of the nerve.

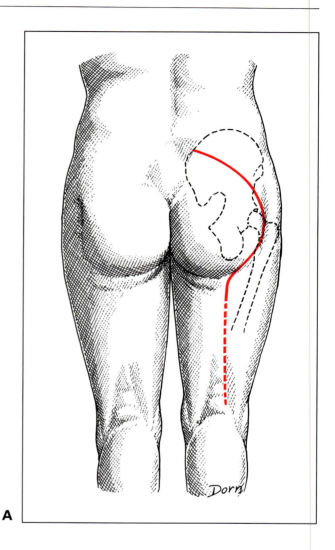

A

Sciatic nerve: exposure in the buttock

Indications

- Repair of lacerations.
- Identification of the nerve in the posterior approach to the hip.
- Neurolysis.

Position of the patient

The patient is prone, the limb being entirely included in the operative field. An alternative is to place the patient on the contralateral side, if the posterior approach to the hip has been used in the past.

Incision

A The incision begins at the posterior superior iliac spine, skirts the lateral margins of gluteus maximus, passes posterior to the greater trochanter and curves into the gluteal fold, before being extended distally in a lazy S fashion along the posterior aspect of the thigh if necessary.

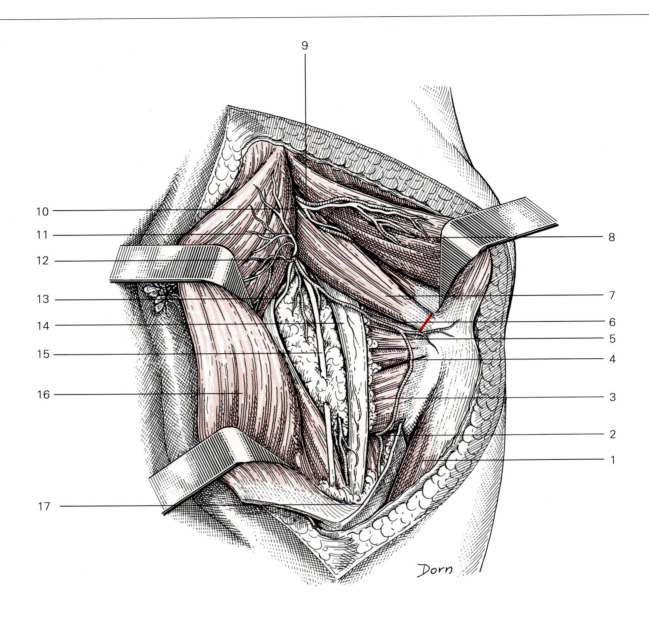

Exposure

B The deep fascia is incised after reflecting the skin margins. Proximally the anterior fibres of gluteus maximus are split and distally the tendinous insertion of the muscle is divided. At this level, several branches from perforating arteries must be diathermied. Gluteus maximus is retracted medially, exposing the insertion of the external rotators of the hip. Lying on these muscles is the sciatic nerve surrounded by loose areolar tissue which is well vascularized.

B

1 vastus lateralis
2 medial circumflex femoral artery
3 quadratus femoris
4 inferior gemellus
5 obturator internus
6 superior gemellus
7 piriformis
8 gluteus medius
9 superior gluteal artery

10 superior gluteal nerve
11 inferior gluteal nerve
12 inferior gluteal artery
13 pudendal nerve
14 sciatic nerve
15 posterior cutaneous nerve of thigh
16 gluteus maximus
17 tendinous insertion of gluteus maximus, cut

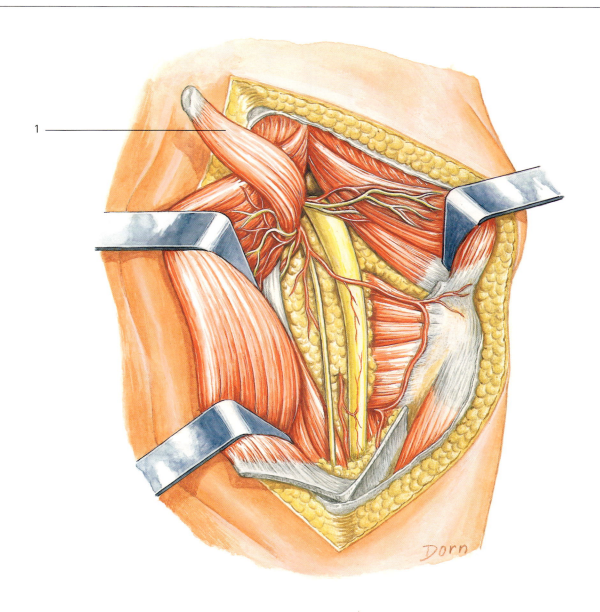

C In the proximal part of the wound, the tendon of insertion of piriformis can be divided and the muscle retracted medially to expose the edge of the greater sciatic foramen and the point of emergence of the nerve from the pelvis.

C

1 piriformis, released from its insertion and retracted

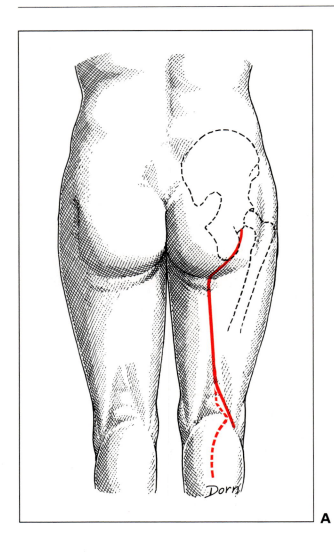

A

Sciatic nerve: exposure in the thigh

Indications

- Repair of lacerations.
- Neurolysis.

Position of the patient

The patient is prone.

Incision

A The incision starts from the gluteal fold and descends towards the popliteal fossa as a lazy S.

Exposure

B The fascia is opened carefully to avoid injuring the posterior cutaneous nerve of thigh which is superficial to the long head of biceps femoris. The plane between semitendinosus and biceps femoris is developed medial to the posterior cutaneous nerve. Then the exposure is deepened by dissecting between semimembranosus and biceps femoris.

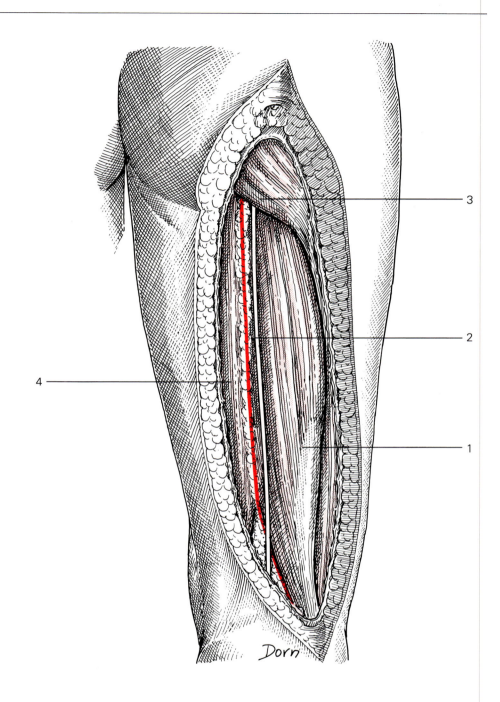

B

1 biceps femoris
2 posterior cutaneous nerve of thigh
3 gluteus maximus
4 semitendinosus

C The nerve is identified and surrounded by loose aerolar tissue. It should be dissected on its lateral border to avoid injuring the muscular branches to the hamstrings. Care should be taken to protect the branch to biceps femoris, which arises from the lateral border of the nerve in the proximal third of the wound. Distally, the bifurcation of the nerve may be exposed at the apex of the popliteal fossa.

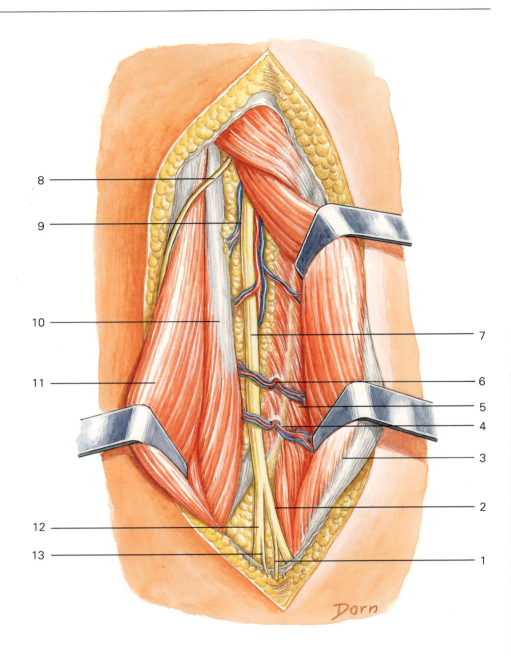

C

1 lateral sural nerve
2 common peroneal nerve
3 biceps retracted (long head)
4 fourth perforating artery
5 short head of biceps femoris
6 third perforating artery
7 sciatic nerve
8 posterior cutaneous nerve of thigh
9 muscular branch
10 semimembranosus
11 semitendinosus, retracted
12 tibial nerve
13 sural nerve

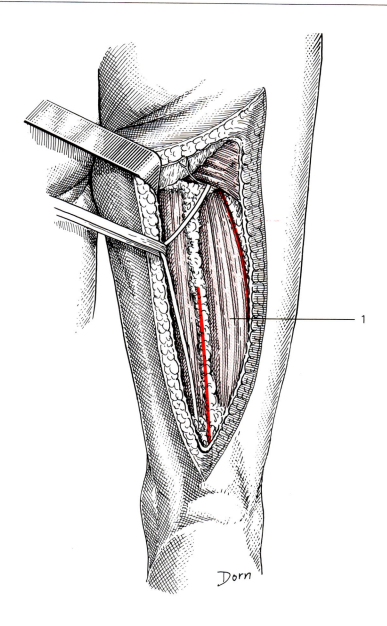

D In the proximal third of the incision the long head of biceps crosses the nerve, and the exposure of the nerve and its continuation into the buttock requires biceps femoris to be retracted medially.

D

1 biceps femoris

E The plane between biceps femoris and vastus lateralis is developed. The proximal segment of the sciatic nerve is thus exposed in the thigh. Care should be taken to preserve the vessels which cross superficial to the nerve.

1

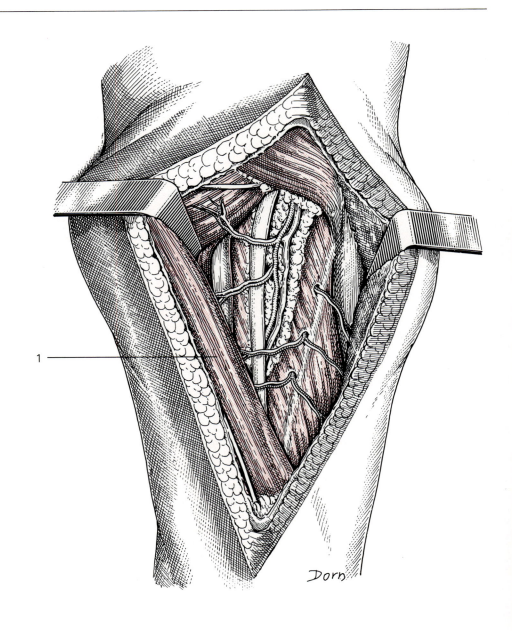

E

1 biceps femoris, retracted medially

Sciatic, tibial and common peroneal nerves: the popliteal fossa

Introduction

The neurovascular bundle in the popliteal fossa is susceptible to damage as follows:

• Traction lesions following dislocation of the knee.
• Compression by haematoma or tumour.
• Lacerations by sharp instruments.

The approach to the popliteal fossa may be extended proximally to expose the main sciatic trunk and distally by splitting soleus and its arcade to expose the tibial nerve. The separate exposure of the common peroneal nerve requires a posterolateral approach.

Anatomy

The sciatic nerve divides into the tibial and common peroneal nerves at a variable level, but usually at the apex of the popliteal fossa. These two nerves are superficial to the vessels.

Indications

• Excision of nerve tumour.
• Repair of laceration.
• Neurolysis.

Position of the patient

The patient is prone with the knee slightly flexed.

Incision

A   A lazy S incision is made over the popliteal fossa with the transverse limb following the flexion crease. The proximal and distal ends of the lazy S should lie in the midline of the thigh and leg respectively, and can be extended as necessary.

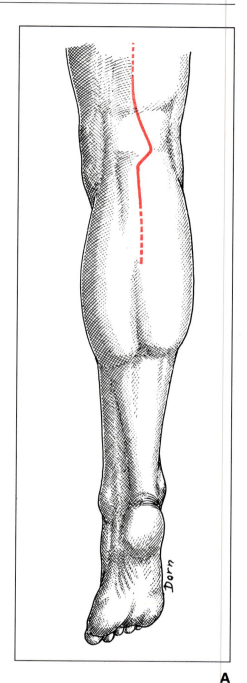

A

Peripheral nerves

Exposure

B The skin flaps are reflected and the short saphenous vein and sural nerve are dissected. The deep fascia is incised lateral to the vein. Proximally, the plane is developed between biceps femoris and semitendinosus. The bifurcation of the sciatic nerve is superficial to the vessels.

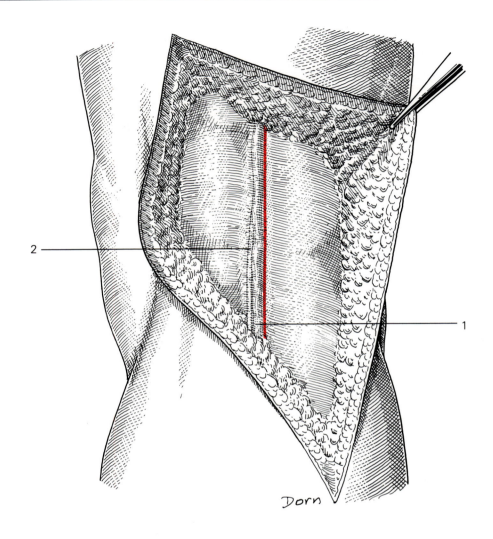

B
1 short saphenous vein
2 sural nerve

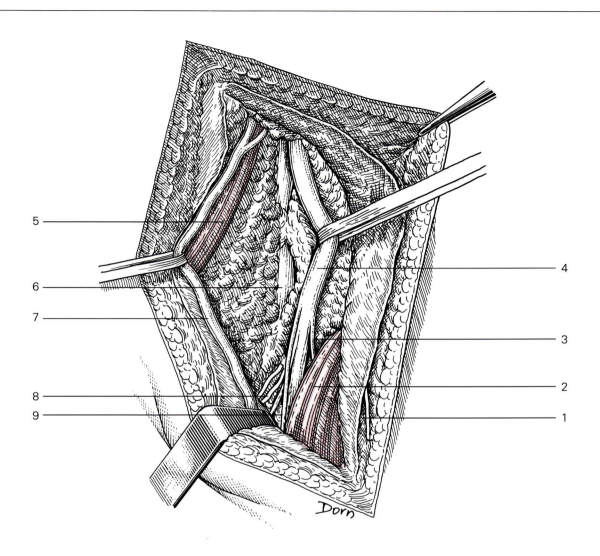

C The common peroneal nerve is followed along the posterior and medial aspect of the biceps tendon. It lies on the lateral aspect of the lateral head of gastrocnemius. The sural communicating nerve runs medial to the common peroneal nerve.

The tibial nerve runs beneath the two heads of gastrocnemius in the distal part of the fossa. These are retracted, protecting the sural nerve. The branches of the tibial nerve to gastrocnemius, soleus, popliteus and plantaris are exposed.

c
1 lateral cutaneous nerve of calf
2 lateral head of gastrocnemius
3 motor branch to lateral head of gastrocnemius
4 tibial nerve
5 semitendinosus
6 popliteal vein
7 short saphenous vein
8 motor branch to medial head of gastrocnemius
9 sural nerve

Peripheral nerves

D The tibial nerve can be demonstrated distally by carefully splitting the arcade and the proximal soleus.

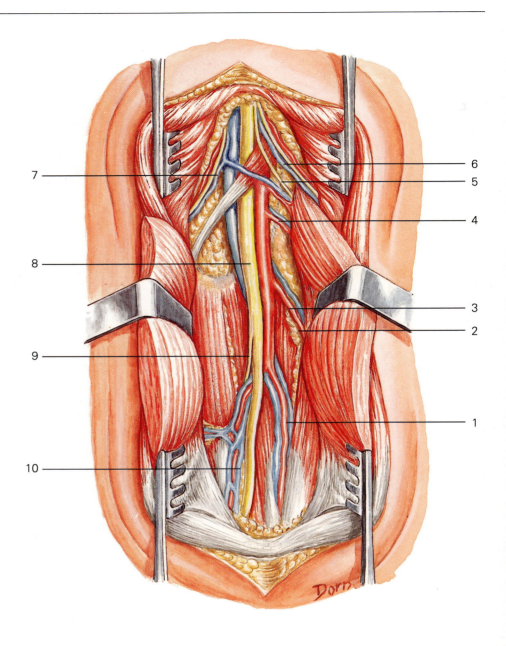

D

1 peroneal vessels
2 motor branch to flexor hallucis longus
3 vascular pedicle to soleus
4 anterior tibial vessels
5 motor branch to soleus
6 motor branch to lateral head of gastrocnemius
7 motor branch to medial head of gastrocnemius
8 tibial nerve
9 motor branch to flexor digitorum longus
10 posterior tibial vessels

Common peroneal nerve: posterolateral approach

Introduction

The common peroneal nerve is the most commonly injured nerve in the lower limb due to its exposed position at the fibular neck. Traction lesions are common, occurring either at surgery or associated with injury to the lateral knee ligaments. The nerve may also be compressed externally by bandages, plaster or splints, particularly in the early postoperative phase. Surgical access to the common peroneal nerve is straightforward.

Indications

- Repair of lacerations.
- Neurolysis.

Position of the patient

The patient is prone, with a small sandbag beneath the ipsilateral anterior iliac spine to facilitate external rotation of the hip. An alternative position is to place the patient on the contralateral side.

Incision

A The two main landmarks are the tendon of biceps femoris and the head of the fibula. The incision commences just medial to the biceps tendon and runs distally along the lateral border of the popliteal fossa and curves forward just distal to the fibular head.

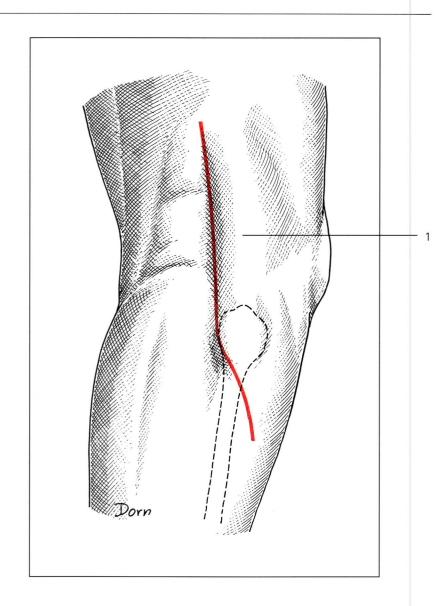

A

1 biceps femoris

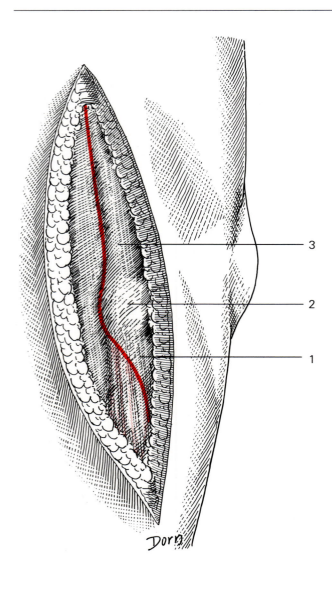

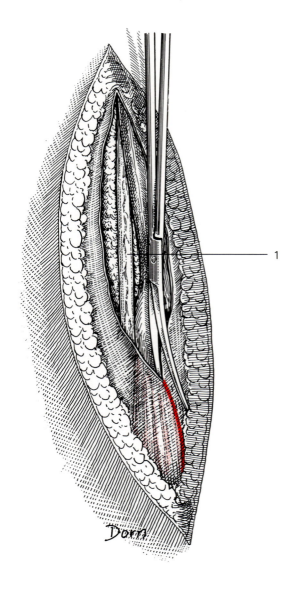

B

1 peroneal muscles
2 head of fibula
3 tendon of biceps femoris

Exposure

B The fascia is opened in line with the skin incision. The nerve is found in the proximal part of the wound, just medial and posterior to the biceps tendon surrounded by loose areolar tissue.

C A plane is developed between the biceps tendon and lateral head of gastrocnemius, and the two muscles retracted to expose the nerve. Care should be taken at this level to avoid injuring the lateral cutaneous nerve of calf and the sural communicating nerve.

D   At the fibular neck, the nerve enters a tunnel beneath the proximal part of peroneus longus, which can be divided to expose the common peroneal nerve as it splits into the deep and superficial peroneal nerves.

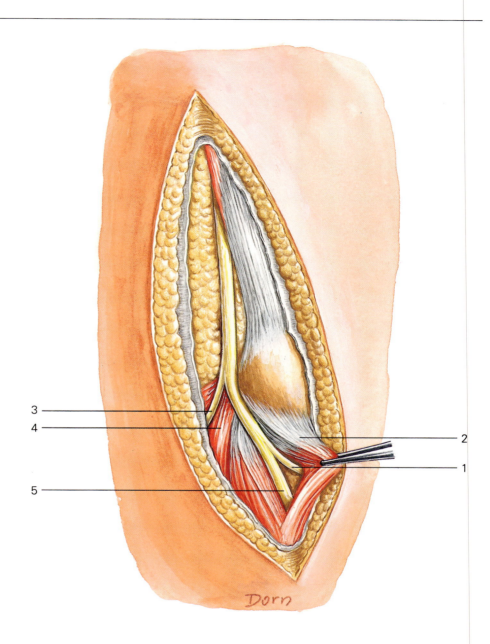

D

1 deep peroneal nerve
2 peroneus longus, cut
3 lateral cutaneous nerve of calf
4 lateral head of gastrocnemius
5 superficial peroneal nerve

The tibial nerve and its bifurcation: medial approach

Introduction

The tibial nerve is rarely injured in the leg. Injuries in the popliteal fossa require a posterior approach which can be extended distally by splitting soleus and dividing the arcade.

In the leg, the medial approach is used by detaching soleus from the tibia. The medial approach is the same as for the posterior tibial vessels (see pages 318–20), and can be extended proximally by dividing the tendon of the medial head of gastrocnemius. The most specific lesion of the tibial nerve is its compression posterior to the medial malleolus beneath the flexor retinaculum.

Indication

- Neurolysis of the distal tibial nerve and its bifurcation.

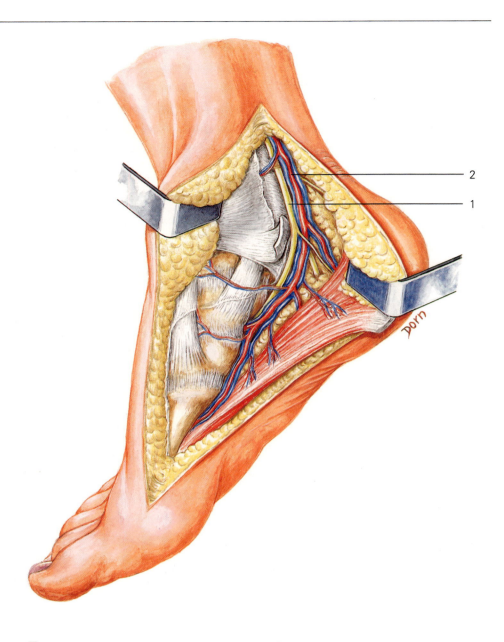

Position of the patient

The patient is supine, with a sandbag under the contralateral hip to facilitate external rotation of the leg.

Incision

The incision commences proximal to the medial malleolus and curves round it posteriorly, running towards the instep of the foot.

Exposure

The superficial veins are cauterized before opening the flexor retinaculum. The nerve is lateral and deep to the posterior tibial vessels, necessitating mobilization of the artery and vein in order to isolate the nerve and its bifurcation into the medial and lateral plantar nerves. Proximally, the exposure of the nerve may be achieved by incising the deep fascia and retracting the Achilles tendon. Distally the medial plantar nerve may have to be released by dividing abductor hallucis.

A
1 tibial nerve
2 posterior tibial artery

Sural nerve

Introduction

The sural nerve is frequently used as a donor nerve graft. To this end it has several advantages. Surgical access is easy and functional impairment secondary to the harvesting is practically non-existent. Moreover, the nerve may be raised as vascularized nerve graft because it is accompanied by a branch of the sural artery or popliteal artery.

Anatomy

The sural nerve descends between the two heads of gastrocnemius and becomes superficial distally in the leg. Sometimes the nerve runs in a fibrous tunnel before piercing the fascia. Commencing medially, the nerve gains the lateral border of the Achilles tendon along which it runs. It winds around the lateral malleolus to supply the lateral border of the foot via several branches. In its superficial course, it is accompanied by the short saphenous vein. The sural nerve is usually joined distal to the belly of gastrocnemius by the sural communicating branch which arises from the common peroneal nerve near the head of the fibula. In other instances, the sural communicating branch may have no connection with the sural nerve and may descend to the ankle on the posterolateral aspect of the leg.

Position of the patient

The patient is placed prone, but this may be incompatible with the exposure of the recipient site for the graft. The sural nerve can be harvested with the patient supine, with a sandbag under the ipsilateral hip, the knee flexed to 60° and the leg in maximal internal rotation.

Incision

A Two types of incision are possible:

1 A long sinuous incision from the flexion crease of the knee to the posterior aspect of the lateral malleolus, thus exposing the entire nerve. This type of incision is necessary in two instances: in babies due to the thickness of the subcutaneous tissue, as long nerve grafts may be required in a brachial plexus repair; secondly, when a vascularized nerve graft is needed.

2 In other circumstances, four or five short transverse incisions are used to release the nerve by subcutaneous stripping. However, some surgeons prefer to harvest the nerve by a continuous longitudinal incision, because this allows a choice to be made in the proximal leg between the sural nerve or the sural communicating nerve. If necessary both branches are harvested.

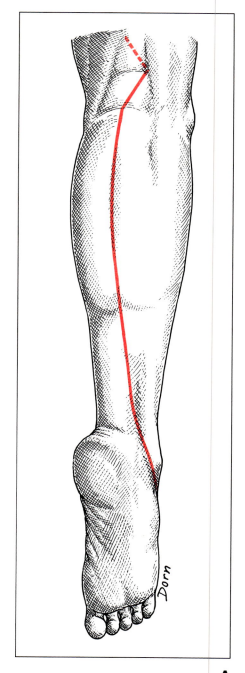

A

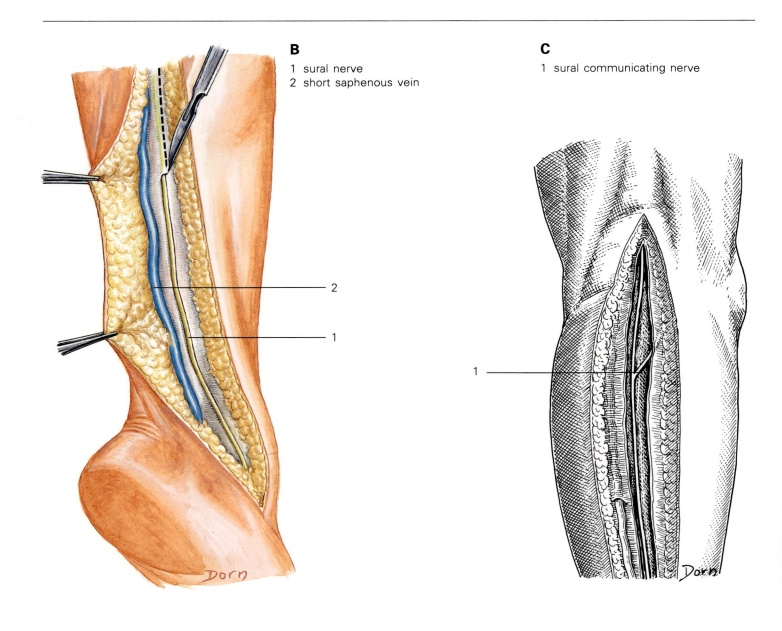

B
1 sural nerve
2 short saphenous vein

C
1 sural communicating nerve

Exposure

B,C The exposure of the sural nerve is shown in its course superficial to the deep fascia in the distal part of the leg and deep to the deep fascia in the proximal half of the leg, between the medial and lateral heads of gastrocnemius. However, if transverse incisions are used, the first is made 2–3 cm above the tip of the lateral malleolus and posterior to it. The superficial fascia is incised longitudinally, and the short saphenous vein identified and retracted to expose the nerve. Small branches of the nerve are divided.

The second incision is located 10 cm proximal to the first one, being slightly more medial. The short saphenous vein is localized superficial to the deep fascia and the nerve identified medial to it. Traction on the nerve through the distal incision will allow the exact location of the course of the nerve and the siting of the more proximal incisions.

The third incision is placed in the midcalf, and at this level both the vein and nerve may be beneath the deep fascia. The most proximal incision is made in the flexion crease of the knee, and the deep fascia is opened transversely and the nerve found medial to the vein. Additional transverse incisions may be necessary to harvest the nerve in order to avoid placing excessive traction upon it.

9

Skin and muscle flaps

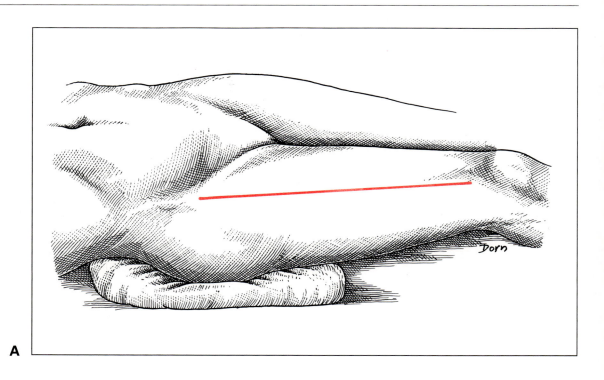

A

Introduction

The development of the use of cutaneous and myocutaneous flaps in reconstructive surgery over the last 10 years has revolutionized treatment of tissue loss. Consideration should be given, during any surgical approach to the deep structures, to whether flap reconstruction may be required subsequently so that the initial incision can be placed satisfactorily.

The principles of raising a flap in the upper limb are different to those in the lower limb. In the upper limb the majority of the muscles are needed for satisfactory function of the hand and limb, and the sacrifice of only one muscle can lead to significant functional impairment. Certain muscles are of lesser functional importance, eg brachioradialis, and this muscle can be used as part of a flap. Thus, in the upper limb most of the flaps are cutaneous rather than myocutaneous.

In the lower limb, several muscles provide the same function. For example, extension of the knee is produced by the four muscle bellies of the quadriceps. The use of one belly as part of a flap will barely compromise active knee extension. The same principle can be applied to the hamstrings and to the dorsi and plantar flexors of the ankle. Even when considering movements of the toes, several muscles provide the same function. Thus, in the lower limb, flaps can frequently be muscular or myocutaneous without leading to significant functional impairment.

Cutaneous flaps alone are less frequently used and should be undertaken cautiously, especially following recent trauma, because the blood supply may be impaired. Soft tissue loss, in both upper and lower limbs, is more likely to require flap cover in the distal part of the limb. Thus, in the lower limb flap cover is most frequently required over the knee, shin and foot.

The vastus lateralis muscle flap

Anatomy

Vastus lateralis is one of the four parts of the quadriceps. It is richly vascularized by numerous pedicles which arise mainly from the profunda femoris. Proximally, the muscle is supplied by the transverse descending branch of the lateral circumflex artery from which a large branch arises that ascends along the medial border of vastus lateralis. The middle third of the muscle is nourished by a perforating artery from the profunda femoris. The distal third receives a sizable muscular branch from the first collateral artery of the popliteal artery. The two proximal branches from the lateral circumflex artery are sufficient to supply the muscle in its entirety, and the motor nerve accompanies the descending branch of the

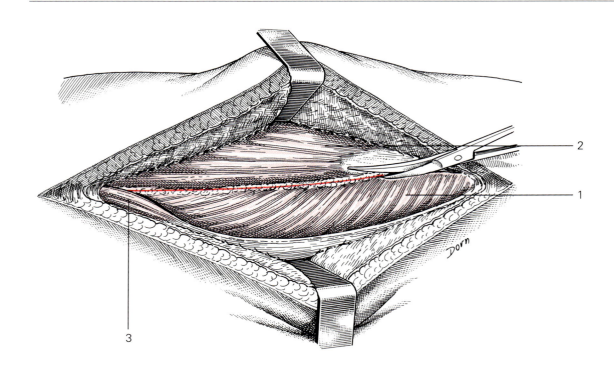

lateral circumflex artery and enters the muscle in its proximal third. The neurovascular pedicle is thus defined.

Indications

● Cover of the proximal portion of the thigh (femoral vessels, trochanteric sore).
● Cover of the pubis and the lower ipsilateral abdominal wall.

Position of the patient

The patient is supine, with a sandbag under the ipsilateral buttock. The whole limb is included in the operative field.

Incision

A The incision is made along a line from the anterior superior iliac spine to the lateral angle of the patella, beginning between 10 and 15 cm distal to the spine. If a trochanteric sore is to be resurfaced, the incision starts from the margin of the defect and runs obliquely towards the patella.

Operative procedure

B The fascia lata is opened, care being taken in the proximal third to preserve the vascular pedicle to tensor fasciae latae. The space between rectus femoris and vastus lateralis is identified and cautiously opened in its middle third.

B
1 vastus lateralis
2 rectus femoris
3 tensor fasciae latae

Skin and muscle flaps

C

1 vastus lateralis
2 rectus femoris
3 major vascular pedicle to the muscle
4 motor nerve to vastus lateralis
5 minor vascular bundle

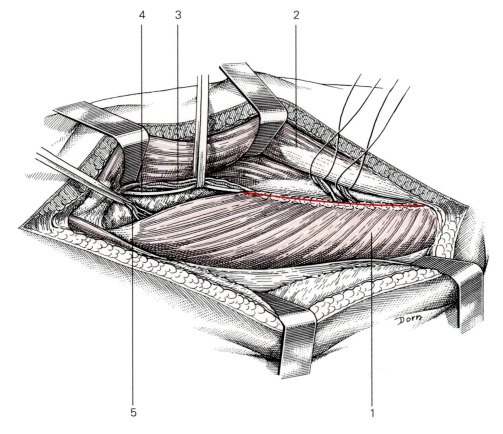

C Care should be taken to preserve the vascular pedicle to vastus lateralis which runs deep to rectus femoris and crosses the operative field in the proximal third. The branch that descends along the medial border of the muscle must also be protected. It lies in thin fatty tissue that should be left in continuity with the muscle.

D In the distal third, the tendon is incised to separate rectus femoris and vastus lateralis. The distal end of the muscle is separated from the extensor apparatus of the knee and the muscle is then released from vastus intermedius which lies beneath it. The aponeurosis on the deep aspect of vastus lateralis should be included to facilitate the dissection between the two muscles.

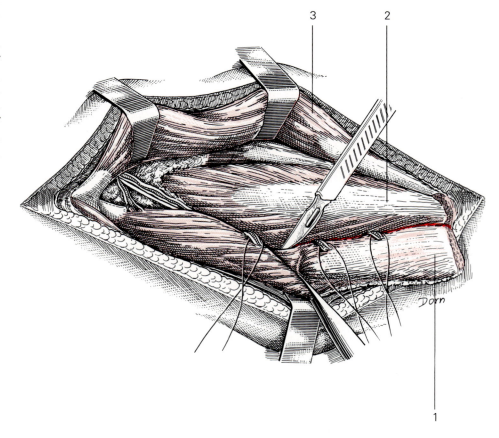

D

1 vastus lateralis, retracted
2 vastus intermedius
3 rectus femoris

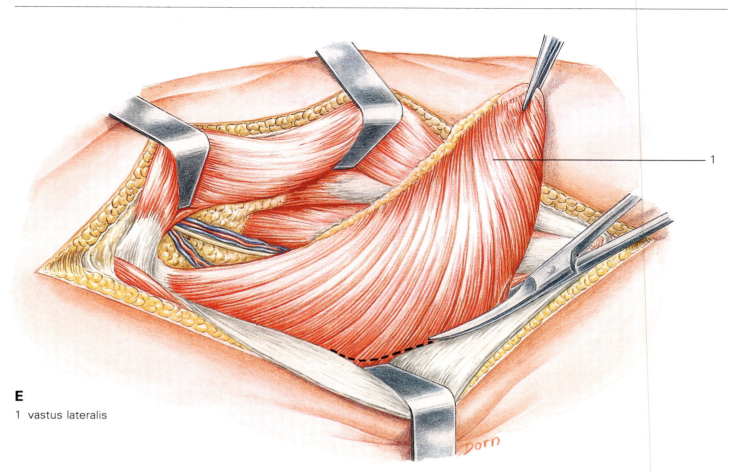

E

1 vastus lateralis

E,F Vastus lateralis is dissected from the linea aspera. Vastus intermedius and lateralis insert into the linea aspera and are not easily separated at that level. The muscle flap is raised from distal to proximal, being carefully released from its insertion into the linea aspera. The muscle can be isolated on its two proximal vascular pedicles, as a true island flap, by releasing its femoral insertion.

F

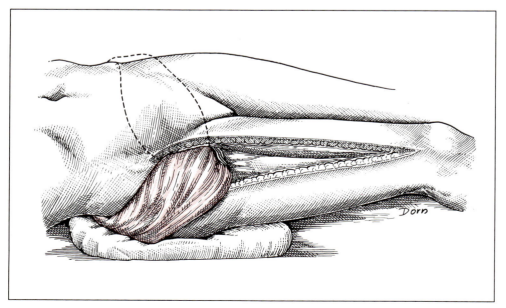

375

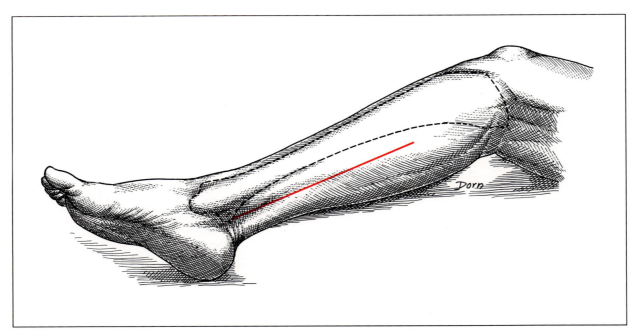

A

The soleus muscle flap

Introduction

Soleus is a very useful muscle for covering defects of the leg. It lies in the superficial part of the posterior compartment and frequently is undamaged in compound fractures of the middle third of the tibia.

Anatomy

Soleus is triangular, but its length is variable and this is important because it determines the total arc of rotation that is possible. The muscle is richly vascularized by the posterior tibial and per-oneal arteries via two main pedicles proximally. Smaller pedicles supply the muscle along its border and can be ligated without impairing the viability of the muscle. Thus, soleus can be mobilized on its proximal pedicles without detaching its origin.

Indication

- Cover of the middle third of the leg.

Position of the patient

The patient is supine, with the limb in external rotation and the knee slightly flexed.

Incision

A The incision commences midway between the medial malleolus and the Achilles tendon, and ascends as far as the proximal quarter of the leg, 1 cm posterior to the medial border of the tibia.

B

1 soleus
2 gastrocnemius

Operative procedure

B The deep fascia is incised in line with the skin incision, preserving the saphenous nerve and vein. Distally, the sheath around the Achilles tendon is incised. The dissection between gastrocnemius and soleus is practically avascular and the separation can be achieved with a finger.

C Distally, the lower part of soleus is separated from the deep posterior compartment. The aponeurosis should not be incised, in order to protect the posterior tibial neurovascular bundle. Numerous pedicles arise from the main vessels and supply soleus, and these should be ligated and divided. The release of the medial and anterior aspect of the muscle is continued. Midway between the medial malleolus and the patella, a large pedicle arises from the posterior tibial vessels, and this should be ligated to allow the flap to be rotated.

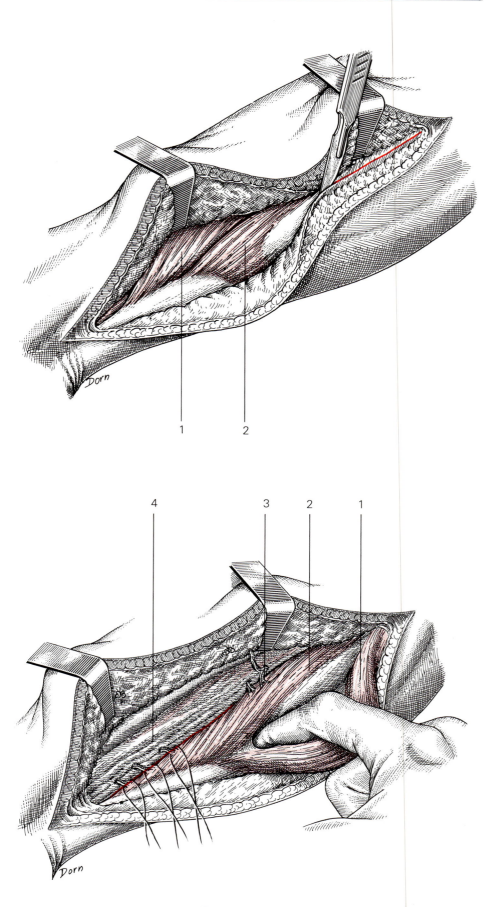

C

1 gastrocnemius
2 soleus
3 vascular pedicle to the muscle midway between the knee and the ankle
4 posterior tibial neurovascular axis covered by the deep fascia

Skin and muscle flaps

D

1 tendo Achillis
2 gastrocnemius
3 soleus

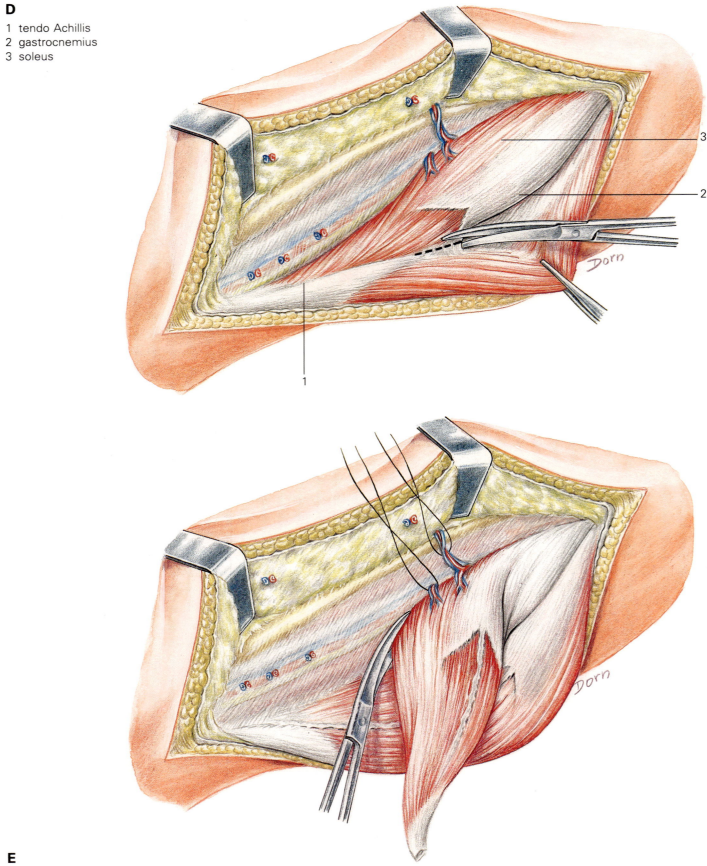

D The second stage is the release of the superficial aspect of soleus. At the middle third of the leg, the superficial aponeurosis of soleus presents a deep, central, intramuscular tendon. The aponeurosis joins the tendon of gastrocnemius to form the Achilles tendon. The aponeurosis of soleus is separated digitally as far as possible from the tendon of gastrocnemius, and is then incised to release the muscle fibres of soleus from the Achilles tendon. It is particularly useful to retain a thin layer of aponeurosis in order to avoid tearing the distal part of the muscle.

E,F The third and final stage is the release of the muscle from its lateral attachments. The distal portion which has been freed is gently drawn out from the wound and the lateral border is progressively released. Numerous small pedicles arise from the peroneal artery and should be ligated. The distal two-thirds are hence mobilized and, when rotated, will cover defects of the anterior shin.

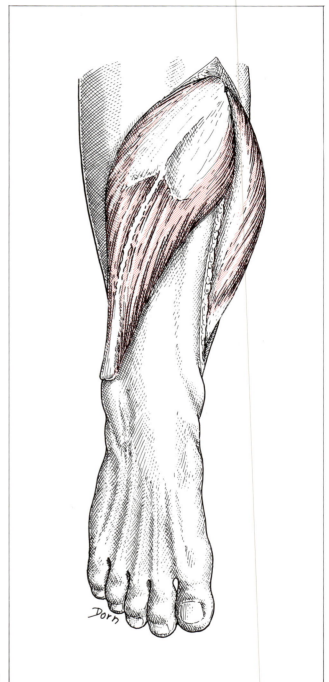

F

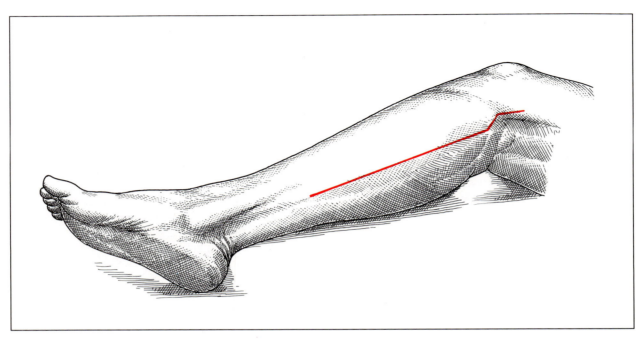

A

Gastrocnemius muscle flaps: introduction

Anatomy

Gastrocnemius comprises both medial and lateral heads and is supplied by the sural arteries, which arise from the popliteal artery and are accompanied by the motor nerves. Each head can be mobilized individually on its own proximal neurovascular pedicle.

Indication

● Cover of the knee and proximal third of the leg.

Gastrocnemius muscle flaps: the medial head

Position of the patient

The patient is supine, the limb in external rotation and the knee slightly flexed.

Incision

A The incision starts at mid-calf 2 cm behind the posteromedial border of the tibia, and curves proximally to reach the popliteal fossa. It can be extended along the thigh if necessary.

Operative procedure

B Care should be taken to avoid injury to the saphenous vein and nerve. The deep fascia is incised in line with the skin incision and a large skin flap, including the aponeurosis, is retracted posteriorly as far as the plane between the two heads of gastrocnemius. The intermuscular plane is developed with a finger between soleus and the medial head after incision of the thin aponeurosis. Often the plantaris tendon is found in this space.

C The sural nerve is identified on the posterior aspect of gastrocnemius. It lies between the two heads on an aponeurotic sheet and is covered by a thin layer of muscle fibres from the medial head. It is dissected free and retracted posteriorly.

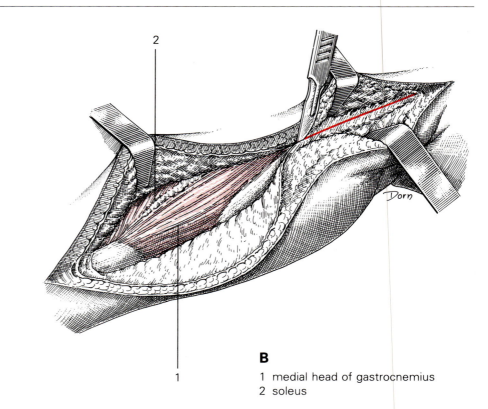

B

1 medial head of gastrocnemius
2 soleus

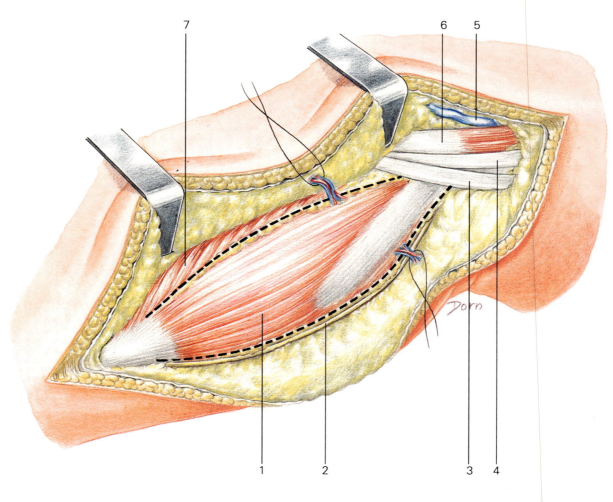

C

1 medial head of
   gastrocnemius
2 sural nerve
3 semitendinosus
4 gracilis
5 saphenous vein
6 sartorius
7 soleus

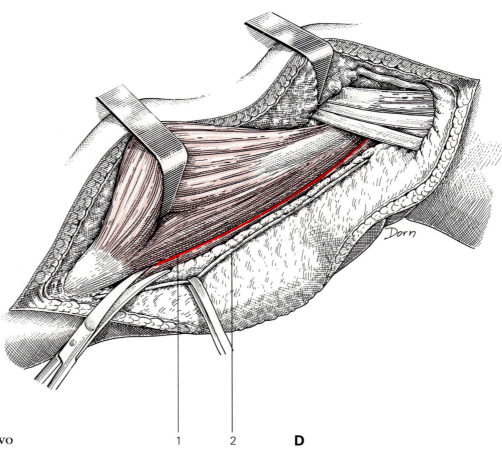

1 2

D

1 aponeurosis between the two heads
of gastrocnemius
2 sural nerve, retracted

D The space between the two heads is identified with care being taken to preserve the neurovascular pedicle. The tendon of the medial head is divided, and the muscle is progressively raised in a distal to proximal direction by cutting the aponeurotic sheet that joins the two heads. The motor nerve should be divided to avoid postoperative pain caused by muscle contraction. It accompanies the vascular pedicle and is found on the lateral side of the proximal part of the muscle.

E,F The arc of rotation may be increased by releasing the origin of the muscle from the femur. The skin incision, extended over the lower part of the thigh, allows the exposure of the tendons of semitendinosus, semimembranosus and gracilis. The medial head of gastrocnemius, isolated on its vascular pedicle, must be passed deep to these tendons in order to reach the anterior aspect of the knee.

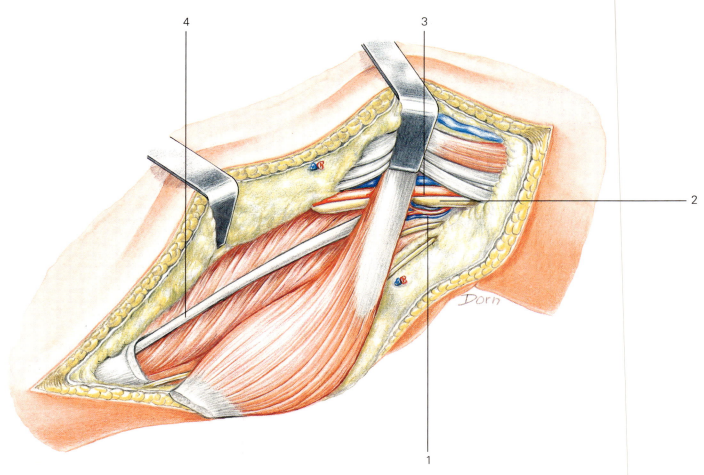

E

1 vascular pedicle to the medial head of gastrocnemius
2 tibial nerve
3 popliteal artery
4 plantaris

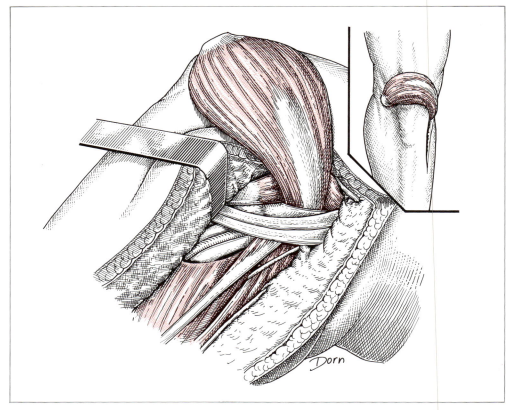

F

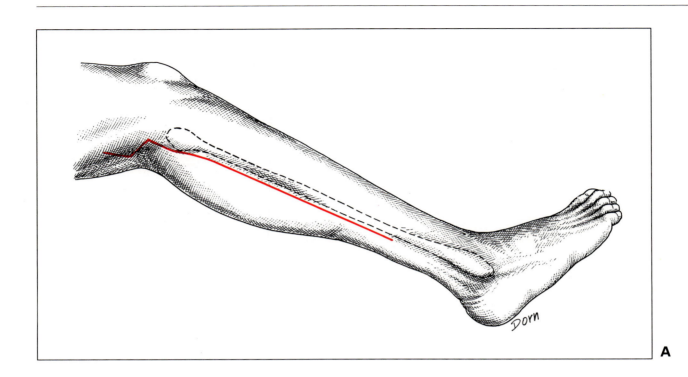

A

Gastrocnemius muscle flaps: the lateral head

Position of the patient

The patient is supine, with a sand-bag under the ipsilateral buttock to maintain the limb in slight internal rotation and the knee semi-flexed.

Incision

A The line of incision lies just posterior to the fibula. It can be extended proximally, crossing the popliteal fossa.

Operative procedure

B,C When extensive mobilization of the muscle is required, the biceps tendon and the common peroneal nerve should be exposed. The fascia is incised in line with the skin incision. Proximally, the tendon of biceps femoris, the common peroneal nerve and the lateral sural nerve are identified. Medially, the sural nerve is dissected and retracted. Laterally, the plane between soleus and gastrocnemius is developed. The transfer is progressively raised after dividing the distal aponeurotic sheet. The common peroneal nerve is mobilized.

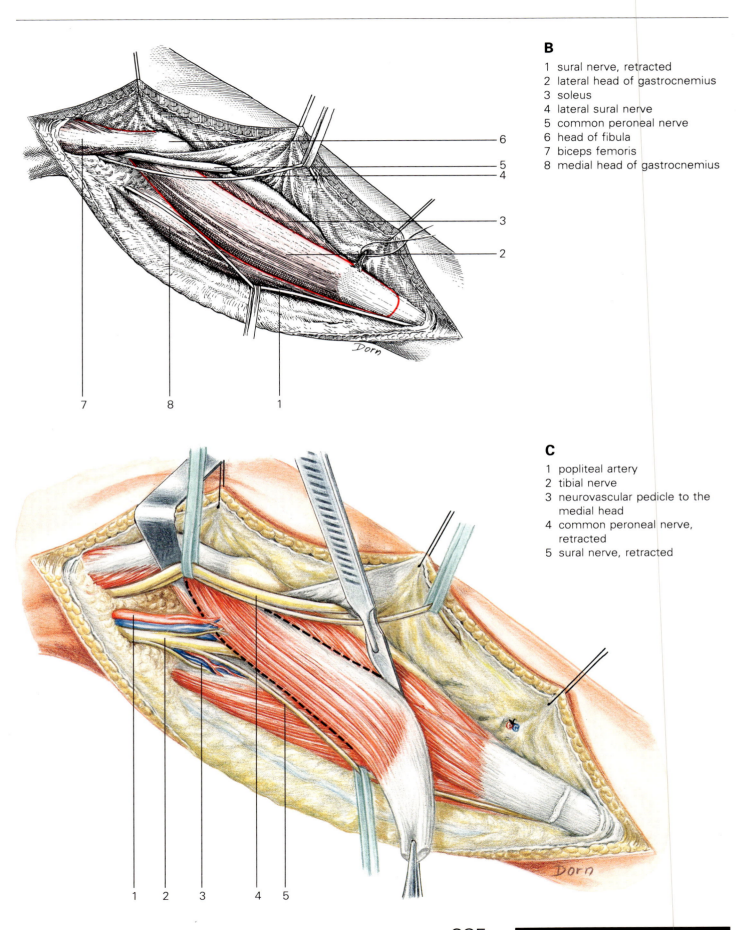

B

1 sural nerve, retracted
2 lateral head of gastrocnemius
3 soleus
4 lateral sural nerve
5 common peroneal nerve
6 head of fibula
7 biceps femoris
8 medial head of gastrocnemius

C

1 popliteal artery
2 tibial nerve
3 neurovascular pedicle to the medial head
4 common peroneal nerve, retracted
5 sural nerve, retracted

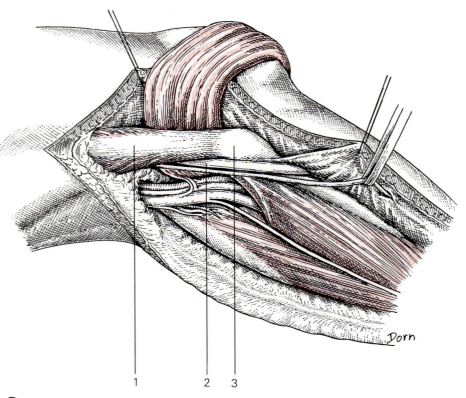

D If the muscle is needed to cover a defect over the anterior aspect of the knee, the muscle transfer is passed deep to the peroneal nerve and sometimes deep to the biceps tendon. This manoeuvre is not necessary when the defect is over the proximal shin.

D

1 tendon of biceps femoris
2 common peroneal nerve
3 head of fibula

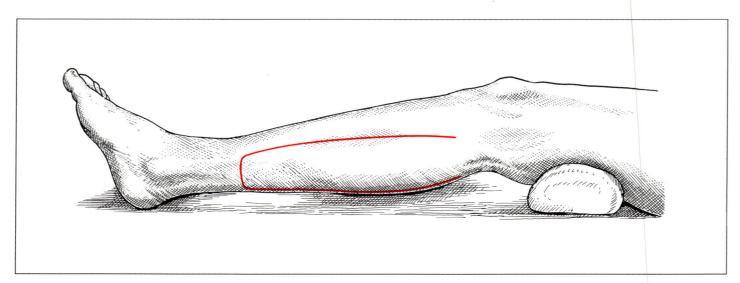

A

The fasciocutaneous saphenous flap

Introduction

This flap is the prototype of a fasciocutaneous flap. It is raised on the medial aspect of the calf. The inclusion of the deep fascia allows the preservation of the suprafascial vascular network and of the multiple anastomoses between cutaneous, fascial and muscular vessels.

Anatomy

The skin of the medial aspect of the calf is supplied by three groups of arteries:

1 The saphenous artery, which accompanies the saphenous nerve, providing numerous small branches to the skin. It can be considered as the axial artery of the flap.

2 The arteries arising from the posterior tibial artery, emerging from the intermuscular space between the superficial and deep flexor compartments of the leg.
3 The short branches arising from the deep surface of the muscles, particularly the medial head of gastrocnemius.

Indications

- Cover of the infrapatellar region of the knee and of the proximal two-thirds of the tibia.
- The cross-leg flap.

Position of the patient

The patient is supine, the knee semi-flexed and the limb in external rotation.

Incision

A   The anterior border of the flap includes the long saphenous vein to preserve the saphenous artery. Posteriorly, the incision is slightly medial to the midline of the calf. The distal end of the flap should not extend further than the distal third of the tibia. Proximally, a fasciocutaneous bridge is preserved at the distal border of sartorius.

Skin and muscle flaps

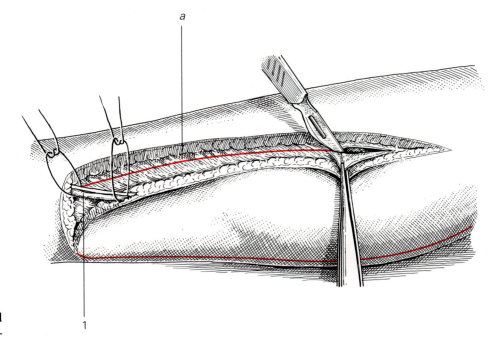

Operative procedure

B,C The deep fascia is incised strictly in line with the skin incision. The long saphenous vein is ligated and divided, and the saphenous nerve divided. The flap is raised from distal to proximal, the dermis being sutured to the fascia. Cutaneous arteries from the tibial or muscular vessels should be ligated or diathermied. Frequently, a large proximal branch arising from the medial head of gastrocnemius can be preserved. The donor site is covered with a split-skin graft.

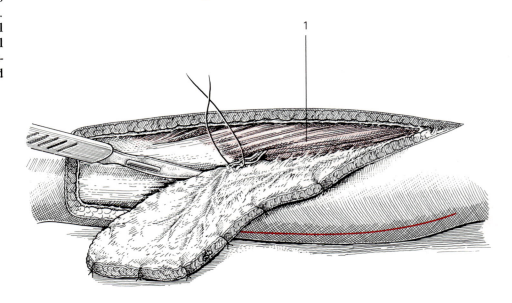

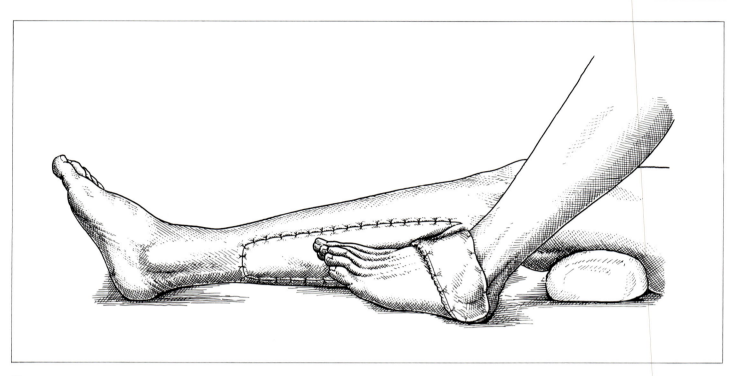

D

D   The saphenous flap is particularly useful in the cross-leg flap to cover soft tissue defects on the opposite leg or foot.

The dorsalis pedis flap

Introduction

This flap is one of the earliest described neurovascular flaps and can be used as a free flap.

Anatomy

The vascular axis of the flap is the dorsalis pedis artery, which is a continuation of the anterior tibial artery and crosses, from proximal to distal, the anterior capsule of the ankle joint, the talus, the navicular and the second cuneiform. The tendon of extensor hallucis longus lies on its medial side, whilst the tendons of extensor digitorum longus and the medial terminal branch of the deep peroneal nerve lie laterally. At the proximal end of the first metatarsal space, it passes into the sole of the foot to join the plantar arch. Its branches are the tarsal, the arcuate and the first dorsal metatarsal arteries. The lateral tarsal artery runs laterally deep to extensor digitorum brevis and supplies this muscle. The cutaneous branches, which will nourish the flap, arise from the short segment of the artery as it lies between extensor hallucis longus and the first head of extensor digitorum brevis. Some cutaneous arteries also arise from the first muscular head of extensor digitorum brevis. The first dorsal metatarsal artery also supplies the skin when it lies superficial to the first dorsal interosseous.

Applied anatomy

Several keypoints must be emphasized.
- Dissection of the flap is difficult because the tissue which connects the artery to the skin is very thin and the artery lies directly on the tarsal skeleton.
- The key for raising the distal portion of the artery is to divide the tendon of extensor digitorum brevis where it inserts into the tendon of extensor hallucis longus.
- A safer procedure is to include the first head of extensor digitorum brevis, leaving the flap with the attached segment of the lateral tarsal artery.
- When a superficial dorsal intermetatarsal artery exists, the territory of the flap can be extended to the base of the toes. A superficial artery may be palpable or identified by Doppler. When this artery lies deep to the muscle, it is safer to limit the distal end of the flap to the middle of the metatarsals.
- The branches of the superficial peroneal nerve which are included in the flap provide sensation.

Indications

- Cover of soft tissue defects of the foot and lower third of the leg.
- A free sensory flap.

Position of the patient

The patient is supine, with a sandbag under the ipsilateral buttock to hold the leg in neutral rotation.

A

Incision

A The incision begins proximally over the distal limb of the inferior retinaculum. The medial border overlaps the tendons of extensor hallucis longus to include the vein on the medial border of the foot, which drains into the long saphenous vein proximally. The lateral border is lateral to the tendon of extensor digitorum longus. When the first metatarsal artery is not palpable, the distal end of the flap is at the level of the middle of the metatarsals.

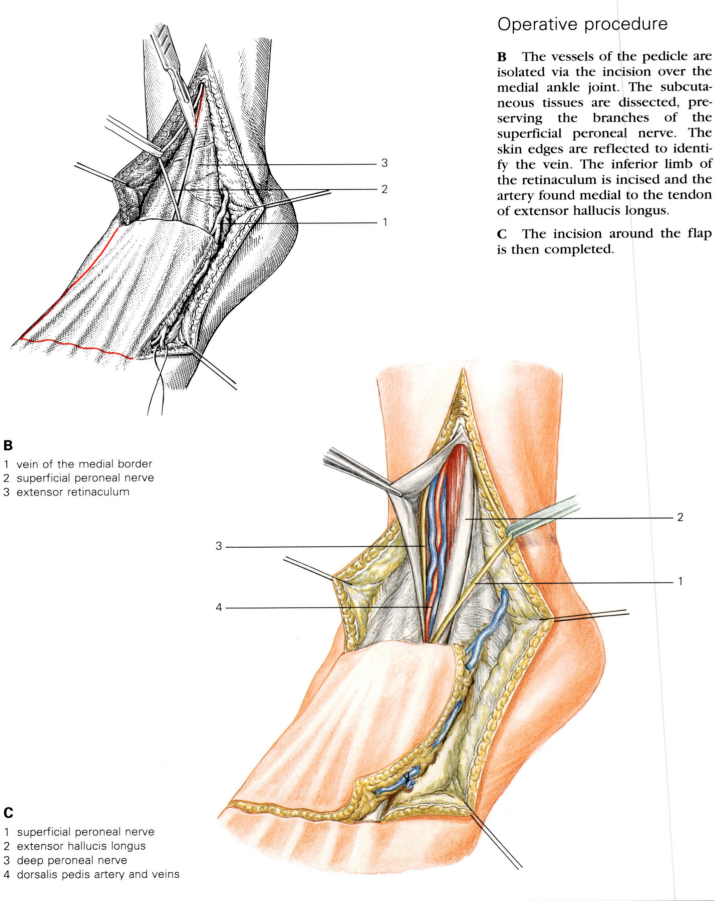

Operative procedure

B The vessels of the pedicle are isolated via the incision over the medial ankle joint. The subcutaneous tissues are dissected, preserving the branches of the superficial peroneal nerve. The skin edges are reflected to identify the vein. The inferior limb of the retinaculum is incised and the artery found medial to the tendon of extensor hallucis longus.

C The incision around the flap is then completed.

B

1 vein of the medial border
2 superficial peroneal nerve
3 extensor retinaculum

C

1 superficial peroneal nerve
2 extensor hallucis longus
3 deep peroneal nerve
4 dorsalis pedis artery and veins

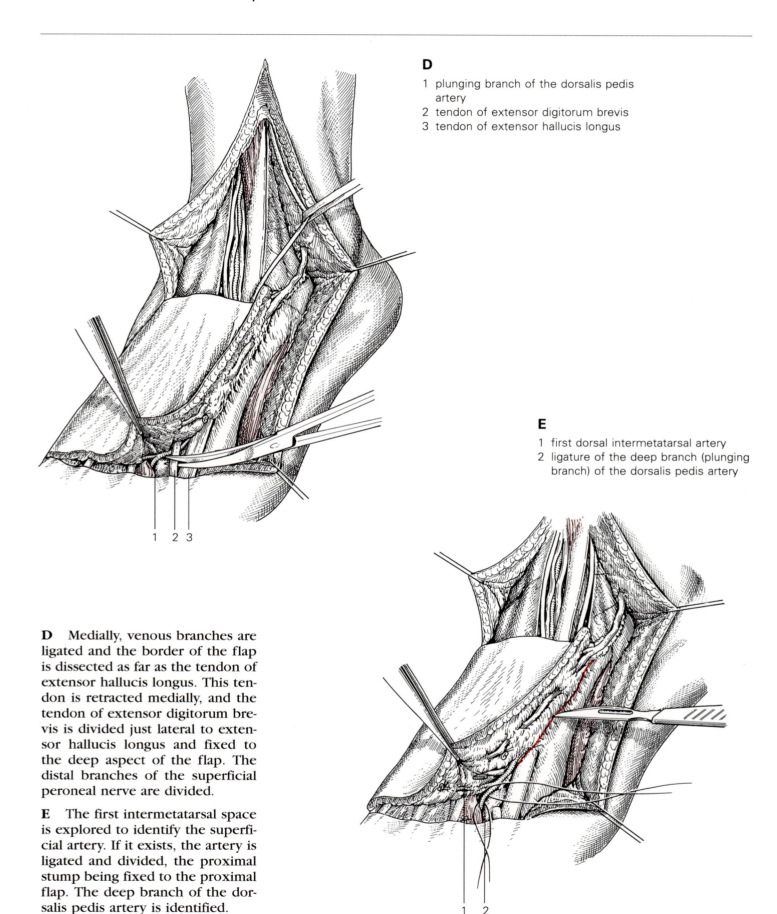

D
1 plunging branch of the dorsalis pedis artery
2 tendon of extensor digitorum brevis
3 tendon of extensor hallucis longus

E
1 first dorsal intermetatarsal artery
2 ligature of the deep branch (plunging branch) of the dorsalis pedis artery

D Medially, venous branches are ligated and the border of the flap is dissected as far as the tendon of extensor hallucis longus. This tendon is retracted medially, and the tendon of extensor digitorum brevis is divided just lateral to extensor hallucis longus and fixed to the deep aspect of the flap. The distal branches of the superficial peroneal nerve are divided.

E The first intermetatarsal space is explored to identify the superficial artery. If it exists, the artery is ligated and divided, the proximal stump being fixed to the proximal flap. The deep branch of the dorsalis pedis artery is identified.

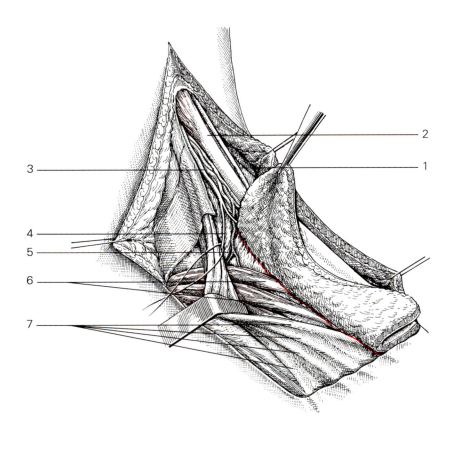

F

1 superficial peroneal nerve
2 extensor hallucis longus tendon
3 deep peroneal nerve
4 motor nerve to extensor digitorum brevis
5 lateral dorsal artery
6 extensor digitorum brevis
7 extensor digitorum longus

F Laterally, the flap is progressively raised and care should be taken to preserve the loose, vascularized areolar tissue over the extensor tendons which provides a bed for the skin graft. Extensor digitorum longus is retracted laterally, exposing extensor digitorum brevis. The first head of the muscle is left connected with the superficial tissues and separated from the rest of the muscle. The lateral tarsal artery is ligated deep to the muscle. When the medial portion of the muscle is not included in the flap, the motor nerve should be spared.

G At this stage of the dissection, the flap remains attached to the foot only by the deep connection of the artery that lies on the tarsal bone and by the distal portion that enters the proximal end of the first metatarsal space to gain access to the sole of the foot. The distal end of the artery is ligated and divided. Finally, the artery is freed from its bed, taking care to leave it attached to the flap. The tendons of extensor digitorum longus and extensor hallucis longus are sutured together and a split-skin graft used to cover the defect.

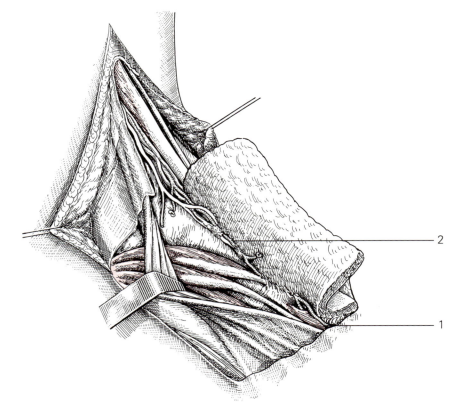

G

1 first dorsal intermetatarsal artery
2 dorsalis pedis artery

H

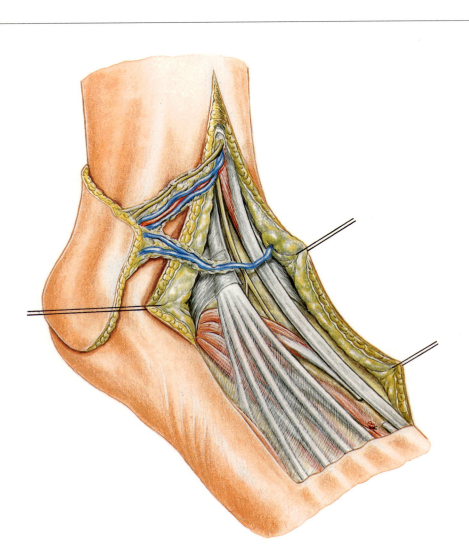

H   The dorsalis pedis flap can be used as a free or as a pedicled island flap.

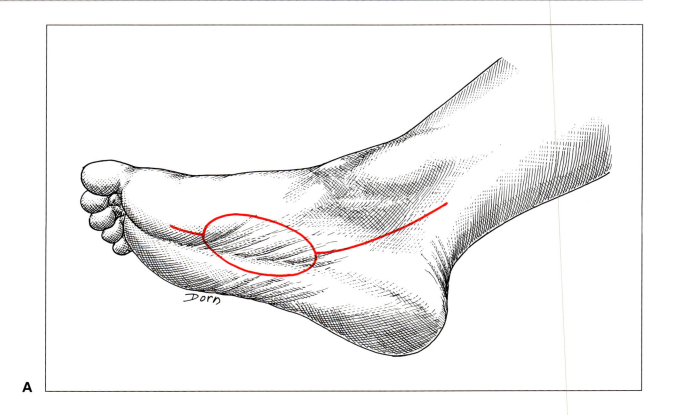

A

The medial plantar flap

Introduction

Soft tissue defects of the foot remain a difficult problem in reconstructive surgery. The medial plantar flap is ideal to cover the heel, although the technique is difficult.

Anatomy

The medial plantar flap is raised from the non-weight-bearing area of the plantar arch. It is based on the medial plantar artery which is a distal branch of the posterior tibial artery. It divides into a deep branch which runs medially adjacent to the tarsal bones and a superficial branch which runs between abductor hallucis and flexor digitorum brevis. Cutaneous branches arise from the intermuscular space; the artery is accompanied by a venous network and the medial plantar nerve, which supplies one or two small branches to the skin of the plantar arch. The medial plantar flap is a sensory flap. Preoperative arteriography is essential as the medial plantar artery can be absent.

Indication

• Cover of the weight-bearing area of the heel.

Design of the flap

A The design of the flap is limited by the boundaries of the non-weight-bearing area of the foot. The weight-bearing areas are the heel, the metatarsal heads, the lateral arch and, medially, the inferior border of the medial arch.

B

1 posterior tibial artery
2 flexor retinaculum

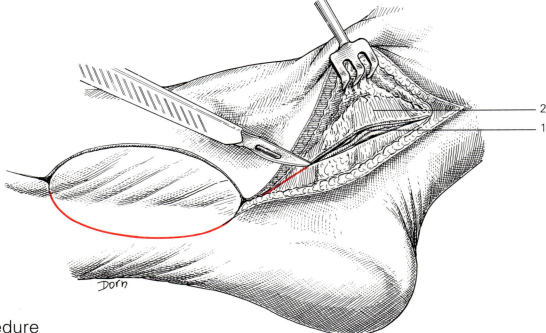

Operative procedure

B   Medially, the incision exposes the fascia which covers abductor hallucis. Posterior to the medial malleolus, the flexor retinaculum is incised to expose the posterior tibial artery. The origin of the medial plantar artery is identified at the proximal border of abductor hallucis.

C   The medial margin of the flap is gently reflected, thus exposing the muscle.

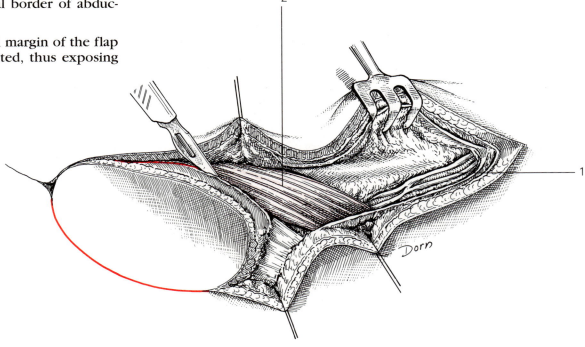

C

1 posterior tibial artery and veins
2 abductor hallucis

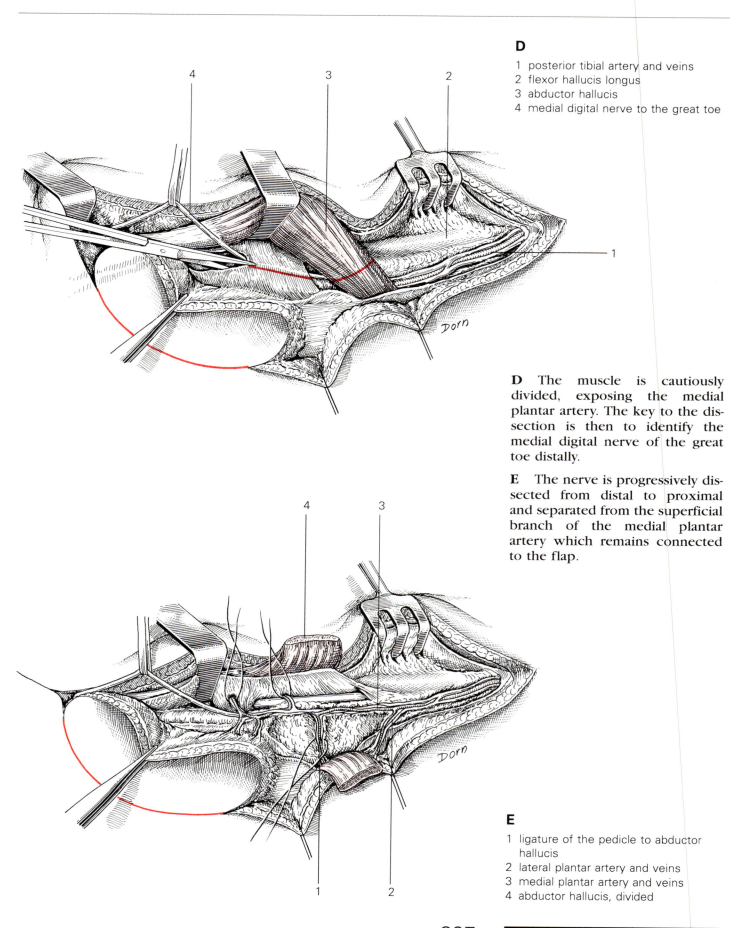

D
1 posterior tibial artery and veins
2 flexor hallucis longus
3 abductor hallucis
4 medial digital nerve to the great toe

D The muscle is cautiously divided, exposing the medial plantar artery. The key to the dissection is then to identify the medial digital nerve of the great toe distally.

E The nerve is progressively dissected from distal to proximal and separated from the superficial branch of the medial plantar artery which remains connected to the flap.

E
1 ligature of the pedicle to abductor hallucis
2 lateral plantar artery and veins
3 medial plantar artery and veins
4 abductor hallucis, divided

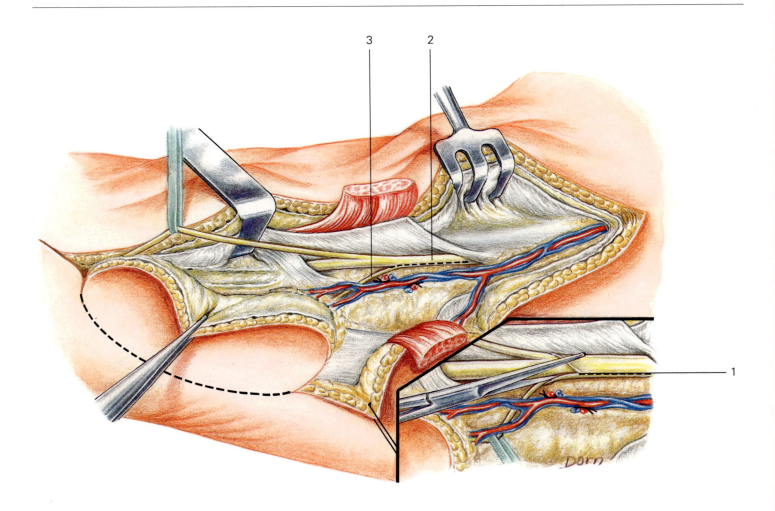

F

1 intraneural dissection of the branch
2 tibial nerve
3 sensory branch to the flap

F Proximally, the common trunk of the medial plantar nerve is also dissected from the artery. One or two branches supply the flap and these are identified. In order to provide a long pedicle, an intraneural dissection of these branches is required. The medial plantar artery is ligated distal to the flap and the proximal end is sutured to the flap; the deep branch of the medial plantar artery is ligated. The neurovascular bundle is released up to the bifurcation of the posterior tibial vessels.

G,H The lateral margin of the flap is freed without necessarily including the plantar aponeurosis. Care should be taken to conserve the loose connective tissue between the neurovascular bundle and the flap.

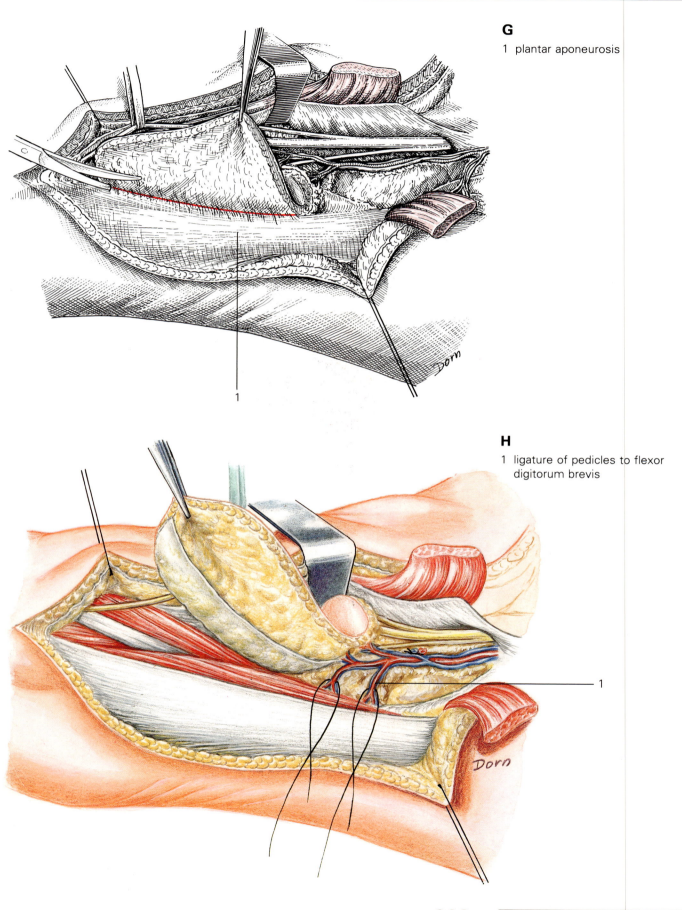

G

1 plantar aponeurosis

H

1 ligature of pedicles to flexor
digitorum brevis

1

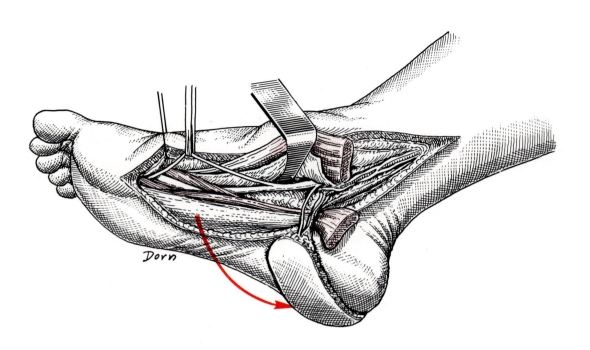

I The arc of rotation provided by the pedicle allows the weight-bearing area and the posterior aspect of the heel to be covered. Closure of the wound is achieved by suturing abductor hallucis to flexor digitorum brevis and applying a split-skin graft, after excision of the exposed part of the plantar aponeurosis.

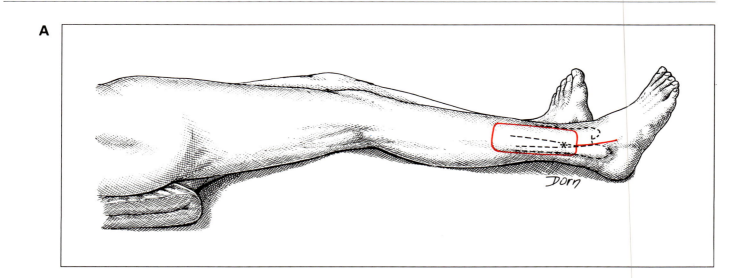

A

The lateral supramalleolar flap

Introduction

This flap is a distally based, pedicled, fasciocutaneous flap raised on the lateral aspect of the lower leg.

Anatomy

The arterial anatomy of the flap is based on the anastomotic arcade of the ankle. The perforating branch of the peroneal artery pierces the interosseous membrane at the distal tibiofibular angle, about 5 cm proximal to the medial malleolus. It anastomoses at a variable level with the anterior lateral malleolar artery which arises from the anterior tibial artery. It then descends anterior to the inferior tibiofibular syndesmosis, and anastomoses with the lateral tarsal artery on the lateral border of extensor digitorum brevis and with branches arising from the lateral plantar artery on the lateral

border of the foot. It is accompanied by a venous network. The perforating branch is sometimes large and may replace the dorsalis pedis. Just after crossing the membrane, the perforating branch gives one or two branches to the skin of the lateral aspect of the leg. Sometimes one branch may arise from the anterior malleolar artery. These cutaneous branches run proximally and anastomose with the artery that accompanies the superficial peroneal nerve, which enters the subcutaneous tissues at the junction of the middle and distal third of the leg; it then divides into medial and lateral branches at the level of the ankle joint. The principle of the flap is as follows: the perforating branch is ligated and divided just proximal to the cutaneous branch and released as far as possible in the foot. The pivotal point of the pedicle is usually the sinus tarsi, the length of the pedicle being approximately 7 cm. The venae comitantes are sufficient to ensure the venous return. The territory of the flap is bounded laterally by the fibular crest, medially by the tendon of tibialis anterior. The outline of the flap should include the origin of the perforating branch. Proximally, the flap may overlap the middle of the leg.

Indications

- The cover of the posterior aspect of the heel, the dorsum of the foot and the stumps of a transmetatarsal amputation.
- The flap is not designed for the cover of weight-bearing areas of the foot.

Design of the flap

A The essential landmark is the perforating branch, as it pierces the interosseous membrane, and the surface marking is the depression in the lower part of the tibiofibular space which can be identified by digital palpation. The outline of the flap must include this landmark. A line of incision is drawn anterior to the lateral malleolus and reaches the depression of the sinus tarsi on the lateral aspect of the hindfoot.

Skin and muscle flaps

B

1 landmark of the perforating branch
of the peroneal artery

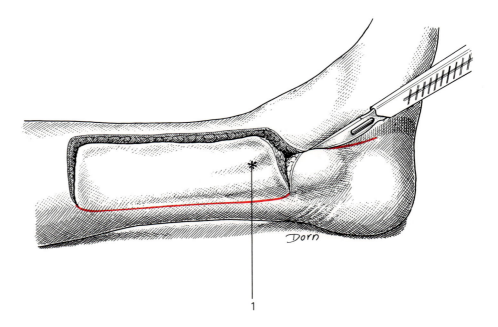

Operative procedures

B,C   The skin is incised in continuity along the anterior margin of the flap and anterior to the lateral malleolus. The pedicle is first exposed. It is deep to the extensor retinaculum which is incised. The pedicle lies on the tibiofibular ligament and is isolated with its surrounding loose areolar tissue.

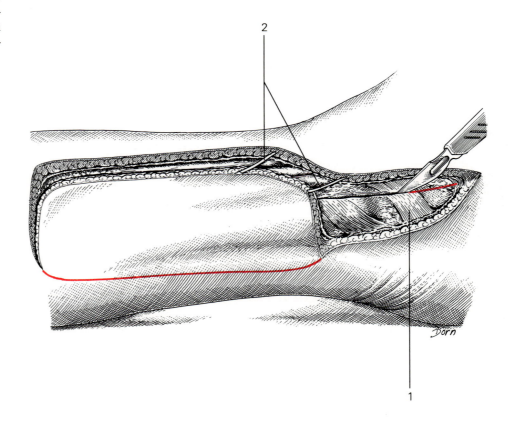

C

1 extensor retinaculum
2 branches of the superficial peroneal
nerve

D,E The anterior margin of the flap is progressively reflected, including the fascia. At the distal end, the superficial peroneal nerve is divided. The posterior margin of the flap is left intact. The extensor compartment of the leg is exposed and the muscles are gently retracted, exposing the lower part of the tibiofibular space. The vascular structures are thus identified: the perforating branch, the cutaneous branches of the flap and the anastomosis with the anterior lateral malleolar artery, which is ligated and divided. Then the membrane is cautiously incised proximal to the foramen to free the perforating branch.

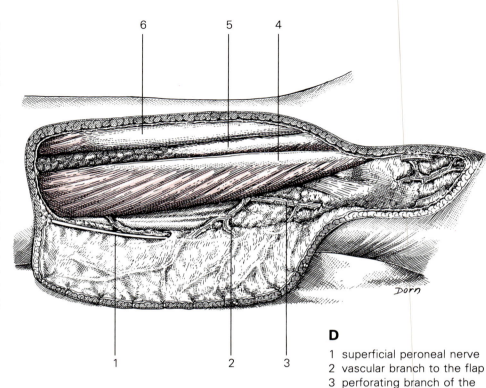

D

1 superficial peroneal nerve
2 vascular branch to the flap
3 perforating branch of the peroneal artery
4 extensor digitorum longus
5 extensor hallucis longus
6 tibialis anterior

E

1 anastomosis with the lateral tarsal artery
2 inferior tibiofibular syndesmosis
3 deep peroneal nerve
4 ligature of the anterior lateral malleolar artery
5 anterior tibial artery

F

1 peroneus longus

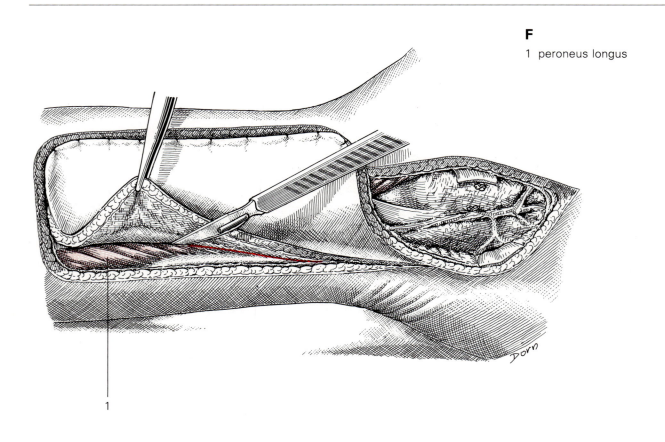

1

G

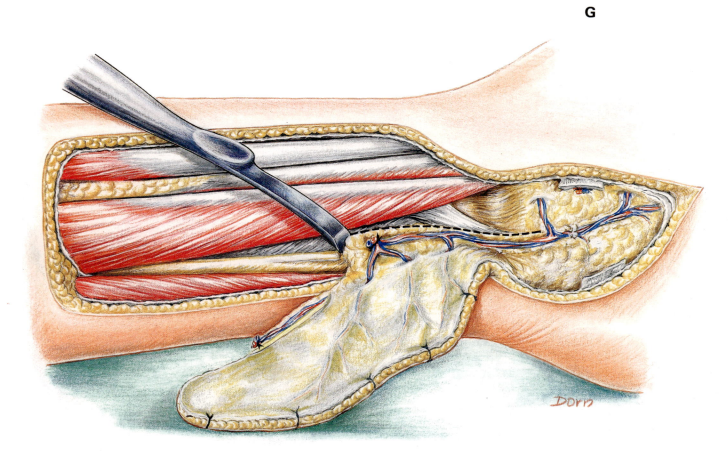

H

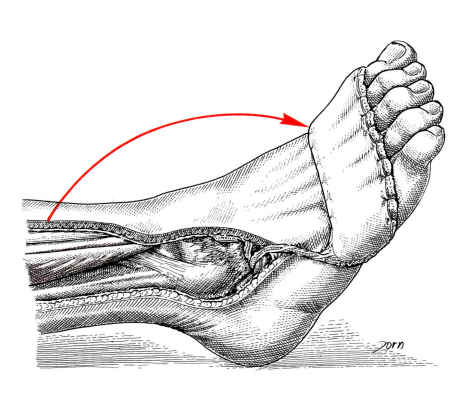

F,G The posterior margin of the flap is then incised, including the fascia, and reflected anteriorly, so exposing the peroneal muscles. Proximally, the superficial peroneal nerve which is subfascial is divided and the proximal end is buried in muscle. At this stage, the flap remains attached only to the septum that separates the anterior and lateral compartments. The septum is divided close to the fibula. Care should be taken in the lower part of the flap to preserve the cutaneous branches that lie on the fibula. The release of the septum should be carried out subperiosteally at that level. The closure of the wound is achieved by suturing the peroneal and extensor muscles together. A split-skin graft is applied immediately.

H The arc of rotation allows cover of the medial aspect of the lower leg, the posterior aspect of the heel and the dorsum, and the borders of the foot.

Select bibliography

Banks SW, Laufman H, *An Atlas of Surgical Exposures of the Extremities*, 2nd edn (WB Saunders: Philadelphia 1987).

Bauer S, Kerschbaumer F, Poisel S, *Operative Zugangswege in Orthopädie und Traumatologie* (Thieme: Stuttgart 1986).

Bosworth DM, Posterior approach to the femur, *J Bone Joint Surg* (1944) **26**: 687–90.

Cadenat FM, *Les Voies de pénétration des membres*, II *Membre inférieur* (Doin: Paris 1933).

Colonna PC, Ralston EL, Operative approaches to the article joint, *Am J Surg* (1951) **82**: 44–54.

De Lestang M, Hourlier H, Warlaumont C, Grodet H, Vives P, La voie d'abord antéro-externe pour le traitement des fractures de l'extrémité inférieure de jambe, *Rev Chir Orthop* (1985) suppl II: 72–4.

Gibson A, Posterior exposure of the hip joint, *J Bone Joint Surg (Br)* (1950) **32**: 183–6.

Gray's Anatomy, 37th edn (Churchill Livingstone: Edinburgh 1989).

Haertsch P, The surgical plane in the leg, *Br J Plast Surg* (1981) **34**: 464–9.

Henry AK, *Extensile Exposure*, 2nd edn (Churchill Livingstone: Edinburgh 1973).

Honnart F, *Voies d'abord en chirurgie orthopédique et traumatologie* (Masson: Paris 1984).

Hoppenfeld S, de Boer P, *Surgical Exposures in Orthopaedics: The Anatomic Approach* (JB Lippincott: Philadelphia 1984).

Letournel E, Judet R, *Fractures of the Acetabulum* (Springer-Verlag: New York 1981).

McMinn RMH, Hutchings RD, Logan BM, *Color Atlas of Foot and Ankle Anatomy* (Wolfe Medical: London 1982).

Masquelet AC, Gilbert A, Romaña MC, *Les Lambeaux musculaires et cutanés* (Springer-Verlag: Paris 1990).

Mathes SJ, Nahai F, *Clinical Applications for Muscle ands Musculocutaneous Flaps* (CV Mosby: St Louis 1982).

Mears DC, Rubash HE, Extensile exposure of the pelvis, *Contemp Orthop* (1983) **6**: 21–31.

Radley TJ, Liebig CA, Brown JR, Resection of the body of pubic bone, the superior and inferior pubic rami, the inferior ischial ramus and the ischial tuberosity, *J Bone Joint Surg (Am)* (1954) **36**: 855–8.

Ruedi T, Von Hochstetter AHC, Schlumpf R, *Surgical Approaches for Internal Fixation* (Springer-Verlag: Berlin 1984).

Salmon M, *Les Artères de la peau* (Masson: Paris 1936).

Sedel L, Voies d'abord des nerfs du membre inférieur, *Techniques Chirurgicales: Orthopédie* (Encyclopédie Medico-chirurgical: Paris) 44530 (4.8.06).

Sénégas J, Liorzou G, Ostéosynthèse des fractures complexes du cotyle par une voie d'abord externe élargie, *XLVIIIᵉ réunion annuelle de la SOFCOT, Paris Nov. 1973* (1974) supp 2: 259–61.

Smith-Petersen MN, Approach to and exposure of the hip joint for mold arthroplasty, *J Bone Joint Surg (Am)* (1949) **31**: 40–6.

Index

Index

Index

Index